THE DEVELOPMENT OF EMOTIONAL COMPETENCE

The Guilford Series on Social and Emotional Development

CLAIRE B. KOPP AND STEVEN R. ASHER, *Editors*

Children and Marital Conflict:
The Impact of Family Dispute and Resolution
E. Mark Cummings and Patrick Davies

Emotional Development in Young Children
Susanne A. Denham

The Development of Emotional Competence
Carolyn Saarni

The Development
of Emotional Competence

Carolyn Saarni

Foreword by Ross A. Thompson

THE GUILFORD PRESS
New York London

© 1999 The Guilford Press
A Division of Guilford Publications, Inc.
72 Spring Street, New York, NY 10012
http://www.guilford.com

Printed in the United States of America

This book is printed on acid-free paper.

Last digit is print number: 9 8 7 6 5 4 3 2

Library of Congress Cataloging-in-Publication Data

Saarni, Carolyn
    The development of emotional competence / Carolyn Saarni.
        p.   cm.—(The Guilford series on social and emotional
    development)
    Includes bibliographical references and index.
    ISBN 1-57230-433-2 (hard). — ISBN 1-57230-434-0 (pbk)
    1. Emotional maturity. 2. Maturation (Psychology)
3. Interpersonal relations. I. Title. II. Series.
    [DNLM: 1. Emotions. 2. Adaptation, Psychological. 3. Social
Behavior. 4. Interpersonal Relations.   BF 531S112d 1999]
BF710.S22 1999
155.2′5—dc21
DNLM/DLC   98-39676
                                                              CIP

*To my large and wonderful "clan,"
presided over by my parents,
Margaret and Walfrid Saarni,
and with very great appreciation
to my husband, Michael Flynn,
and our children, Heather and Matthias.*

About the Author

Carolyn Saarni received her PhD from the University of California at Berkeley, specializing in developmental psychology. She began her academic career at New York University, but after a number of years returned to the West Coast. Since 1980, she has been on the faculty of the Department of Counseling at Sonoma State University in California, where she trains prospective marriage, family, child, and school counselors.

Dr. Saarni's research has focused on how children learn that they can adopt an *emotional front;* that is, what they express emotionally need not match what they really feel. She has also investigated how children use this knowledge strategically in their interpersonal relations with others as well as when coping with aversive feelings. Her research has been funded by the National Science Foundation and the Spencer Foundation, among others. In addition to *Lying and Deception in Everyday Life* (with Michael Lewis), Dr. Saarni's other edited volumes include *The Socialization of Emotion* (also with Michael Lewis) and *Children's Understanding of Emotion* (with Paul L. Harris). She has also written numerous chapters and articles on children's emotional development. Dr. Saarni is a licensed clinical psychologist and is regularly consulted by the popular media on topics concerning emotional development in children and youth.

Foreword

*E*motion animates life. It accounts for the depths and peaks of daily existence, the memorable richness and darkest moments of individual experience. Throughout human history, philosophers, poets, playwrights, sages, and (most recently) psychologists have reflected on how to live with the experience of emotion. From the ancient admonitions of St. Paul that we should tame our passions to Hamlet's summoning the courage to act rightly, from Freud's portrayal of the irrational emotional unconscious to e. e. cumming's claim that "love is a deeper season / than reason," they have each sought to characterize emotional competence, the theme of this remarkable book by Carolyn Saarni.

Emotional competence is revealed when an infant seeks the solace of a parent's lap when surprised by an overly friendly stranger. It is reflected in a 9-year-old's capacity to respond to a peer's provocation in a manner that either maintains the friendship or solicits the assistance of peers (depending on her goal). Emotional competence is reflected in a child's ability to talk about the events of her day so that her father can understand the feelings they evoked, and it is shown in the parent's empathic response to his child's report. It is revealed in an adolescent's ability to respond appropriately when opening a disappointing birthday gift (even if that means masking disappointment at receiving underwear from Mom). Emotional competence is involved in how emotions are shared in marriage, parenting, and other close relationships so that they enhance rather than deter intimacy. It is, in short, efficacy in accomplishing adaptive goals in emotionally arousing situations.

The theme of emotional competence was first amplified by Carolyn Saarni in a presentation to the Nebraska Symposium on Motivation in 1988 when, borrowing the term from sociologist Steve Gordon, she described the skills that contribute to the growth of self-efficacy in emotional transactions. Her insightful research leading up to that presentation—and her studies since then—have contributed to a better understanding of those skills, including children's grasp of the nature of emotional dissemblance, their understanding of the origins and outcomes of emotional expressions, their strategic capacities to manage others' emotional experience, and their emotional coping capacities. At the same time, colleagues in developmental and clinical psychology have explored other topics related to emotional competence, including the development of emotion regulation capacities, the emergence of empathy and its prosocial correlates, emotion-related discourse in parent–child relationships, and the emotional dynamics of close relationships. This long-awaited book synthesizes this exciting work in the context of a compelling theoretical account of the development of emotional competence that integrates emerging research insights, perspectives from emotions theory and developmental psychology, the author's clinical experience, and her background as a skilled teacher, therapeutic supervisor, and keen observer of human behavior and development.

One of the central themes of *The Development of Emotional Competence* is the intimate connection between relationships and emotional development. If you ask "How could it be otherwise?" you have not been attending to a long tradition in emotions theory that portrays emotions as inward, biologically based experiences that are played out on a social stage. By contrast, Carolyn Saarni's portrayal of the development of emotional competence draws on functionalist and social constructivist perspectives to affirm that relationships help to define the meaning of emotional experience. In immediate contexts, social responses are central to the situations that elicit emotion and the goals that are relevant to emotional arousal. Considered more broadly, social partners help to define what it means to be "emotionally competent," whether this involves empathic responsiveness, facility with emotion terms and emotional scripts, or the capacity to convey emotion or to cope adaptively with arousal. From the wide view of human development, moreover, relationships are crucial to emotional socialization by which children appreciate the significance of emotion to themselves, others, and their culture, and learn the behaviors that are appropriate to emotional expression. In Saarni's view, therefore, the skills of emotional competence—like emotion itself—are constituted through a developing person's transactions with others throughout life.

The social construction of emotional competence also includes the culture. With refreshing perspective, Saarni reminds us that familiar emotions carry significantly different meaning in different human cultures. To illustrate, the reader is introduced to the early child-rearing practices of !Kung bushmen in northwestern Botswana by which the expression of aggression is channeled in ways much different from middle-class norms in the United States. She also presents Western and non-Western conceptions of self that shape children's feelings of shame and guilt, examples of adult teasing in Mexican-American and lower-income south Baltimore families that socialize emotion and self-awareness in children, and varieties of cultural display rules that guide the emotional expressions of children in Japan, India, Britain, and the United States. Indeed, each chapter that presents a component skill of emotional competence also includes a discussion of cultural differences in how that capacity is socialized in different cultural systems.

A second theme of *The Development of Emotional Competence* is the intimate connection between emotional development and the self. Emotional competence is built on self-understanding. An emerging sense of self defines many of the goals underlying emotional experience. Self-understanding also underlies the awareness of emotional states, the perception of self in a social context that guides emotional communication and self-presentation, and the strategies for emotional management that have personal and social consequences. As it develops, however, emotional competence alters self-understanding. Skills of emotional competence enhance self-esteem, and a sense of self-efficacy derives from accomplishing one's goals in emotional transactions. When a child manages social anxiety to make friends in a new school, an adolescent offers empathic support to a distressed peer, or an adult deters conflict by thoughtful emotional communication, the skills of emotional competence contribute to social success and self-confidence.

Viewed in this light, emotional competence is an important contributor to psychological well-being. This is thoughtfully elucidated in the author's discussion of how emotional competence is relevant to the growth of coping and resilience. Because personal well-being is a function not just of the vagaries of life's challenges but of one's capacities for effectively managing these challenges, the skills of emotional competence provide valuable personal resources. But in Saarni's view, emotional competence is a personal resource whose efficacy is significantly affected by the demands of the immediate context, the support of significant relational partners, and the values of the culture. Children acquire emotional competency not as a universally applicable, trans-contextual capability, but in relation to the relationships and contexts in which they live and develop. The author thus offers fascinating hypotheses concerning how, for example, the individualism of Western cultures may rob children of the coping skills that depend on well-established collective practices, and the possibility that children who are emotionally incompetent in certain social contexts may be extremely competent in others. In doing so, the author thoughtfully reminds us that individual capacities for emotional competence are a function of both the person and the context.

This leads to a final theme of *The Development of Emotional Competence*, which is the practical relevance of these issues to policy and practice. Throughout this book, developmental processes contributing to emotional self-efficacy are reexamined through the prism of developmental psychopathology, troubled family ecologies, and other challenges to human development. Each chapter that profiles a constituent skill of emotional competence includes attention to individual differences in "social maturity" that may derive from emotional disturbances, social incompetence, domestic conflict, child maltreatment, behavior problems, or other reasons, and the final chapter is devoted to a focused exploration of these issues in the context of emotional incompetence and dysfunction. In so doing, the author reminds readers of the broad range of developmental challenges and capacities that are relevant to the growth of emotional competence, and the applicability of these formulations to clinical intervention.

The author's clinical heart is also revealed in the first-person narratives, case studies, and vignettes that illustrate facets of emotional competence in each chapter. Like most readers, these stories linger in my memory as they exemplify the developmental influences Saarni discusses. I think of the comparison of Alex and Takeo, who each experience shame in the context of their culture's values concerning the self and the collective. C's acute sensitivity to the feelings of a troubled peer that might have escaped the detection of any other eighth-grader is an evocative portrayal of emotional competence in a young adolescent. Fred tries to protect his mother and younger sister from an abusive stepfather through hypervigilance and deception, with the same tendencies having disastrous consequences in his second-grade classroom. There is also the remarkable sequence of narratives and stories by Heather, Carolyn Saarni's daughter, gathered by her mother at different ages to illustrate children's developing facility with emotional communication through language (and the evocative poem by Mei Yao Ch'en in the same chapter). The author's clinical insight and skill as a teacher make these narratives and case studies extraordinarily powerful illustrations of the practical implications of the processes of emotional development she unfolds.

There is, in fact, much to ponder in this book. The influence of moral character on the development of emotional competence is a fascinating (and somewhat unexpected) theme that will, it is hoped, stimulate new research interest in this issue. I found other questions occurring to me as I read these provocative chapters. How do older adults achieve emotional self-efficacy, especially in relation to changes in their physical capacities and living circumstances (such as retirement and nursing homes)? In what ways are the challenges to emotional competence in adolescence unique to that stage of life? Can interventions be tailored to foster the development of specific skills in emotional competence for troubled individuals? The author's thoughtful discussion provides a wealth of research questions for future study.

The Development of Emotional Competence advances our understanding of the rich tapestry of human emotion, and of the skills that emerge as we learn to live with its influence in daily life. It is a valuable resource to students (advanced undergraduate and graduate) as well as professionals in psychology, counseling, social work, and education. As a developmentalist, clinician, parent, and astute observer of human emotion, Carolyn Saarni has presented a complex and essential feature of human experience in a comprehensible and compelling manner.

Ross A. Thompson
University of Nebraska

Preface and Acknowledgments

I had been intrigued for some time by children's sophistication in dissociating how they felt from what they expressed behaviorally, and with the support of the Spencer Foundation, the National Science Foundation, and assorted small grants from Sonoma State University I was able to carry out several key studies on children's emotional dissemblance. But children's skill at this sort of emotional–expressive maneuvering turned out to be just the "tip of the iceberg," so to speak. What I became fascinated with was that this facile strategy for managing one's expressive behavior, especially in challenging social interactions, was really a reflection of larger issues such as what do children need to be able to take into account in order to participate in this dance of emotion-laden exchange, and, on a more abstract level, what role do context and culture play in generating the meaningfulness of emotion?

Fortunately, I had the opportunity to enjoy many a good conversation with Paul L. Harris, who challenged me to think carefully about how cognition interfaces with the more social and expressive aspects of emotional experience, and for many years I had had the privilege of "arguing and debating" with Michael Lewis. As can be seen in this volume, both of these astute (and very productive) individuals have had considerable influence on my thinking. We have also worked together on several edited books, yielding *Children's Understanding of Emotion* (with Paul L. Harris), *The Socialization of Emotion,* and *Lying and Deception in Everyday Life* (both with Michael Lewis). More recently, Joe Campos has also influenced how I look at emotion and culture, and through him I have immersed myself in Richard Lazarus's work. The functionalist–relational view of emotion that these two individuals espouse added depth to my thinking about how our interpersonal relationships permeate our emotional experience and vice versa. This friendship yielded a productive outcome as well; the chapter with Joe Campos and Donna Mumme on "Emotional Development: Action, Communication, and Understanding" in the most recent edition of the *Handbook of Child Psychology* presages in many ways what this volume is about.

However, there were three things that seemed sorely missing in what had been written about emotional development. One was that most of the thoughtful essays and books focused on the first two or three years of life; this volume intends to fill that gap by focusing on childhood and early adolescence. The second omission was the role of cultural differences in emotional development. The approach I have taken in this volume is that culture is the "master narrative" which ideally we should make more explicit in our research on emotional development. The third and final missing feature was more personal: Every time I read an essay or book about emotion in general or emotional development in particular, I felt as though the writers had diabolically "killed" emotion. It seemed extraordinary that something so rich, pervasive, and socially nuanced could be rendered by our psychological science into something so lifeless. Since I am also trained as a clinician, I could not help but notice that clinical writing was a lot more engaging to read and did not put me to sleep quite so fast. The difference between the two lies in the use of cases, which we as developmental researchers have been loathe to use to illustrate our thinking. In recent years there has also been a resurgence of fascination with narratives, essentially stories, and how we all learn from them. As a consequence of my exposure to this growing field and, frankly, in order to have more fun writing this book, I have incorporated many cases and vignettes into the volume. I hope that readers will in turn enjoy reading about children's emotional experiences accompanied by lively examples.

The cases are composites, based on children I have worked with clinically or whom I have come to know through my students' counseling internships; the real children have been sources of inspiration for thinking about emotional competence and resiliency. Although they must remain anonymous, I very much appreciate their gift to this book. Lastly, I must acknowledge my own children, Heather and Matthias, who have taught me more than any book ever could about emotional competence.

In closing, I want to extend heartfelt thanks to Claire Kopp for her unfailing support and encouragement as Coeditor of The Guilford Series on Social and Emotional Development. Her splendid critique of multiple drafts has contributed in very substantial ways to making this volume a more professional endeavor. She deserves some sort of editorial gold medal to acknowledge the time and energy she gave to this enterprise. Earlier partial drafts were also scrutinized by Marion Underwood and Michael Lewis, and I am grateful to both of them for their extensive input.

Contents

What Is Emotional Competence?

*A*n effective way to grasp just what is involved in emotional competence is to look inside oneself. Think back over the last week about a couple of situations in which you were very much aware of having had feelings about an issue, a relationship, an exchange with someone. Was there a sense of justification for how you felt? Did you feel at the end of the episode that there was some degree of closure or of understanding between yourself and the other person? Did you get what you wanted or at least manage to avoid what you really did not want?

Perhaps you contemplated situations that evoked in you a sense of coming to terms with your feelings about yourself, about others, about your efforts and aptitudes, and so forth. Overall, in each of these situations you might have felt that you emerged from them in ways that felt as though you got what you wanted *within a realistic context.*

On the other hand, perhaps as you thought back about the last few days, you thought of occasions that stymied you, you were convinced your awkwardness was visible to all, but eventually you resolved the difficult transaction and felt that given its potential for disaster or excruciating embarrassment, you came out pretty well, dignity more or less intact, and the relationship perhaps more realistically defined or enhanced by additional coping skills.

As you contemplated this recent emotional episode, consider how you also responded in light of your *character,* which you might think of as your disposition to act with a sense of justification, of "doing the right thing." Granted your feelings reflected self-interest, which is clearly the adaptive reason for having emotions, but your self-interest is also defined by your moral sense on which I elaborate in the first chapter.

Emotional competence entails resilience and self-efficacy (and self-efficacy includes acting in accord with one's sense of moral character). When one is emotionally competent, one is demonstrating one's self-efficacy in emotion-eliciting transactions, which are invariably social in nature. Our emotional response is *contextually anchored in social meaning,* that is, the cultural messages we have absorbed about the meaning of social transactions, of relationships, and even our self-definitions. Emotional competence sounds straightforward and simple, but in fact it is subtle, complex, and sometimes downright elusive. This is because the ideas behind each of these concepts, namely, emotion, competence, resilience, self-efficacy, character, emotion elicitation, and social transaction, represent whole sets of theories and assumptions, all of them very much anchored in cultural context.

As you proceed through this book, you will gain understanding about each of these concepts and, I hope, considerable appreciation for how marvelously adaptive and intensely emotional people are. I make liberal use of narratives, vignettes, and cases throughout the volume to render more "alive" the emotional experience that is inherent in all of the skills and capabilities that make up emotional competence. These cases and examples also illustrate my theoretical emphasis on the social context of emotional experience, which is further elaborated on in Chapter 1.

Finally, to make things even more complicated, consider how emotional competence develops in the individual. We are born with some impressive affective capacities and innate responses, but if you think of this as the basic "skeleton" of emotional experience, where does the "flesh and blood" come from? I concur that our biological evolution has endowed us to *be* emotional (e.g., Plutchik, 1980), but I argue that it is our embeddedness in relationships with others that provides the diversity in emotional experience, the challenges to emotional coping, and the immensely rich array of ways in which we communicate our emotional experience to others. Thus, our relationships influence our emotions, and our emotions reciprocally influence our relationships.

❧ *Chapter 1*

The Inseparability of Emotional and Social Development

INTRODUCTION

In this first chapter I lay the foundation for emotional competence: its antecedents or contributing elements, its components, and its effects on how we adapt to the challenges of our lives. As described in the Prologue, we demonstrate emotional competence when we emerge from an emotion-eliciting encounter with a sense of having accomplished what we set out to do. *Self-efficacy* is the psychological concept that refers to this sense of accomplishment, and Bandura (1977, 1989) is credited with having elaborated on the notion of self-efficacy as meaning that the individual has the capacity and skills to achieve a desired outcome. The emotion-eliciting encounter derives its meaningfulness from the *social context* in which we have grown up, and thus emotional experience is developmentally embedded in social experience; indeed, the two are reciprocally influential (Saarni, 1989b, 1990a). The theme of inextricability of emotional and social development is evident throughout the book, not only in the research described but also in the emphasis given to cultural influence.

Contributing Elements

The primary contributors to emotional competence include *one's self* or ego identity, *one's moral sense* or character, and *one's developmental history*—with this last element an especially significant factor. I elaborate on the role of the self in emotional competence in Chapter 2, and I return to the role of one's moral character in the present chapter as well as touch on its relevance in other chapters. One's developmental history is addressed in summary form later in this chapter, in Chapter 3 from the standpoint of the socialization of emotion, and in each of the remaining chapters with considerable detail.

Components

The components of emotional competence are those *skills* needed to be self-efficacious, particularly when we are in emotion-eliciting social transactions, for interpersonal exchange is the crucible in which meaningfulness is established (Mead, 1934) and identities negotiated (Swann, 1987). The notion of self-efficacy in regard to emotion-eliciting *social* transactions considers how people can respond emotionally yet simultaneously and strategically apply their knowledge about emotions and their emotional expressiveness to negotiate their way through interpersonal exchanges. To some extent, the notions of competence and efficacy are redundant. The notion of competence has been defined as the capacity or ability to engage with a variable and challenging social–physical environment, resulting in growth and mastery for the individual (White, 1959). However, by using the term "emotional competence," we can begin to articulate the emotion-related capacities and abilities an individual needs to deal with that changing environment such that he or she emerges as more differentiated, better adapted, effective, and confident. Throughout the text I frequently refer to these emotion-related capacities and abilities as skills to emphasize the effective functioning that is implicit in the notion of emotional competence.

Table 1.1 lists eight skills of emotional competence. Chapters 4 through 11 elaborate on each skill with relevant research and illustrative examples. These eight skills are not necessarily exhaustive; there may be others.

The derivation of these eight skills is pragmatic: In surveying the field of emotional development, the first six of these skills reliably appear in empirical investigations. The last two are more subtle and probably reflect my clinical training as well as my role as a developmental psychologist. They are my attempt to capture the fact that we live in social–emotional *systems* (skill 7) and that emotional competence should ultimately address *wisdom,* namely, that we can discern what works best

TABLE 1.1. Skills of Emotional Competence

1. Awareness of one's emotional state, including the possibility that one is experiencing multiple emotions, and at even more mature levels, awareness that one might also not be consciously aware of one's feelings due to unconscious dynamics or selective inattention.

2. Ability to discern others' emotions, based on situational and expressive cues that have some degree of cultural consensus as to their emotional meaning.

3. Ability to use the vocabulary of emotion and expression terms commonly available in one's (sub)culture and at more mature levels to acquire cultural scripts that link emotion with social roles.

4. Capacity for empathic and sympathetic involvement in others' emotional experiences.

5. Ability to realize that inner emotional state need not correspond to outer expression, both in oneself and in others, and at more mature levels the ability to understand that one's emotional–expressive behavior may have an impact on another and to take this into account in one's self-presentation strategies.

6. Capacity for adaptive coping with aversive or distressing emotions by using self-regulatory strategies that ameliorate the intensity or temporal duration of such emotional states (e.g., "stress hardiness").

7. Awareness that the structure or nature of relationships is in large part defined by how emotions are communicated within the relationship, such as by the degree of emotional immediacy or genuineness of expressive display and by the degree of emotional reciprocity or symmetry within the relationship; for example, mature intimacy is in part defined by mutual or reciprocal sharing of genuine emotions, whereas a parent–child relationship may have asymmetric sharing of genuine emotions.

8. Capacity for emotional self-efficacy; the individual views her- or himself as feeling, overall, the way she or he wants to feel; that is, emotional self-efficacy means that one accepts one's emotional experience, whether unique and eccentric or culturally conventional, and this acceptance is in alignment with the individual's beliefs about what constitutes desirable emotional "balance"; in essence, one is living in accord with one's *personal* theory of emotion when one demonstrates emotional self-efficacy as well as in accord with one's moral sense.

for us relative to our values (skill 8). These skills of emotional competence also reflect a Western cultural bias, which is of concern to me, and thus for each of the respective skill chapters I include a section on cultural influence for how the emotional competency skill might manifest itself in other societies.

Effects

The effects of emotional competence may be seen in the *ability to manage one's emotions,* which is critical to the idea about being able to negotiate one's way through interpersonal exchanges; other important effects of emotional competence are *enhanced self-esteem* and adaptive *resilience* in the face of stressful circumstances. I briefly discuss these topics here; however, these effects are revisited in several subsequent chapters.

Emotion Management

As you contemplate your own recent emotional experiences, consider how you managed your emotions internally and externally, that is, how you coped with your emotional state "on the inside" and also how you managed your emotional–expressive behavior "on the outside" with others. Weber and Laux (1993) use the phrase *presentation of emotion* to describe how we cope with both our interpersonal interaction and our emotional experience. Depending on whom we are with and what we are feeling, we express our emotions with communicative intent, that is, our emotional–expressive behavior is meaningful to others. By adulthood we carry out these strategic displays almost too automatically, yet children have to learn these expressive strategies. Impressively, by the time they enter school, many children have acquired some of our society's expectations about how emotional–expressive behavior is to be regulated vis-à-vis particular social situations (e.g., children may readily show their anger at peers, but expressing it toward their teachers may give them pause; Saarni, 1989b; Underwood, Coie, & Herbsman, 1992). In Chapter 8 I review the expanding body of research on managing one's emotional–expressive behavior. However, some research evidence suggests that not until a few years later do children recognize and become able to verbalize how to strategically maneuver their *internal* emotional states so as to cope more effectively (Harris & Lipian, 1989). I return to this topic in greater detail in Chapter 9 as part of the discussion on coping with aversive emotions and distressing circumstances.

Self-Esteem

Self-efficacy has also been linked with self-esteem (e.g., Harter, 1982), and implicated in such an umbrella construct as emotional competence is self-esteem. But I foresee a chicken-and-egg problem here: Which comes first, emotional competence or high self-esteem? If they are correlated but one does not "cause" the other, does something else bring their concordance about? My hunch is that as one develops the skills of emotional competence, one also feels better, which serves to reinforce or validate one's self-esteem and confirms one's competence (mastery) in some situation. The more one feels that one's self-esteem is resilient, I suspect one then also becomes more likely to risk one's as yet untested competence in some new situation. If the situations to which we are referring are social ones, then resilient self-esteem facilitates trying out new interpersonal negotiation strategies. Resilient self-esteem also makes the job of managing one's emotional experience easier because anxiety about self-evaluation is reduced (cf. Thompson, 1990). A case borrowed from a colleague who supervises school counselors illustrates this point:

> Julie, age 9, was approached by her teacher to join a children's separation and divorce counseling group that met during the lunch hour once a week at the elementary school. The teacher was concerned by Julie's withdrawal from peers and mediocre academic performance; she had also heard that Julie's parents were recently separated. The school counselor met with Julie individually and learned that Julie felt ashamed by her parents' impending divorce. Julie felt she was somehow stigmatized and viewed as strange and weird in the eyes of the other children (despite a number of them living in single-parent homes).
>
> However, she did join the support group, and after several weeks began to participate in some of the "sit-coms" (skits) in which the kids acted and which allowed them to disclose and/or ventilate their anger, sadness, and, in Julie's case, feelings of shame. Not long after, Julie developed a firm friendship with another girl in the group, and the two of them, with the school counselor's guidance, formed their own "crisis outreach team." If another child in their class was unhappy about something (e.g., "So-and-so said she wouldn't be my friend anymore"), Julie and her new friend would go to the rejected and/or otherwise miserable feeling child and offer comfort and willingness to listen. At the end of the school year she confided to the school counselor that she felt sad about her parents' divorce but she really enjoyed coming to school. Her teacher confirmed the positive changes, and Julie finished the school year with excellent grades.

We see in this vignette that as Julie acquired greater emotional coping skills to deal with her own source of anguish, she became more able to try out previously unfamiliar interpersonal strategies that involved peer leadership, listening skills, and collaborative teamwork. Julie's sense of isolation was reduced by joining the support group, and as a result, we can infer that she began to feel better. This in turn allowed her to feel more effective with peers, and she risked "exposing" herself by beginning to participate in the mock sit-coms. As that activity further enhanced her sense of belonging and positive peer feedback fostered her self-esteem, she felt still better and arrived at a point where she felt emotionally ready to risk getting hurt or rejected in allowing a friendship to develop. The friendship flourished, and by that time Julie was well into her upward spiral toward developing further emotional competence and greater resilience in her self-esteem. In addition, her social skills had probably become more sensitive and complex, permitting her to fine-tune her negotiations with others. Her worries about what others might think of her family situation seem to have diminished or be replaced by more self-affirming attributions.

Resilience

Although the preceding vignette reflects a "successful" intervention with a distressed child, resilient or invulnerable children are also a source for learning how self-esteem and emotional competence may mutually develop. When we speak of resilience, we are talking about the capacity to recover after experiencing adversity, but this suggests to me that we return to some set point. I contend that psychological resilience in conjunction with emotional competence yields greater gains or growth following the recovery from adversity or trauma. Nowhere is this more evident than in Murphy and Moriarty's (1976) volume on children's vulnerability, coping, and growth (see also Anthony & Cohler, 1987). Their exquisitely sensitive insights into children's coping with stressors and coming to terms with losses suggest that children become more resilient when exposed to stressors that are within their coping capacity yet push them just a bit to deal with the emotional challenge. They are also clear that there is no such thing as a completely invulnerable child: Trauma, social exploitation, and lack of developmentally appropriate support from attachment figures create havoc in an otherwise temperamentally healthy child.

Murphy and Moriarty (1976) followed a number of children from birth to early adulthood. What they repeatedly found was that seemingly vulnerable infants began to develop abilities in the preschool years to increase their capacity for maintaining *integrity* in the face of pressures or threats to their adaptive functioning. Those children who were effective tended to progress through their childhood and adolescence with resilience. They were the "good copers," and in many respects what they demonstrated was emotional competence: They were self-efficacious in their social transactions with others, showing a range of emotional expressiveness and responsivity to others. These children also revealed what has been called healthy narcissism; in short, they liked themselves. Even when faced with serious setbacks and episodes of distressing emotional experience, they were able to "ride out the storm," handle anxiety and tolerate frustration, seek help when needed, and adapt flexibly to alternatives.

In Chapter 9 I return to this important effect of emotional competence and explore coping and emotion regulation in depth. However, before I proceed further, I think it is also important to provide an overview of my theoretical assumptions regarding emotional experience.

THEORETICAL PERSPECTIVES ON EMOTION

I can best describe my viewpoint in this volume on "what is emotion," "what causes emotion," "what do emotions consist of," and "where do emotions come from" as a blend of Lazarus's (1991) relational model of emotion, Campos and Barrett's (1984) functionalist model of emotion, and Lewis and Michalson's (1983) social constructivist model of emotion. Each model is briefly described; however, I see emotional experience and social experience as reciprocally influential. Thus, when I use Lazarus's or Campos's thinking about how emotion episodes reflect the individual's "goal-directed encounter with the environment," I couch my examples in the human relationships experienced by the individual, whether they were "encountered" in the present or in the past. In important ways, we are the products of our relationships, which are always transactional, whether we think of the outcome as working models of attachment that influence our subsequent close relationships (Cassidy, 1994) and style of emotion regulation (Thompson, 1990) or simply the pervasiveness of cultural context in how we think and construe our world. Another way to think about this is to see ourselves as deriving meaningfulness—without which we would not have a consciousness of experience—from the people who have loved us, spent time with us, taught us, or spurned and perhaps even exploited us.

Relational Model of Emotion

Lazarus's research spans decades and his definitive volume on emotion, *Emotion and Adaptation* (1991), has been a wonderfully rich source for my own thinking about the development of emotional competence. The brief summary offered here cannot do justice to the depth and breadth of his relational model of emotion. Pivotal to Lazarus's model is the idea that each category of emotion (see Table 1.2 for a list of the 15 emotions he discusses) has associated with it a *core relational theme,* and by this he means that each emotion has allied with it an appraisal process in which the relationship between the individual and the environment is construed as harmful or beneficial. Lazarus notes that there

TABLE 1.2. Core Relational Themes for Each Emotion

Anger	A demeaning offense against me and mine.
Anxiety	Facing uncertain, existential threat.
Fright	Facing an immediate, concrete, and overwhelming physical danger.
Guilt	Having transgressed a moral imperative.
Shame	Having failed to live up to an ego ideal.
Sadness	Having experienced an irrevocable loss.
Envy	Wanting what someone else has.
Jealousy	Resenting a third party for loss or threat to another's affection.
Disgust	Taking in or being too close to an indigestible object or idea.
Happiness	Making reasonable progress toward the realization of a goal.
Pride	Enhancement of one's ego identity by taking credit for a valued object or achievement, either our own or that of someone or a group with whom we identify.
Relief	A distressing goal-incongruent condition that has changed for the better or gone away.
Hope	Fearing the worst but yearning for better.
Love	Desiring or participating in affection, usually but not necessarily reciprocated.
Compassion	Being moved by another's suffering and wanting to help.

Note. From Lazarus (1991, p. 122). Copyright 1991 by Oxford University Press. Reprinted by permission.

are different kinds of harmful and beneficial relationships; for example, harmful ones might involve loss as in sadness and others might involve threat as in anxiety. Thus, the appraisal process is not merely dichotomized into positive or negative; indeed, Lazarus discusses at length primary and secondary appraisal processes, the former including goal relevance, goal (in)congruence, and degree of ego involvement and the latter including blame or credit, coping potential, and future expectations. Each kind of emotion derives its unique experiential pattern from this complex appraisal and in addition includes an action tendency or motivating disposition. For Lazarus, motivation is inseparable from emotion, regardless of whether the motives are considered conscious or unconscious. Indeed, we *feel* when we have a stake in the outcome of our encounter with our environment, and it does not matter whether we can verbalize what that stake is. But it is this dynamic process of engagement with an environmental encounter that yields the goals we strive for and which provides the texture to the different sorts of emotions we feel.

Another critical component of emotional experience that Lazarus stresses—as do I—is the *self* that experiences the feelings, makes sense of things, attributes varying degrees of importance to events, copes with circumstances, considers the degree to which one has control over outcomes, and so forth. Lazarus refers to this coordinating role of the self as *ego identity*, and he too views the self as inextricable from emotional processes. I see us as having composite selves, or what has been referred to as a self-system, and we may find that part of us wants one thing and another aspect of ourselves wants another. The resulting multiple emotions may result in ambivalence, procrastination or indecisiveness, or even self-deception about what one desires and seeks to do because of conflict with other goals and beliefs about the self. The self-system plays a central role in the construct of emotional competence, as is elaborated on in Chapter 2.

Functionalist Model of Emotion

The functional approach to emotion is closely aligned with Lazarus's relational model, although it may be somewhat more "radical" in that particular categories of emotion are not addressed as noted in Table 1.2 for Lazarus's core relational themes. To quote Campos, Kermoian, and Campos (1994), emotion is "the attempt by the person to establish, maintain, change, or terminate the relation between the person and the environment on matters of significance to the person" (p. 285). Indeed, Campos (1994) says that four things give significance to our experience and thus evoke an emotional response from us: (1) the relationship of the event to our goals (and this includes what we want in our transactions with others), (2) the social responses others give to us (e.g., their emotionally expressive reactions which we may view as evaluative of ourselves), (3) the hedonic tone of the event (e.g., consider the hedonic differences in an excruciating social exposure versus a tenderly affectionate exchange), and (4) our memories of similar earlier events (e.g., our interpersonal history surrounding this sort of event). Note that in the functionalist approach to emotion there is no need to resort to constructs such as "basic (or primary) emotions" or "emotion prototypes." The former are typically used by those researchers concerned with the bioevolutionary continuity of emotions (e.g., Ekman, 1989; Izard, 1993), the latter by social psychologists who typically studied verbalized emotional experience in adults (e.g., Shaver, Schwartz, Kirson, & O'Connor, 1987). Use of dimensions, such as a positive–negative continuum or degree of arousal (e.g., Russell & Bullock, 1985), would be descriptively relevant to a functionalist position insofar as the hedonic tone of the emotional experience is a notable marker and will influence subsequent behavior (e.g., avoidance or approach). Likewise, Frijda's (e.g., 1986) important contributions to emotion theory are consistent with a functionalist perspective: He too emphasizes emotion as the dynamic interface between the individual and the environment. For Frijda, that interface is by definition transactional and is most readily seen in people's plans and actions vis-à-vis their environment.

Because Campos and his associates are developmental researchers, they appear to give greater weight than Lazarus (or Fridja, for that matter) to the importance of social influences on the generation of emotion. Specifically, infants and toddlers, through a process called social referencing, learn from their caregivers the *emotional meaning* of many otherwise ambiguous transactions (discussed further in Chapter 4, in this volume; see also Saarni, Mumme, & Campos, 1998; Sorce, Emde, Campos, & Klinnert, 1985). Social contexts can also lead to the generation of emotion through contagion (e.g., Haviland & Lelwicka, 1987), as when several babies in a day-care center start to cry and the rest all join in. Finally, powerful social influences on the generation of emotion stem from others' approval or disapproval of our actions. Shame, pride, and embarrassment are "*self-conscious emotions*" because of the social exposure involved and the accompanying approval or disapproval from others that we experience. These self-conscious emotions become powerful motivators for subsequent behavior; that is, either we try to avoid these feelings, as in shame and embarrassment, or we try to promote feelings of pride upon the accomplishment of a significant achievement. (I return to a discussion of self-conscious emotions in Chapter 2.) The combined social influences on the generation of emotional experience are perhaps seen in their most complex outcome in the attachment relationship between child and parent, which appears to affect profoundly subsequent peer relations in childhood and even adult romantic relationships (e.g., Hazan & Shaver, 1994).

Social-Constructivist Model of Emotion

Similar to a functionalist model of emotion, which emphasizes the context in which emotion is experienced, a social-constructivist approach also views emotional experience as embedded in the conditions that justify it; that is, we do not have emotions in a vacuum, nor can we decisively tell what we are feeling based *solely* on introspection (Armon-Jones, 1986). But this perspective also emphasizes that we *learn* to give meaning to our context-dependent experience via our social exposure and our cognitive developmental capacities. In this sense, a social-constructivist approach to emotion is highly individualized: One's emotional experience is contingent upon specific contexts, unique social history, and current cognitive developmental functioning. Our unique social history includes our immersion in our culture's beliefs, attitudes, and assumptions; our observation of important others (as in social referencing described above); and the patterns of reinforcement from those with whom we are significantly involved. All these factors contribute to our learning what it means to feel something and then do something about it. The concepts we assign to emotional experience are saturated with nuance and context-dependent meaning, including the social roles we occupy (e.g., gender and age roles).

As for our current cognitive developmental functioning, Lewis and Michalson (1983), in their landmark volume, use the metaphor of a musical *fugue* to describe the interweaving and inseparable processes of cognition and emotion in human development. (Think of emotional experience as a melody which loses its identity if you begin to isolate and remove its various strands or musical subthemes.) Based on their research with 6-month-old infants, Lewis and Michalson found that the infants showed cycles of emotional expressivity interspersed with instrumental behaviors as they learned to pull on a strap attached to their arms to make a picture of another infant appear on a screen in front of them along with a recording of the *Sesame Street* theme song. Analyses of the infants' learning curves across 3-second intervals revealed rich patterns of waxing and waning instances of surprise, fear, interest, pleasure, and sadness, with considerable variation in patterning yet apparently coordinated with the infants readily learning to master the task. From this close-grained analysis of infants' learning, Lewis and Michalson concluded that the processing of information that was apparently involved in the infants' learning how to get the picture and music "to work" for them was inextricably linked with their affective responses to the stimuli. For these young infants cognition and emotion formed an integral system that functioned motivationally and thus facilitated the infants' learning how to get the desired picture and music to play.

When we think about Lewis and Michalson's cognition–emotion "fugue" model and extend it to older children who have access to verbal concepts, we can see how emotion learning expands phenomenally. With access to emotion-laden language, children are no longer dependent solely on direct exposure to immediate emotion-eliciting circumstances and on having to perceive directly others' emotional responses as in social referencing. They can now traverse time and space to learn about emotional experience, be it about others' emotions or in response to their own feelings. Books, media, narratives and other family "stories," the Internet (and maybe the all-important telephone, especially for young adolescents) can become powerful sources of emotional influence and learning. Chapter 6 addresses this topic in detail.

The sociologist Steve Gordon (1989) takes the idea of emotion learning a step further and contends that children are active *creators* of their own emotional experience. Through exposure to others, they learn the emotional behaviors, norms, and symbols of their culture (or subculture) as unintended consequences of social interaction. He states, "Having understood the cultural meaning of an emotion, children become able to act *toward* it—magnifying, suppressing, or simulating it in themselves, and evoking or avoiding it in other people" (p. 324). Thus, Gordon firmly embeds emotional experience in relationships and emphasizes the social *process* aspects of emotion in ways that developmental psychologists have only more recently begun to investigate explicitly. This emphasis on one's own active creation of emotional experience, integrated as it is with one's cognitive developmental functioning and one's social history, also underlies my use of the term "constructivism" and differentiates it from the more commonly encountered term, "social construction of emotions." The latter is related in that it poses that all emotions are sociocultural products, but it does not allow for the vagaries of human development (e.g., Armon-Jones, 1986).

In summary, my "theoretical roots" for the construct emotional competence take something from each of these three theoretical models, and I have synthesized my theoretical perspective toward emotional development by using these models as converging approaches to understanding emotion rather than as distinctly different perspectives. Specifically, the idea that the dynamic and organizing features of the self in relation to a social environment yield motivated behavior, is distinctively Lazarus's and reflects his social psychology orientation. When I combine this emphasis with the functionalist (Campos and colleagues) and social constructivist (Lewis and colleagues) approaches to examine emotional competence, I can anchor more firmly how motivation links up theoretically with emotion to yield self-efficacy. We are motivated to be efficacious (Bandura, 1977, 1989), and our emotions provide us with an ongoing experiential flow of information as to our degree of efficacy or sense of justification for feeling the way that we do. Chapter 2 elaborates on the self as a system, and Chapter 11 further addresses the notion of subjective well-being, a concept also studied by Lazarus.

The emphasis on cognitive development and learning that is evident in much of Lewis's and his colleagues' research has influenced not only my work but also much of the research cited on children's understanding of their own and of others' emotions (Chapters 4 and 5, respectively). All three theoretical models emphasize the social embeddedness of emotions, and that view is fundamental to my thinking about all of the emotional competence skills. Certainly the acquisition of an emotion lexicon and emotion scripts (Chapter 6), the experience of empathy (Chapter 7), and the recognition of emotions as definitive of relationship quality (Chapter 10) reflect the child's social nexus as inextricable from her or his emotional functioning. Lazarus's emphasis on ego identity and Lewis's concern with self-awareness are also evident in my interest in self-presentation strategies (Chapter 8). Lazarus's contribution to the literature on coping is also enormous, and much of the literature and theory that I review in Chapter 9 has been directly or indirectly influenced by the work of Lazarus and his colleagues. The functionalist view has also explicitly emphasized the significance of cultural context and exposure for how emotional responses are assigned meaningfulness (e.g., Saarni et al., 1998). In each of the emotional competence skill chapters (Chapters 4–11), I consider how culture may affect the skill in question. Let us now return to a further discussion of two of the other contributing elements to emotional competence, one's moral disposition and one's developmental history. As noted, the third contributing element, the self, is taken up in Chapter 2.

MORAL DISPOSITION AND EMOTIONAL COMPETENCE

We cannot talk about a construct such as emotional competence without addressing moral behavior. I do not intend to address moral development in this volume (the reader is referred to Kurtines & Gerwitz, 1995, 1991), but I do think that if we are functioning in an emotionally adaptive and balanced fashion, we invariably also live in accord with our moral *disposition*—not necessarily, however, with our moral code or rules. The latter are quite frequently relativistic and change with development and context, but the former is embedded in such concepts as sympathy, self-control, fairness, and a sense of obligation (Campbell & Christopher, 1996; Flanagan, 1991; Wilson, 1993). Personal integrity comes with a life lived in accord with one's moral sense or disposition, and concomitantly, such a life reflects emotional competence. Perhaps it is no accident that the individuals studied in Colby and Damon's (1992) case-oriented research on moral action and moral ideals were characterized by their commitment to truth-seeking, open-mindedness, compassion for others, flexibility toward change, and a sensitivity to "doing the right thing" in their daily lives and relationships with others. These adults demonstrated the sort of personal integrity that Blasi

(1983) had earlier described as characteristic of a moral self or identity, wherein one's self-concept is centrally defined by moral commitment. A moral self, a commitment to moral understanding and action, is synonymous with moral character.

The qualities noted previously by Wilson (1993) and others as being essential to moral disposition are not new; they are similar to and overlap with those espoused by Aristotle as constituting virtues (*Nichomachean Ethics,* trans. T. Irwin, 1985): courage (which was also viewed as necessary for sustaining community), justice (fairness in equity, reciprocity, and impartiality), temperance (or self-control), and wisdom (a felt knowingness of what is a right choice). The philosophers Wilson (1993) and MacIntyre (1981) echo Aristotle in their analyses of what is significant about honorable character, and Wilson in particular relies on developmental theory and anthropological findings to buttress his claim that character lies at the heart of a balanced life that is well-lived. Walker and Hennig (1997), in their analysis of moral development as part of personality, echo a similar theme; indeed, in reviewing their own and others' research on moral development (e.g., Haan, 1991; Walker, Pitts, Hennig, & Matsuba, 1995; Walker & Taylor, 1991) they emphasize that moral commitment and personal integrity are inextricable from one's social–emotional experience. I claim as well that such a balanced, well-lived life, characterized by personal integrity, is one that reflects emotional competence. I do not see how they can be separated from one another.

The idea that character is embedded in emotional competence also reveals that emotional competence is something we get better at as we mature. Young preschool children demonstrate sympathy, some degree of self-control (or compliance), and occasionally a sense of equity in their sharing. Duty, obligation, or conscience require more maturity, and this moral sense becomes evident in school-age children. But it is probably not until adolescence that we see an emerging personal integrity, or "character." I suggest that with mature adolescents, we see well-developed emotional competence. Indeed, when we encounter immature adolescents (i.e., for their age, they are acting like younger children), we are apt to *distrust* their personal integrity. In short, their character is still unformed, and I wager that our response to their emotional functioning indicates that we experience them as less than emotionally competent. I think that well-adjusted school-age children may be good candidates for emotional competence as well, but because they have not yet gone through the challenges of puberty to their self-definition and emotional experience, I suggest instead that they are well on their way to demonstrating emotional competence, albeit not yet at a mature level. If the past more or less predicts the future, they will make it.

EMOTIONAL COMPETENCE AND DEVELOPMENT

Traditionally, the major conceptual influences on developmental views of emotion have been derived from psychoanalytic or object relations theory (e.g., A. Freud, 1965; Mahler, 1968), evolutionary or psychobiological views (e.g., Izard & Malatesta, 1987; Panksepp, 1982), social learning (e.g., Cairns, 1979), or a Piagetian cognitive developmental perspective (e.g., Case, Hayward, Lewis, & Hurst, 1988; Fischer, Shaver, & Carnochan, 1988; 1990). The views espoused by Lewis and Michalson (1983) and my social-constructivist perspective reflect strong contributions from both social learning and cognitive developmental theory. I also approach emotional development with an emphasis on the individual's learning connections between felt emotions and the interpersonal transactions experienced by that individual (see also Saarni, 1978, 1989b), which is consistent with a social systems approach. Lewis (1997) recently elaborated the relations among context, social systems, and individual development, and I concur with his view that the social environment (broadly defined) and developmental processes are mutually influencing.

For the sake of brevity, Table 1.3 presents a brief descriptive summary of the developmental "milestones" in emotional experience relative to social interaction. This summary also portrays the inseparability of emotional and social development in that each of the broad organizing themes that I have used (regulation/coping, expressive behavior, and relationship building) assumes that social context is an inherent feature of emotional development. Indeed, these organizing themes capture for me the essence of what is important in emotional development: Consider what happens when there are deficits in emotion regulation, anomalies in expressive behavior, or difficulties in developing relationships (and Chapter 12 does just that). These organizing themes are also interactive with one another; I think of them as the multidimensional threads that constitute a dynamic fabric's weft and warp, yielding the woven pattern of adaptive emotional functioning. The developmental progression illustrated in Table 1.3 begins with birth and extends through adolescence, but the "fabric of emotional functioning" is indeterminate in length and may even extend its influence across generations.

As noted earlier, developmental issues and research outcomes are included in each of the chapters addressing the individual emotional competence skills. Concerns about methodology and measurement are also discussed in these chapters as they affect what we know about the development of the skills of emotional competence. Readers should also be aware of what I do *not* address in the context of emotional de-

TABLE 1.3. Noteworthy Markers of Emotional Development in Relation to Social Interaction

Age period	Regulation/coping	Expressive behavior	Relationship building
Infancy: 0–12 months	Self-soothing and learning to modulate reactivity. Regulation of attention in service of coordinated action. Reliance on caregivers for supportive "scaffolding" during stressful circumstances.	Behavior synchrony with others in some expressive channels. Increasing discrimination of others' expressions. Increasing expressive responsiveness to stimuli under contingent control. Increasing coordination of expressive behaviors with emotion-eliciting circumstances.	Social games and turn-taking (e.g., "peek-a-boo"). Social referencing. Socially instrumental signal use (e.g., "fake" crying to get attention).
Toddlerhood: 12 months–2½ years	Emergence of self-awareness and consciousness of own emotional response. Irritability due to constraints and limits imposed on expanding autonomy and exploration needs.	Self-evaluation and self-consciousness evident in expressive behavior accompanying shame, pride, coyness. Increasing verbal comprehension and production of words for expressive behavior and affective states.	Anticipation of different feelings toward different people. Increasing discrimination of others' emotions and their meaningfulness. Early forms of empathy and prosocial action.
Preschool: 2½–5 years	Symbolic access facilitates emotion regulation, but symbols can also provoke distress. Communication with others extends child's evaluation of and awareness of own feelings and of emotion-eliciting events.	Adoption of pretend expressive behavior in play and teasing. Pragmatic awareness that "false" facial expressions can mislead another about one's feelings.	Communication with others elaborates child's understanding of social transactions and expectations for comportment. Sympathetic and prosocial behavior toward peers. Increasing insight into others' emotions.

Age			
Early elementary school: 5–7 years	Self-conscious emotions (e.g., embarrassment) are targeted for regulation. Seeking support from caregivers still prominent coping strategy, but increasing reliance on situational problem-solving evident.	Adoption of "cool emotional front" with peers.	Increasing coordination of social skills with one's own and others' emotions. Early understanding of consensually agreed upon emotion "scripts."
Middle childhood: 7–10 years	Problem solving preferred coping strategy if control is at least moderate. Distancing strategies used if control is appraised as minimal.	Appreciation of norms for expressive behavior, whether genuine or dissembled. Use of expressive behavior to modulate relationship dynamics (e.g., smiling while reproaching a friend).	Awareness of multiple emotions toward the same person. Use of multiple time frames and unique personal information about another as aids in the development of close friendships.
Preadolescence: 10–13 years	Increasing accuracy in appraisal of realistic control in stressful circumstances. Capable of generating multiple solutions and differentiated strategies for dealing with stress.	Distinction made between genuine emotional expression with close friends and managed displays with others.	Increasing social sensitivity and awareness of emotional "scripts" in conjunction with social roles.
Adolescence: 13+ years	Awareness of one's own emotion cycles (e.g., guilt about feeling angry) facilitates insightful coping. Increasing integration of moral character and personal philosophy in dealing with stress and subsequent decisions.	Skillful adoption of self-presentation strategies for impression management.	Awareness of mutual and reciprocal communication of emotions as affecting quality of relationship.

velopment, namely, the domain of neurophysiological development of emotional experience, which is a rich and exciting area of research and warrants its own separate volume (for an overview of this topic, see Greenberg & Snell, 1997).

NARRATIVES OF EMOTIONAL EXPERIENCE: ILLUSTRATIONS FROM CHILDREN'S LIVES

I believe that altogether too much has been written *about* emotion that is stultifyingly devoid of any feeling, even as the given essay or book purports to inform us about emotion. I am not convinced that this is the best way to communicate what we know about emotion (this is where novelists and poets probably have an edge on social scientists). I hope to provide my readers with enough *narratives of emotional experience,* such as the case of Julie described earlier, throughout this volume so that the construct of emotional competence takes on vividness and is "knowable" beyond just the meaning of the words on the paper in front of them.

In recent years there has been considerable interest in how we use narratives, essentially stories, as ways to teach, to comprehend, to influence, and to develop self-understanding as well as an understanding of our unique social worlds (e.g., Haden, Haine, & Fivush, 1997; Hudson, Gebelt, Haviland, & Bentivegna, 1992; McCabe & Peterson, 1991; Neisser & Fivush, 1994; Oppenheim, Nir, Warren, & Emde, 1997). Metaphorically speaking, narratives are mirrors of individual experience, rich in personal detail, but they also reflect cultural meanings. Throughout this volume I try to capture the cultural meanings of emotional experience by using relevant narrative vignettes. Use of narratives (i.e., case illustrations, vignettes, and descriptive anecdotes) also helps to contextualize in *a planful manner* the diverse threads of meaning that need to be coordinated. We see in research on preschool children's learning to talk about themselves, using a narrative structure, that their conversations reveal their beginning to use multiple perspectives for both planning and coordinating their social interaction (e.g., Wolf, 1990). Play therapists have long used the narratives told by children as they "play out" conflicts and traumas as important indicators of how the children are constructing their understanding of events as well as regulating their emotional response to events (e.g., Slade, 1994). Thus, my use of narratives in this volume is both to facilitate the reader's understanding of what at times may seem like a great deal of abstract detail and to engage the reader affectively.

Parallel to my approach for communicating an otherwise abstract set of constructs are the investigations pursued by psychologists studying children's self-concept development. They too have found narratives to be a useful tool for looking at how children come to acquire *understanding* about complex events (e.g., Eder, 1994; McCabe & Peterson, 1991; Miller, 1994; Miller, Mintz, Hoogstra, Fung, & Potts, 1992). Fivush (1991), for example, found that the narratives that are told *to* the children and *by* the children typically involve an organization that sets the contextual stage (orientation), describes the crucial event, and provides a way for how to think about or evaluate the event. Similarly, both to facilitate readers' understanding and to make more graphic and vibrant what the components of emotional competence "look like" (and I hope "feel like") in the emotional experience of children at different ages and in different contexts, I include next two "narratives," the first from one of my students and the second from personal experience with children well-known to me. Similar to the investigative approach used by Fivush, Miller, and others, these cases also provide a contextual orientation, describe an emotional event, and provide an affective framework *for the reader* that gives a more personal meaning to the emotional experience of these children. (Names and circumstances have been modified to preserve the privacy of the children and their families.)

A 6-Year-Old's Emerging Emotional Competence

In this first vignette, the reader should note the young girl's emotional competencies of awareness of emotions in herself and expectations of emotions in others. In addition, she was aware of social standards and thus was capable of experiencing self-conscious emotions such as shame.

> Six-year-old Rachel's grandfather, George, regularly picked her up from school and walked her home past an old Petaluma neighborhood grocery store, where they regularly dropped in to chat with the owner, Mrs. Barkan, who was recently widowed, and Rachel would get a treat to eat. George was also a widower. Sometimes Rachel felt quite impatient at how long their chats lasted, and she would whine at him to hurry up and leave, because, frankly, after finishing her treat, standing around in the shop was boring.
>
> One day she waited around for Grandpa, and he didn't come. Rachel waited and waited, growing angry and feeling aware of her full bladder. Urgency finally propelled Rachel toward Mrs. Barkan's store, and she hoped she could ask Mrs. Barkan if she could go inside and use the toilet; but how embarrassing! Maybe Mrs. Barkan would know where Grandpa was too.

The store was quiet except for the bell over the door that jangled when she pushed it open and walked through; where was Mrs. Barkan? Rachel felt nervous about being in the shop alone, and she felt her insides tighten; for the moment she forgot her bladder's pressure. She walked past the candy counter where she usually selected her treat when she was with Grandpa. Rachel's eyes paused longingly on the Sugar Daddy lollipops and her hand reached out and seemed to go of its own accord to take one of the Sugar Daddies. As she thought of him, she felt mad, why had he forgotten her? That was mean of him, that he didn't care to come and get her and had just left her. And Mrs. Barkan was mean too; why didn't she come downstairs and let her use the toilet? Rachel decided that she deserved to keep the Sugar Daddy because Grandpa and Mrs. Barkan had been mean to her. But maybe Grandpa was angry with her and hadn't come to get her because she usually complained in the shop that she wanted to go and Mrs. Barkan was always reminding her to say thank you for the treats because she often forgot. Maybe they decided she was too much bother and too rude to care about!

Just then a familiar noise from upstairs caught her ear; why, it was Grandpa's coughing! What was he doing up there? She moved away from the candy counter, the Sugar Daddy tight in her hand. Suddenly Mrs. Barkan appeared, her hair down and her face flushed, and, quite startled, Rachel's bladder let loose.

Mortified tears flooded her face next, and she handed over the Sugar Daddy to the approaching Mrs. Barkan, sure that she was going to be rebuked for stealing and for messing up the floor. But Mrs. Barkan was laughing and saying something about teaching old dogs new tricks. Rachel felt confused and ashamed. Then Grandpa appeared, looking sheepish and smiling all the while, and Mrs. Barkan said, "George, here are my car keys, go ahead and take Rachel home, and then come on back and stay for supper." She tucked the Sugar Daddy back into Rachel's hand and with a wink at George, she said, "We all deserve some treats today." Rachel felt forgiven, relieved, but still a bit confused. Why weren't they mad at her?

Rachel's mother entertained me as she told me what her father had revealed and what little Rachel had also tearfully described about the incident. In looking at Rachel's emotional experience, her various "emotional contortions" involved a couple of the emotional competency skills listed earlier. She was aware of her own emotional state ("mad") and righteously believed she was entitled to the candy because the adults had not done what they were "supposed to." Subsequently, Rachel made attributions about her grandfather's emotional state that included believing he was angry with her because she was rude and bothersome to him when she should not have been, that is, he did not deserve her "meanness" in a reciprocal sense. Rachel's shame over violating social propriety (wetting herself) and moral standards (taking the candy) were seen by her as having causal value for others' to have an emotional response toward her; she expected them to become angry with her. When they weren't, she felt confused, and it was here that her ignorance showed itself, for she was unable to read subtle situational cues and expressive behavior and combine them to yield hunches about what Mrs. Barkan and George may have been doing. For our present purposes this vignette also anchors the notion that emotional experience is firmly embedded in relationships, and that understanding contextual nuances—if this had been available to Rachel—can make all the difference in the world in one's emotional experience.

Preadolescent Emotion Management Used to Influence Others

The next vignette, involving two preadolescent boys from my extended family, illustrates the emotional competency of being able to dissociate one's emotional state from one's expressive behavior. The two brothers, identical twins Ned and Jack, adeptly maneuvered through a difficult social situation with an older bully, Steve, by dissembling how they really felt; thus, they managed their emotional reactions for the sake of self-presentation and thereby strategically gained advantages and avoided disadvantages in their interaction with Steve.

> Ned and Jack looked dismally at the gray-colored bologna inside the sandwiches their dad had packed for them while they were attending "Marine Adventures Daycamp." They were enrolled in a class to learn how to kayak on the San Francisco Bay during their summer vacation. The stiff breeze blew one of their sandwich wrappers away, and the camp counselor barked at them, "Hey, no garbage dumping around here!" Then the older know-it-all kid, Steve, puffed himself up and called out to all the other would-be kayakers, "yeah, if that four-handed, two-headed creature over there can't even hang onto its lunch, I wonder how it's going to be able to hang onto the paddles." He sat back smirking at the twins. Ned and Jack bit into their tasteless sandwiches, chewed, and swallowed without missing a beat and, without awareness, in complete unison. Their faces registered nothing of the insult.
>
> Later, as they donned their wet suits in preparation for going out into the bay, they muttered assorted threats and curse words to one another about Steve and vowed vengeance. As the week went on, Steve kept up his needling remarks and even shoved Jack

at one point. Even the camp counselor seemed a bit intimidated by the arrogant and hostile youth. Finally, Ned and Jack got their chance for revenge. They had spent part of a lunch break exploring the tide pools along the rocky edge of the bay and had found a small rock crab, which they caught and bagged in one of their sandwich wrappers, of course. Ned opted to engage Steve in some berating and putdowns while behind Steve's back Jack dropped the crab into the bully's wetsuit pull-on pants.

The twins fairly leapt into their wetsuits and paddled out onto the water to watch what Steve would do. He donned his wetsuit, seemingly nothing amiss. He too paddled out, and then let out a scream that revealed his adolescent changing voice as it oscillated back and forth between a young boy's soprano shriek and a youth's guttural bellow. He clutched his crotch, rocking the kayak violently, and dumped it over. As he bobbed up and down in the water, furiously trying to loosen his wetsuit under water (which is nearly impossible to do), the twins paddled over, with great effort suppressing their laughter and substituting expressions of concern and worry, and asked what was wrong and if they should get help. Steve said he was pretty sure a scorpion was in his wetsuit or perhaps it was a yellow jacket that got in there. Yeah, he needed to be towed back to shore because his kayak had also drifted away.

Ned and Jack artfully played out their rescue role, and Steve's performance in the water became the source of much comic repetition by the other boys on shore. Steve looked balefully around for the perpetrator of the trick and not finding a ready target, he vented his anger and chagrin by making a great show of offering the squashed crab that had been retrieved from his wetsuit to the ever-hovering seagulls.

He never suspected the twins; after all, they had been right in front of him because he had been arguing with them before getting into his wetsuit. For once, it paid off for Jack and Ned to be perceived as one, and they nodded with astute commiseration over Steve's ostensible suffering, and added sympathetically with perhaps just a trace of ruefulness, "What a terrible thing to do to that crab, too."

This story shows both emotional competence and incompetence, the former illustrated by the twins and the latter by the bully, Steve. Ned and Jack were aware of how they felt but strategically did not show their anger upon being insulted on the first day of daycamp by an older and bigger boy; similarly, they concealed their glee at the success of their "revenge" on Steve and adopted an emotional front of a concerned expression to prevent retaliation from the bully. Steve's emotional competence was rather limited: He coped with aversive emotion such as shame by taking it out on a hapless creature (the crab); he was not sensitive to emotional response in others, and empathy was presumably not one of his strong points.

These narrative examples provide an experiential sense of the more obvious aspects of emotional competence as well as the more subtle components and skills of emotional competence. My intention with these stories was also to further emphasize emotions as inextricably connected to social relations (Saarni, 1989b). We may have a biological base for our emotions, but social experience, whether conveyed by media or in real-life interpersonal exchange, provides the full range of complexity of emotional experience. That growth in complexity of emotional experience is also represented in the construct of emotional competence.

THE BOOK'S PLAN

In the next chapter I consider how the development of the self-system is intimately linked to emotional development within the individual. In Chapter 3 I map out the theoretical context for how the socialization of emotion is linked to emotional competence. An important ingredient in that linkage of emotion socialization with emotional competence is how we acquire our culture's (or subculture's) view of what emotion is all about and how it works; I refer to these cultural beliefs as the individual's naive or *folk theory of emotion.* Folk theories of emotion are also discussed from a cross-cultural perspective and are embedded in narratives. For example, consider how often people in the United States recount some anger episode using the "volcano theory" of emotion—a belief that unexpressed emotions if not somehow "vented" will build up inside an individual and "explode" in some intense fashion, presumably also with a high likelihood of being destructive, much like a volcano. But other non-Western societies do not necessarily view emotions as accumulative or explosive. In Chapters 4 through 11 I elaborate on each of the eight skills of emotional competence previously listed in Table 1.1 relative to empirical research conducted by myself and others. Each of the eight skills is discussed in terms of how it is further influenced by gender and culture. For the most part, my focus is on children and young adolescents, although infant emotional development is occasionally considered. In the final chapter of this volume I consider distortions in emotional development that result in emotional *in*competence and discuss implications for developmental psychopathology and clinical practice.

Chapter 2

The Role of the Self in Emotional Competence

GOALS AND EMOTIONS

Given that emotional competence, by definition, entails a sense of *self-efficacy*, we need to address the role of the self in emotional experience and in emotional development. In the discussion that follows I lay the foundation for why one of the primary contributors to emotional competence is one's self or ego identity and how one of the more significant effects of emotional competence is resilient self-esteem. My views on the role of the self in emotion are consistent with both Lazarus's relational model of emotion and Campos's functional model in that I see the self as the "contact point" between environment and biological organism. This contact point or interface functions to *coordinate and mediate in an adaptive fashion the meaningfulness of the environment for the individual.* Thus, the self plays the role of coordinator and mediator of experience. (For a comprehensive literature review on the development of self-representations, see Harter, 1998.)

A critical consequence of the self's playing its coordinator and mediator roles is that *values* are assigned to the context we are engaged in. When we differentially respond to the particular context facing us because of its relative significance to us, we are also acting in a goal-directed fashion. In turn, our goals are multifaceted: For example, our goals may be concerned with matters of greater or lesser importance, be oriented toward the short or long term, or be premised on avoidance (self-protection) or approach (self-enhancement). In short, to be goal-directed is to function with motives vis-à-vis a particular context. The connection between emotions and motives comes about because when we are engaged in an encounter with our environment, we have a personal stake in this encounter (Lazarus, 1991). That is, we have construed this encounter as meaningful for us in either a generally beneficial or a harmful way, and as a result we become motivated to do something about our involvement in the emotion-eliciting situation. It is in this sense that emotions are *functional*: They goad us into action whereby we initiate, modify, maintain, or terminate our relationship to the particular circumstances in which we are engaged (Campos et al., 1994). Stein and Trabasso (1993) also emphasize the centrality of goals to emotional experience and subsequent action. They state succinctly, "When a change in goal maintenance occurs, and emotions are experienced, plans are mobilized" (p. 282). Lazarus's core relational themes noted in Table 1.2 (Chapter 1, this volume) are also designated as such because they describe a *goal relationship* between the self and its involvement in a particular encounter.

I want to highlight further the role of the self in emotional competence by emphasizing that goals are individualized. The aphorism "different strokes for different folks" captures the variability and unique preferences or values that are invested in the goals we have vis-à-vis our encounters with our environment. When we recall that this environment invariably involves other people interacting with us as well (all of whom also have their unique goals), then we truly have an interesting and highly dynamic mélange of emotions, goals, and motives. It surely feels at times as though we must act as though we are on the right track toward attaining our goals, even as self-doubt nibbles at us from behind or we recognize, belatedly, that once again we have acted according to one of our emotional foibles. We are not guaranteed that our goals will be met in each individual emotional encounter with our environment; rather, we have a probabilistic belief in our self-efficacy to attain our goals (Bandura, 1989).

Self-efficacy is clearly served when we attain adaptive goals, and we infer, in hindsight, that emotional competence was manifested in those encounters. But how does the "self" recruit emotionally competent strategies and thus facilitate effective adaptation to the emotion-eliciting interpersonal encounter? And just "who" is it that is doing this ascription of meaning to a context and deriving appropriate and planful goals for the self? This is where we get into some fascinating theoretical discussion about the very nature of the self, which is itself a Western cultural construction. The remainder of this chapter addresses the hypothesized nature of the self, cultural constraints on the beliefs we ascribe to a "self," implications for self-esteem, and emotional development involving awareness of the self (i.e., self-conscious emotions such as embarrassment, shame, pride, and guilt; Lewis, 1992a, 1992b, 1993a). Relative to this last topic I also revisit the connection between moral disposition and emotional competence.

THE SELF-SYSTEM

Although we find it easy to talk about what is a "self" in Western cultures, it is quite a different story when one tries to undertake empirical research on the self. There are all sorts of questionnaires designed to get at self-esteem and the self-concept, but the interesting question is, *Who* is rating the self on these questionnaires? Clearly it is one's self observing and evaluating one's self, and ultimately checking a box on a questionnaire that refers to some characteristic quality about oneself. In short, the self is not unitary: It can act and reflect on itself. Theoretically, I believe the self to be multidimensional, and some theorists use the term "self-system" to indicate the many interrelated parts of the self. In this chapter I describe our culture's historical view of the self as consisting of two aspects. However, to link this dual self to emotional development, I have to complicate things a bit, for the dual self is globally conceived and does not permit us a fine-grained description for how the self can be aware of experiencing multiple feelings or ambivalence, feelings about feelings, or emotional defenses. Specifically, I add Neisser's (1988, 1992) view of a triple self (the ecological self, the self extended in time, and the evaluative self) and Markus and Kitayama's (1991) analysis of the self as independent and individualistic (typically a Euro-American view) as opposed to a construal of the self as interdependent or social interaction-based (more commonly encountered in non-Western cultures).

A multifaceted self also permits a discussion of the cognitive and emotional processes involved in self-deception, a topic I find most intriguing. Our capacity to deceive ourselves is usually motivated by our having fairly intense feelings about something we do not want to deal with. A multifaceted self can make sense of phenomena such as selective attention, distorted reasoning, and self-serving biases. But I see these self-deceptive processes as attempts at coping with feelings and distressing circumstances (Saarni & Lewis, 1993; Taylor, 1989). By having this complex self-system at our disposal, we can more readily "park" our unwanted, conflict-producing, feared, or shame-inducing thoughts, feelings, and experiences in a part of ourselves where we do not have to be aware of them, at least not when we are confronted by our sense of our own vulnerability. Indeed, self-deception may be useful in reaching some goals, such as those that require profound conviction and unwavering confidence in one's talent, mission, or quest (e.g., Gollwitzer & Kinney, 1989). However, many self-deceptive strategies for coping with negative emotions and distressing circumstances are ultimately maladaptive, even self-destructive. Horney's (1950) early clinical work is relevant to this sort of destructive self-deception, and toward the end of this chapter I comment briefly on connections between her work and the role of the self in emotional experience.

Subjective and Objective Selves

Subjective Self

There is a long tradition in psychology to look at the self as a duality (e.g., Cooley, 1902; James, 1892); that is, the self is composed of a subjective part and an objective part. The subjective self is that aspect of the self without awareness of itself; it is the self that processes experience. The subjective self can be described as that facet of the self-system that acts on the world. When we use such phrases as "I am feeling challenged," or "I am skiing," or "I am working on a book," we can capture that processing aspect of the subjective self. Parenthetically, when we use verbs as gerunds we imply that processing of experience (see also Table 1.2 in Chapter 1 on the use of gerunds to describe core relational themes in common Western emotions). The subjective self has also been referred to as the existential self, the "I" in English language (Lewis, 1992a).

Think of the subjective self as your active, agentic self: You jump on your bicycle and ride to the post office; you are able to pedal and ride without much thought about the specific actions you undertake, and assuming you are in a familiar community, you know without having to reflect where you are going. But imagine your confused state if you climbed onto your bicycle without any reason for doing so! There you are, astride your bicycle, with nowhere to go and wondering why you are sitting on it. If your self had no agency, there would be no volition, direction, or intentionality. With an agentic self, you get on your bicycle with an intention of going some place or simply with the intention to go out and get some exercise with no particular destination or route. But you still had an intention about what to do with that bicycle.

The subjective self possesses what we might call intuitive or practical knowledge of oneself that is most readily revealed in our well-rehearsed ordinary routines, or scripts as they have sometimes been called. The subjective self's practical knowledge is probably most clearly revealed in our intentional behavior, and it is in this area that developmental psychologists studying young infants believe that the foundation of a subjective self emerges. When an infant learns to control some sequence of action or some interesting event, she learns a contingent relationship between an action stemming from her own body and an outcome she desires. This begins very early in infancy (Lewis, 1992b) and suggests a simple discrimination of self versus not self. When infants are given the opportunity to develop contingent play routines or contingent interactions with caregivers, they do so with relish and endless enthusiasm. For example, I can remember my daughter learning how effective she could be in getting one of us to her bedside during the night. She would throw her pacifier on the floor, then she would begin to fuss and, finally, wail. One night, when she was about 6 months old, I stayed in her room for a while after comforting her and retrieving her pacifier for her. She sucked on it noisily, then took it out of her mouth and vigorously threw it through her crib bars onto the floor again. Her fussing started within seconds. (She had us so well trained with her pacifier trick that we kept getting up in the night to retrieve it for another year longer.) The sense of efficacy that accompanies learning to control a contingent relationship is probably inherently reinforcing, and thus we gradually develop intentionality or a sense of agency. Supportive research by Lewis, Alessandri, and Sullivan (1990) showed that infants as young as 2 months appeared to acquire expectations about controlling a contingent relationship, and when their expectations were thwarted, they displayed negative "angry" affective behavior. Apparently, even infants do not like to lose control.

Objective Self

The objective self is that aspect of the self that does include self-awareness. The objective self has also been referred to as the categorical self, the self concept, and the social self; it is the "me" in English language. The objective self has been aptly termed the categorical self because it is with our lexical concepts that we describe ourselves according to categories (e.g., gender). But the categories can be more complex than age group or gender, and, indeed, they can be dimensionalized as in possessing more or less of a personality trait. For example, if we announce to another, "I consider myself to be quite sensitive to others' feelings," we are selecting the category (i.e., trait) of sensitivity as relevant to our self-concept and then ranking ourselves as high in that dimension. Obviously the objective self requires self-awareness: "I" look at "me" and categorize what is seen. Thus people may describe themselves according to all sorts of personality traits, likes, and dislikes or simply list the social roles they occupy (e.g., student, woman, wife, and scientist). The categories applied to the self by the self may be accurate or inaccurate, specific or global, positive or negative, clear or vague, but they are meaningful to the self and contribute significantly to whether we experience low or high self-esteem (see especially Baumeister, 1993a, for papers addressing the "puzzle of low self-regard").

In a sense, we possess a subjective self from an early age: Infants act on the world, have emotional states, and respond to social and physical stimuli. It is not until we develop the capacity to *reflect* on ourselves that we begin to develop objective self-awareness. The sociologists Cooley (1902) and Mead (1934) both emphasized that our relationships with others are pivotal to how we come to describe ourselves—and thus develop a self-concept. Others give us feedback: For example, parents tell their children, "You are a good girl," or "You are a brat," and perhaps later with their adolescents, "I can't believe how selfish you are!" As children come to be able to adopt the perspective of another, they can begin to reflect on their feelings and behavior as viewed by others. Higgins, Loeb, and Moretti (1995) reviewed how children develop this increasing attentiveness to others' responses to themselves and how this attentiveness comes to have a regulating function on one's behavior. With increasing maturity, older children and adolescents can selectively choose whether or not to concur with others' views of themselves. Indeed, a common conflict experienced by many North American adolescents is whether to go along with their parents' expectations for themselves or whether to pursue those activities preferred by their friends but not by their parents. I suspect that adaptive resolutions of such conflicts require self-reflection and goal striving, which take into account one's *moral disposition* and one's sense of emotional self-efficacy. Interestingly, social psychologists have determined that those individuals who rely excessively on others' evaluations of themselves rather than on their own self-reflections are more prone to experience low self-esteem. As a result, they also experience more frequently mood swings and negative emotions (for relevant reviews, see Baumeister, 1993a). In sum, their sense of subjective well-being is fragile.

Self-Development

Lewis (1992b) suggests that the self as an object emerges between 12 and 16 months of age; the toddler can point to pictures of himself and responds distinctively when confronted by a mirror image of himself with a smudge on his nose (he touches his nose or peers closer to examine intently his "dirty" nose). Prior to this age, babies look with interest at their reflections in mirrors, but their behavior does not suggest that they know that it is themselves portrayed in the mirror. After touching the hard surface of the mirror, some have even crawled behind the standing mirror to see who was there! Coyness or early forms of embarrassment may also emerge at this time, and such emotional responses require a self-awareness that demonstrates a tacit understanding of "I am aware that you are aware of me."

By 18 months many toddlers use self-referential language, most noticeable in their highly accomplished use of the word "mine." Siblings and peers are probably the most common communication targets of such self-referential possessive language, but gender labels also begin to emerge and use of their own name to refer to themselves may be heard as well. By 24 months we may also begin to see in some children the attribution of value-laden qualities to the self as in "good boy/bad boy." In sum, the objective self requires cognition capable of self-reflection; however, it is the subjective self that is doing the *reflecting* (note that gerund verb again). Thus, an objective self cannot exist without a subjective self to entertain the concept of itself.

Neisser's Ecological, Extended, and Evaluative Selves

Neisser's (1988, 1992) typology of the self reflects his interest in cognition, perception, and the acquisition of skillfulness as a general way to examine the adaptiveness of humans to their variable environments. I focus on his later typology here; the earlier version proposed five components in the self-system, which he subsequently revised to reflect his interest in the acquisition of consciousness and skillfulness (Neisser, 1992). His theory of a self-system is emphatic about the inseparability of the individual and his or her context, and although contexts can change, the individual continues to experience a sense of continuity within her- or himself.

The Ecological Self

Neisser's notion of the ecological self is premised on how we perceive our environment in terms of what it affords us as opportunities for interaction. He gives us an example: Ceilings afford flies an opportunity to walk on them; they do not for humans. For a young infant, a rattle with a narrow midsection affords an opportunity to grasp it; handing that same baby a tennis ball would not. Thus, the individual interacts with an environment that is bidirectional: What happens is a joint function of what we can do with the environment and what the environment provides us as an accessible structure (i.e., its *affordances*; Gibson, 1982).The ecological self is also much like a subjective self in that the emphasis is on the self's phenomenological awareness of the self interacting with those features of the environment that permit or afford interaction. Perhaps Neisser's phenomenological awareness is equivalent to what I referred to earlier as a practical knowledge demonstrated by individuals as they pursue their daily activities. However, *not* included in such a phenomenological awareness of the self-in-interaction-with-the environment is the self-consciousness that typically includes a sense of exposure to others or of evaluation of whether the self is somehow measuring up.

The ecological self is significant for the development of emotional competence because of its emphasis on the self *in relationship to an environment*. That environment includes other people, which means that the social environment can also be looked at as presenting an array of *affordances* or opportunities for functional interaction to the individual. Consider the following two contrasting examples:

Five-year-old Laura had always been a reserved and somewhat cautious child when faced with new situations. Her father had some trepidation as to how she'd fare during the first few days of starting kindergarten at the local elementary school. It had taken her weeks to get comfortable with her preschool, but she had been younger then. He hoped this time it would only be days.

The morning of the first day for kindergarten arrived, and sober Laura clung to her father as they walked into the classroom. She didn't greet the teacher, despite her father's prompting. Trying to engage her, he pointed out the table with assorted small pets on it, but she only looked more distressed. She avoided the other children as they made their way to her group table where her name card was placed. Her father tried to reassure her that he'd be back in the afternoon to take her home and that she'd have a good time here, just like at her preschool. Laura broke into tears. Another girl at the group table announced pointedly, "she's a baby," and Laura got up and ran after her departing father.

Five-year-old Susan was "Miss Energy" herself, much to the exhaustion of her mother. Susan had given up naps by 9 months of age, according to her mother, and generally was a live wire at preschool as well, much to the exasperation of the caregivers. Her mother was looking forward very much to kindergarten at the local elementary school as perhaps providing more stimulation and challenge for her daughter; Susan was excited too.

The morning of the first day for kindergarten arrived, and the bubbly Susan broke away from her mother as they walked into the classroom. She didn't greet the teacher, despite her mother's prompting, because she had already raced over to the table containing the classroom's pets: a fish tank, a turtle aquarium, and a cage of gerbils. She banged on the side of the gerbil cage to wake them up. Her mother retrieved her and led her to her group table where her name card was placed and told her she'd be back in the afternoon to take her home. Her mother didn't bother to say anything about Susan having a good time; what she did say was, "Susan, please listen to your teacher and try to follow directions, OK, honey?" But Susan had already turned to some other children at the table and was asking them their names. Her mother sighed and left the room unnoticed.

Think of the different sorts of social environments encountered by Laura and Susan. Opportunities for interaction with the social environment are probably as variable as personalities are. When you contemplate Laura's ecological self-awareness—as opposed to Susan's—on being faced with kindergarten, Laura's awareness is oriented toward the threatening and scary newness of the kindergarten room, and she is filled with apprehension. Thus, her strategies for self-protection are aroused and staying close to her attachment figure is the outcome. In contrast, Susan's awareness is oriented toward opportunities for exploration and the stimulation of novelty in the kindergarten room, and she responds with zest and affability toward her peers. Her strategies for self-enhancement are aroused and approaching her environment is the outcome.

The Extended Self

Neisser's concept of a self extended in time is intended to address the fact that we are not only in a relationship to a present environment but also concerned with the past and the future. The extended self permits us to imagine the possible, not just the actual. Very likely the preschooler's imaginary pretend play is an early example of an extended self. For example, the young child might imagine herself in positions of power, strength, and authority and temporarily disregard her relative powerlessness and dependency as she acts out the behavior of "Kimberly, the Pink Power Ranger" or whatever other action figures enjoy current popularity among 4- to 7-year-olds.

Expectations are especially powerful influences on which opportunities we seek out (or avoid) in our social and physical environments, and such expectations can be based on past experience of ourselves in some transaction, or they can be based on communications from others or observations of others as to what to expect. For example, a child who witnesses his *admired* older brother reacting to an injection with fearful anticipation and, upon getting the shot, cries, is much more likely to fear shots and react to them with greater emotional intensity. I stressed in this example that the older brother was held in high esteem by the younger child, because credibility of the model or informant is an important variable here in whether children take in others' emotional experience as reliable guides for what they themselves will also come to expect (see also Saarni, 1985, for elaboration of how others' emotional expectations are internalized as personal expectancies).

The extended self also facilitates the development of schemata and scripts: We have a readiness for how to respond to a new environment based on some of its similarities to what we have learned as interaction strategies in former environments. An example is when you rent a car. You may not have ever driven this particular sort of car before, but your schemata for driving are fluid enough to generalize to different sorts of car design. However, if you only know how to drive an automatic and find yourself having to drive a stick shift, your schemata for dealing with this driving challenge may be sorely tested. The person who is accustomed to driving a stick shift, upon renting an automatic, may find herself madly stomping on the floor with her left foot to depress the clutch pedal.

Children also demonstrate the influence of expectations acquired in previous interactions on their behavior in similar but novel situations. As an illustration, consider 6-year-old Kelly's experience:

> Debra, Kelly's mother, had been divorced since Kelly was 2. She had dated a few men, and had lived with a couple of them, but the relationships ended after a year. Now she was involved with Mac, and they were moving into an apartment together with Kelly. Debra's previous partner, Bill, had been emotionally abusive and had often threatened to or indeed broke Kelly's toys when he perceived her as somehow not complying with his wishes. Now in the new apartment with Mac, Kelly became panic-stricken about the whereabouts of her toys and struggled to keep them hidden from Mac. Mac was puzzled, and after buying her a box of Lego blocks, he offered to help build something with her. Kelly burst out crying and said, "You'll break it, won't you!" Debra witnessed the exchange and realized what was happening. She explained to Mac

what Kelly's experience had been with Bill, and together they sought to try to reassure Kelly and pointed out to her on subsequent occasions how different Mac was from Bill.

This illustration also shows the extended self as having anticipations about how to cope with some emotionally challenging situation. The degree to which we have had efficacious experiences in similar earlier situations influences the sense of self-agency or self-confidence we bring to bear on the new situation. In contrast, if preceding similar situations had tended to end poorly for us, as in Kelly's experience, then we would be less likely to feel self-confident in approaching the new situation. False bravado is an alternative response, and avoidant behavior is an especially common response to such anxiety-laden challenges.

The Evaluative Self

With this feature of the self Neisser highlights the feelings people attach to their interactions with the physical and social environments: We like or dislike parties, we are provoked or dejected by social injustices, we are entertained or scared to death by horror movies. The evaluative self is a goal-directed self, and, as a consequence, our environmental interactions are motivated toward some outcomes and away from others. As Neisser (1992) aptly phrases it, "The ecological self does not have a motivational dimension. Babies know what they want, but they do not know who wants it." When the evaluative self develops, as it commonly does between 18 months and 3 years of age (Lewis, 1992b), toddlers *know* how they feel. They are able to use language to communicate their feelings, to self-refer to their own experience. Toddlers also become conscious of others' feelings about them and in conjunction with their self-extended-in-time, they can begin to maneuver their interactions with others to attain certain advantages or avoid disadvantages.

Lewis, Stanger, and Sullivan (1989), with research on young children's lying, provide a good example of young children's learning to maneuver through "risky" social interactions. The children were just under 3 years of age and were told not to peek at an attractive display; then they were left alone. The majority peeked, but only a minority "confessed" when the experimenter returned and asked whether they had looked. Thus, a majority of 2- to 3-year-olds were quite capable of attempting to avoid potential disadvantages to themselves in their interaction with the experimenter by not telling the truth. Of further interest is that already by 2+ years children have acquired a generalized script or expectancy that if an adult tells them not to do something and they go ahead and do it, they are in for trouble. In other words, this was not their parents telling them not to peek, it was just some other adult, and yet the children employed an extended self that revealed this script-related expectancy and an evaluative self that chose to avoid getting into trouble (and therefore feeling badly, e.g., ashamed) by opting for deceptive behavior. Given the aversiveness of feeling ashamed or being punished, children adaptively opt for manipulating their own behavior to mislead another's thoughts and feelings toward them.

The young children in the preceding research were demonstrating practical knowledge; I am not suggesting that these 2- to 3-year-olds could verbalize what the strategy was that they used. Observational research by Stipek, Recchia, and McClintic (1992) also suggests that self-evaluation for positive mastery of a task appears in children's behavior after 33 months. In their study, the 3- to 5-year-olds were more likely than those less than 3 years of age to smile, show an open posture, and utter "prideful" comments when they won at a competitive task. Essentially the inference made here was that positive emotions resulted when the self evaluated the self's functioning as "good" or desirable in some way. Thus, when children won at the competitive game, they showed positive emotionally expressive behaviors with greater frequency than when they lost at the competitive game.

Kopp (1992) has also noted that with the capacity for self-evaluation comes the ability to regulate or monitor the self in relation to others' expectations for appropriate behavior. For young children, compliance with societal or parental standards requires the minimal skills of being able to think about and remember how mommy and daddy want them to behave. Kopp and Wyer (1994) have argued that self-regulation problems in developmentally delayed children (most often manifested in noncompliant behavior) are functionally related to deficits in these children's self-systems. They have consolidated the rich and diverse research on the development of the self according to significant themes that recur in various theoretical perspectives. Their useful summary of these themes is reprinted in Table 2.1, and they use these themes to compare normally developing children with those with developmental disorders.

In summary, the concepts of the ecological, extended, and evaluative self permit us to look at functional interactions between individuals and their social and physical environments. This triple concept of self also gives us a conceptual tool to look at how individual differences may manifest themselves in why person *A* feels self-efficacious in a particular social situation whereas person *B* feels overwhelmed in seemingly the same social situation (e.g., the comparison of Laura and Susan on their first day in kindergarten). The point here is that the ostensibly similar social situation is not experienced *transactionally* as uniform.

The social situation becomes a dynamic experience and functionally varies according to how person *A*'s multifaceted self engages in it as opposed to how person *B*'s multifaceted self engages in it. Emotional competence then becomes linked to how a particular multifaceted self experiences self-efficacy in particular transactions. This implies some degree of inconsistency or variability in emotional competence. We may demonstrate emotional competence in 99 different interactions, but in the 100th we may encounter that situation for which we are not prepared or with which we do not have the skills to cope, and we experience a sense of diminishment, stress, or inadequacy. We may also find that we would rather deceive ourselves about our negative experience than deal directly with our emotional incompetence (see also Baumeister, 1993b, for an excellent discussion).

Neisser's model of the tripartite self is one that helps us to look at emotional experience within the individual as it unfolds (1) in a physical and social environment (the ecological self), (2) relative to a temporal framework (the extended self), and (3) in response to the standards and values of the family and societal context (the evaluative self). But how applicable is this model of "self" in other cultures? This is an im-

TABLE 2.1. Themes in the Early Self-System

Social interaction precursors/maintainers of the self-system	Refers to the importance of caregiver–infant/toddler interactions such that the infant gathers emotional strength from others, learns to trust others' actions, and becomes tuned into others' wishes, desires, values, and affective states.
Physical elements	Refers to the young child's recognition and knowledge of own body parts and body schema; awareness of own actions on objects and with other people.
Cognitive aspects	Refers to the young child's elemental beliefs about the self (e.g., gender), memories of one's own self activities, roles (e.g., a child, a sibling) the self is involved in, and knowledge of rules/routines one is supposed to follow.
Evaluative/motivational	Refers to *good* and *bad* feelings the young child has about his or her actions, the way he or she looks, or an event in which he or she participated. Feelings presumably influence the child's desire to reengage with others or in an activity.

Note. From Kopp and Wyer (1994, p. 47). Copyright 1994 by University of Rochester Press. Reprinted by permission.

portant issue to consider about emotional competence, for recall that the definition given for emotional competence stressed *self*-efficacy in emotion-eliciting social transactions. If another culture did not have the same views as our own about a "self," how would that affect the demonstration of emotional competence in emotion-eliciting social transactions within such societies? We turn next to consider non-Western societies and how the self might be differently conceptualized.

SELVES AS INDEPENDENT OR INTERDEPENDENT

Markus and Kitayama (1991) provide us with a succinct contrast between Japanese and American constructions of the self with the following two proverbs: "In America 'the squeaky wheel gets the grease.' In Japan, 'the nail that stands out gets pounded down' " (p. 224). Selves are viewed differently in different cultures; indeed, a notion of self may not even be especially evident in some societies in which the culture firmly embeds the individual in a complex and enfolding web of kinship, status, gender role, and age role. Markus and Kitayama are particularly interested in the Western self that is construed as individualistic (think of all of our John Wayne-type of western movies, or worse yet, Sylvester Stallone movies) as compared to the Japanese self that is construed as inextricably interdependent with others (think of the movie *Rashomon*).

Control and Separation

The significance of Markus and Kitayama's analysis for emotional competence lies in their description of beliefs held in Western societies about the self. Americans and many Europeans assume that their actions stem from internal motives, drives, desires, and feelings; that is, they believe they operate as they do *because they are in control*. Thus, we believe we exercise choice and autonomy, and in so doing, we operate as individuals or *separate* selves. The independent self is motivated to express itself, its skills, its distinctiveness, its unique achievements (e.g., who is the smartest, who makes the most money, who is the most beautiful). When the independent self has to exert control, it is often over the external situation or one's external expression so as to gain advantages or avoid disadvantages (recall those little 2- to 3-year-olds who could already lie). The implication for how an independent self regulates emotional upheaval, stressful interpersonal interactions, or difficult demands is that we are thrown back on our own inner resources to cope; we are alone. Indeed, it is conceivable that this Western cultural emphasis on the individual might make emotional competence all the more elusive. The phrase that comes to mind is "sink or swim," with the implication that we do not have available a rescue ring or a lifeguard to help us should we get into the emotional equivalent of "deep water."

Connection and Collective Well-Being

In contrast, the interdependent view of the self emphasizes a view of the person as connected to others. Such a connected self certainly experiences internal feelings, drives, desires, and so forth, but they are viewed as secondary, situation-specific, and not as the defining characteristics of the connected self. Regard for collective well-being and sympathetic concern for others (or at least for those in one's clan or kinship system) is a significant value, and much of one's behavior is motivated to maintain a harmonious equilibrium with others. When one is faced with a difficult and trying situation, one has emotional support, sympathy, and often direct assistance. Particularly during times of sadness or distressed vulnerability, considerable social support and ritual may be available to the *individual* as a way of facilitating the return of harmonious *interpersonal* relations. Self-control or internal emotion regulation is more often directed at controlling those feelings or dispositions (e.g., envy and anger) that would disrupt social bonds. Some cultures also have rituals to appease disturbing feelings that are attributed to the influence of spirits on oneself. For example, G. Harris (1978) described the elaborate rituals of the Taita society in Kenya in which reading the entrails of sacrificed goats or sheep was carried out to determine which spirit or living person one had offended; afterwards the sheep or goat provided the fare for a celebratory feast for the village, an obvious cohesion-promoting activity.

Relative to feelings, Markus and Kitayama contend that emotions such as anger, sadness, and fear are *ego focused* because they are diagnostic of the independent self; that is, they are direct pathways to what is going on in the internal self. Disregarding, ignoring, or discounting such feelings is frequently assumed in our Western culture as "being in denial" and therefore somehow compromising ourselves or our self-respect. However, for the self construed as interdependent, such feelings may simply refer to private transitory reactions that require controlling or deemphasizing to promote interpersonal harmony and sense of community. For the independent self, self-esteem is often predicated on "being true to oneself," that is, one "ought" to express one's inner qualities and attributes, whereas for the interdependent self, self-esteem may be a somewhat meaningless concept. Instead, happiness or contentment is sought and is found by effectively promoting the well-being of others and being in relationship to others.

In summary, for the interdependent self, being embedded in reciprocal relationships is taken for granted, and enhancing others' well-being rebounds to one's own enhancement. Self-restraint and control of disruptive thoughts and feelings are valued because they allow for adjustment to the nuances and vicissitudes of social interaction. Indeed, such self-control is viewed as a marker of maturity and moral status.

For the independent self, a positive bias is experienced relative to the self: One believes oneself to be better off, more accomplished, and more likely than others to have a bright future. Harter (1990) suggests that already by 4 years of age American children demonstrate this self-favorability bias. What function is served by the self-positivity bias? I suspect it has to do with coping. When one experiences stress or anguish, such a positivity bias serves as a buffer as one endures the emotionally difficult time, and it may help to keep one's self-esteem resilient. Two possible rationales emerge in the sorts of expectations held by people with independent self-constructions: (1) eventually the situation will improve and the individual will emerge the stronger for it (stoicism) and (2) the situation was anomalous, the individual did not deserve it, or it was not characteristic of the self, and thus it will not *recur* ("it was an accident, but it won't happen again, i.e., I'll be in control, and I'm still a good person"; Sigmon & Snyder, 1993). Again, we see some elements of self-deception in this positivity bias that clearly has *self-serving* features for those individuals who have independent self-constructions.

An Oversimplification?

The preceding comparisons of independent and interdependent self construction presented a dichotomized perspective, and I think that view needs to be tempered. The description of the independent self may be a view that is primarily held by middle-class Caucasian males in Western societies, and it may be anchored historically in late industrial capitalism. Some ethnographers do indeed challenge the preceding dichotomized view as at odds with people's emotional experience, although when people are asked to give verbal attributions about themselves, they may indeed appear to invoke the self as an autonomous entity (Murray, 1993). Holland and Kipnis (1995) argue that there is not a single model of the self in Western societies but rather many variations, and I concur with their point of view. Indeed, we experience self-conscious emotions such as pride, shame, embarrassment, and guilt as well as responsive feelings such as a sense of communion, sympathy, and caring because we do have an awareness of and a regard for ourselves *in relationship* to others' opinions and feelings toward us.

Experiencing these feelings promotes socially responsive and cooperative action, and it is not difficult to think of examples of how caring or sympathy would do so. But it may be more difficult to think of how feeling shame would promote "cooperative" action. Feelings like shame, envy, and embarrassment tend to result in compliance or going along with social conventions. Consider the following example:

> Lorna spilled chili down the front of her shirt in the school cafeteria. She felt quite embarrassed and tried to wipe up the mess; while she mopped with paper napkins at her shirt front, she *smiled* at the other students around her as she also bemoaned her klutziness. She felt somewhat comforted by one person who pointedly gestured at a stain on his shirt, and her friend Joan offered some assistance ("should I go ask in the kitchen if they've got any soap?"). And thank goodness that cute guy from her science class just politely avoided looking at the splotch on her chest!

These social consequences to an experience of embarrassment can promote a sense of belonging to the group (note Lorna's smiling, the subsequent sympathetic responses as well as polite avoidance of staring, nor were humiliating comments made). Yet the aversive nature of feeling embarrassed is also an experience that is more likely to cue the individual the next time to comply with etiquette "requirements," in this case, eating with greater care. The social exposure of our awkwardness or social gaffes (and we must be aware that we have blundered) is usually sufficiently painful that we tend to learn quickly to avoid committing such mistakes in the future. In short, there is nothing like a strong dose of embarrassment to get someone to conform to the collective norms of a group.

Self-conscious emotions and socially responsive emotions such as empathy and caring invoke a conception of the self that is *sociocentric*, and it is clear that the very vast majority of people in Western societies experience such feelings. In sum, the alleged autonomous Western self-system is just as capable as the alleged non-Western interdependent self is for being concerned with everyday social contexts involving relationships and the opinions of others. Our selves are not wholly egocentric, and it is also just as likely that non-Western self conceptions also include concerns about individual attributes and choices. Given our increasingly global "awareness," we may well be on our way to recognizing our mutual similarities with those who live in very disparate societies.

I turn next to the topic of self conscious emotions, which are particularly well-suited to a discussion of how the self is integral to emotional competence, particularly given the controversy about self-conceptions. In addition, the contributing element of moral disposition to emotional competence also becomes evident in self-conscious emotions, for it is with the awareness of transgression of a moral standard that feelings of guilt can be stimulated. We feel guilt over our violations of fairness, loss of self-control in a destructive fashion, disregard for our obligations, and callousness toward those who deserve our sympathy; these would all constitute a breach of one's moral disposition according to Wilson (1993). Yet pride can be elicited by meeting a challenging moral standard, by fulfilling these moral expectations in spite of circumstances that make it difficult to do so. It is in this sense that self-conscious emotions have been referred to as the "moral emotions:" They contribute to the child's growing sense of personal responsibility in an intensely interpersonal world (e.g., Hoffman, 1982; Zahn-Waxler & Robinson, 1995).

THE DEVELOPMENT OF SELF-CONSCIOUS EMOTIONS

What makes the emotional experience involved in embarrassment, shame, pride, and guilt distinct is that they require that the self reflect on the self, and it is that process of self-reflection that elicits these emotions. In other words, yes, there certainly are situational concerns in each of these emotions, but the "active ingredient" for our feeling them is really how we *evaluate ourselves* relative to acknowledged *social standards.* Thus, Neisser's evaluative self would be a necessary component in the self-system for experiencing such emotions, but the capacity to access both an autonomous self and a sociocentric self would appear to be prerequisite as well. This latter requirement manifests itself in children's being able to examine their *responsibility* in some behavior, tantamount to recognizing autonomy in making a choice, and yet at the same time believing themselves obligated to try to live up their family and community standards and expectations, which is a sociocentric orientation of the self. In short, these emotions are often uncomfortable to experience, yet they function to keep us oriented toward our connection with others (as in the earlier example of Lorna's embarrassment) by motivating us to comply with societal expectations for behavior, thought, and feeling.

In the case of pride, which is not at all an uncomfortable feeling (unless we become the target of another's envy or are accused of boasting), it too manifests itself most clearly when there is an audience that values the nature of the achievement. Task accomplishment when alone feels good, as in a sense of mastery or the satisfaction of completing a challenging job, but I suspect for children pride is felt most clearly when they can *share* with someone else what they have accomplished. Parenthetically, Rimé (1995) makes a similar argument in his fascinating paper: People are absolutely incorrigible when it comes to telling others about their emotional experience, particularly, as I suspect, if it makes a good story, gets them sympathy and attention, or puts them in a good light (as in pride—shame and contempt stories were much less frequently shared, according to Rimé). In sum, these three concepts—self-evaluation, valued societal standards, and attribution of self-responsibility for success or failure at meeting the standard—are critical components in what are called the self-conscious emotions, and I turn next to an elaboration of them from a developmental perspective.

Standards

Lewis's work (1992a, 1992b, 1993a) on the development of pride, hubris, shame, embarrassment, and guilt constitutes a cognitive appraisal view of how such emotions come about. These emotions require that an objective self has developed; that is, children can refer to themselves and have conscious awareness of themselves as distinct from others. At around the time children are acquiring this objective self-awareness, they also become aware of parental standards for behavior, of the rules they are expected to follow, and of desirable goals for their comportment. They learn about these standards through their family's disciplinary practices as well as through their growing appreciation of what makes others feel the way they do. Obviously the sorts of standards a young child learns about are rather simple and concrete; for example, "You should say 'please' if you want something," "Big boys don't poop in their pants," "How terrible of you to bite your little sister!" As we mature, we acquire more subtle beliefs about the standards and rules we believe we should follow and the goals we think are worthy of striving for. In fact, we follow a lifelong process of adding and deleting standards, rules, and goals for ourselves as the contexts of our life change. Meeting these standards typically contributes to our feeling positive, both because we feel a sense of mastery in our accomplishments and because we receive social approval from others for fulfilling their expectations about standards (e.g., Harter, 1978; Hunt, 1965; Reissland, 1994). From a developmental standpoint, it appears that younger children (under age 8) associate feeling guilt with failure to meet a standard, even under uncontrollable circumstances, whereas older children begin to recognize the greater significance of controllability of their action and that *their failure to do so when they could* have will likely yield feelings of guilt (Graham, Doubleday, & Guarino, 1984).

Attribution of Success or Failure

Children also develop an appraisal of self-agency or responsibility: Have they failed or succeeded at reaching the goal, or at living up to the standard, or performing according to the rule? Although Lewis does not directly address issues of controllability here, Weiner's work certainly informs us of how perception of controllability is directly implied in whether or not people feel responsible for events (e.g., Weiner, 1985). To use a rather graphic illustration, if a child feels defecation is under her control, she is more likely to attribute to herself success or failure at toileting "accomplishments." She will respond to encouragement to using her "potty" and will show positive emotion upon successful use and distress or other negative emotion (e.g., shame and displaced anger) at failed efforts. If she does not feel as though her bowel movements have any relationship to her sense of control over her body, toileting is better dealt with by using diapers and not exhorting her to use her "potty" or scolding her for soiling herself.

However, I must also stress that young children may believe that they "cause" things to happen, that is, that they are in control of events when in fact they are not, due to their cognitive egocentrism, which blurs desire and reality. On a simple level, a 2-year-old may believe and act as "if I want a cookie, then I should have a cookie." But if that same young child believes that "if I want Mommy to love me, then I have to be a good girl for her," she may then egocentrically conclude she must have been a "bad girl," when her mother simply expresses negative feelings that are unrelated to her child's behavior. Research by Zahn-Waxler and her associates (Zahn-Waxler, Radke-Yarrow, & King, 1979; Zahn-Waxler & Kochanska, 1990; Zahn-Waxler & Robinson, 1995) suggests that young children growing up with depressed mothers may be particularly at risk for developing excessive "accountability" for their mothers' feelings and mood state. Such children were very careful in their interaction with others, as though others were quite fragile, and their behavior included higher levels of appeasement, apologizing, and suppression of negative emotion than comparable children of non-depressed mothers. Thus, these 2- to 3-year-old children appeared to believe unrealistically that they had control over events and over their mothers' emotional responses and/or were responsible for them. Such an early and chronic exposure to viewing oneself as responsible for another's functioning may well contribute to what Janoff-Bulman (1979) has referred to as characterological self-blame, a stance often implicated in helplessness and passivity.

Self-Evaluation

Lewis contends that a focus on one's self from an evaluative standpoint has to develop before self-conscious emotions are experienced: Either the whole self or a particular aspect of the self is considered the focus of the success or failure at living up to the standard or rule or reaching a goal. Lewis contends that the more that the whole self is globally assumed to be responsible for the success or failure, the more that either hubris (arrogance) or shame is felt, respectively. When specific aspects of the self are seen as leading to the success or failure, then pride or guilt will be felt, respectively. The former emotional responses have maladaptive aspects to them: Arrogant, hubris-filled individuals are often socially preemptive, harsh, oppressive; they are self-inflated. Shamed individuals are deflated; they avoid and hide from the presumed condemnation they think they deserve; their humiliation fills them with self-disgust. The emotional responses of pride and guilt are specific self-attributions as in "my effort paid off" or "it was my mistake and I'll deal with this fiasco." The prideful feelings of accomplishment and pleasure allow the individual to undertake still further challenges; the guilt one feels upon failure at a particular event or in a particular situation allows for interpersonal repair and future improvement. With shame one just "crawls into a hole and pulls it in after oneself," thus making future amends impossible. With arrogance one distances others and cannot genuinely share the pleasure of accomplishment; one savors it alone and in isolation.

Empirical research with children that has investigated their self-conscious emotions is limited. It does include a series of studies on pride and shame by Heckhausen (1987) on preschool-age children's winning or losing at a competitive game; research by Stipek et al. (1992) on preschoolers' self-evaluations and subsequent emotions of pride and shame following task success or failure; Lewis, Alessandri, and Sullivan's (1992) work, also with preschoolers, on tasks that differed in difficulty of accomplishment; Lewis, Sullivan, Stanger, and Weiss's (1989) work on young children's self-conscious emotions; Ferguson, Stegge, and Damhuis's (1991) investigation of children's understanding of guilt and shame, and Zahn-Waxler and Kochanska's (1990) examination of the origins of guilt. Tangney and Fischer's (1995) volume on self-conscious emotions is an excellent source and includes good reviews of shame and guilt in childhood (Ferguson & Stegge, 1995), embarrassment (Lewis, 1995), and cognitive developmental changes in understanding pride, shame, and guilt (Mascolo & Fischer, 1995). Recently Reimer (1996) sought to integrate research with young children's self-conscious emotions with clinical work on adolescents and adults to examine the development of shame in later childhood and adolescence. The development and functioning of self-conscious emotions clearly needs more attention at all age levels. It would appear that the development of self-conscious emotions is especially relevant to clinical practice, whether it be the treatment of depression that occurs with a greater frequency among female adolescents or the development of effective interventions to facilitate a child's coping with the emotional aftermath of sexual abuse.

Socialization's Influence

Barrett's (1995) arguments of how the self-conscious emotions come about are similar to Lewis's model, but their theoretical positions differ in the emphasis placed on cognitive development. Lewis believes that there are significant cognitive developmental prerequisites for the development of self-conscious emotions (as do Mascolo & Fischer, 1995), whereas Barrett emphasizes the effects of caregivers' socialization and early disciplinary practices on infants' and toddlers' early experiences of self-conscious emotions, in particular shame. Barrett argues that shame may appear quite early in infancy as a way to avoid overarousal when experiencing negative affect in interaction with a significant caregiver.

She hypothesizes that these emotion-laden caregiver responses to the infant contribute to the infant's sense of efficacy or inefficacy, the former experienced on gaining caregivers' pleasure and positive emotional responses and the latter on being confronted with caregivers' anger and negative emotional responses. Presumably, if these emotional exchanges occur in situations in which the infant tries to exert contingent control, the infant will come to associate the feeling of either efficacy or inadequacy with his or her action. Barrett suggests that the feeling of efficacy contributes to a sense of mastery and inadequacy to the experience of shame.

"Amenders and Avoiders"

Barrett, Zahn-Waxler, and Cole (1993) undertook a fascinating naturalistic study with 2-year-olds in which they explored how these young children would react after playing with the experimenter's "favorite doll" only to have its leg fall off after the experimenter left the room. Upon the experimenter's return, she looked at the leg, then verbally mentioned it to the child, and only after a couple of minutes did she tell the child that he or she had not actually broken the doll's leg. During these 2 minutes the child's behavior was videorecorded and coded for how the child either tried to resolve the situation (the "amenders") or sought to avoid the experimenter. Interestingly, more of these latter children smiled while averting their faces from the experimenter, which is reminiscent of the response that we as adults make when we are embarrassed (recall Lorna's smiling upon spilling food on herself while eating).

Barrett suggests that the amenders were demonstrating behavior that is consistent with feeling guilt; they sought to repair the doll and quickly "confessed" that the doll had broken. The avoiders were presumably feeling something like shame, manifested in their gaze avoidance, their withdrawal from the experimenter, and their neglecting to tell the experimenter about the broken doll. In a later paper, Barrett (1995) suggests that this research might be indicative of how young children view themselves either as inadequate or as having good intentions in regulating social exchanges.

Barrett also believes that the experience of shame contributes to the emergence of self-awareness, whereas Lewis argues that some degree of self-awareness must have already been developed for shame to be experienced. My view is that Lewis has more stringent criteria for the definition of when shame as an emotional experience is displayed; Barrett is willing to accept a wider array of negative emotional behavior on the part of the infant as constituting early forms of shame. Both theorists, however, agree that self-conscious emotions develop in *social* contexts, even though when shamed we respond by pulling away from social contact, and when guilty we reach out and try to make amends. Barrett highlights the functional consequences of shame and guilt for promoting social cohesion, compliance, and harmony, and Lewis emphasizes the development of the self in the self-conscious emotions. Given the complexity of human emotional experience across development, both views are valid for making sense of some of our most intensely aversive emotions.

Cultural Context

It is not difficult to imagine that our own responses to children will differ if we think they are behaving with a desire to make amends as opposed to conveying to us that they have been inadequate. My hunch is that people in Western cultures tend to respond more positively to guilt-oriented children who communicate that their intentions were good but that they will try to make amends for the (unexpected) bad outcome. Indeed, Walbott and Scherer (1995) suggest that guilt is more typical (or more acceptable) in Western cultures, whereas shame is felt as more aversive and disturbing than what is described as shame in non-Western collectivistic cultures. Collectivistic societies appear to view shame benignly and as having little disruptive influence on relationships; in short, it is not as aversively experienced as in individualistic societies. Shame functions to facilitate social bonds and compliance in collectivistic societies, which is viewed as desirable and beneficial. (See also the excellent discussion of self-conscious emotions by Kitayama, Markus, & Matsumoto, 1995.)

Emotional Competence and Self-Conscious Emotions

Both Lewis's and Barrett's views on the development of self-conscious emotions are relevant to the development of emotional competence: Regardless of whether we grow up in an individualistic or a collectivistic society, an early awareness of our society's standards and the frequent experience of mastery in contingency learning facilitates both our development of self-efficacy in emotion-eliciting exchanges and our moral disposition. In the collectivistic society, that self-efficacy would be felt as cohesion and belonging; in the individualistic society self-efficacy would be felt as success in reaching one's goals. Both societies would have their moral values and dispositions embedded in that sense of cohesion or in the nature of the sought-after goals. Consider the following two case illustrations of self-conscious emotion, one drawn from our own culture and the second from Japanese culture. Both demonstrate an emerging emotional competence:

> Alex, a fifth grader at ABC Elementary School, had looked at a copy of the teacher's spelling test that had been stolen by Jake, another kid in his class. After lunch, the teacher noticed that the test was missing from her desk. She glanced silently around the room, and Alex felt ashamed. He looked down, felt his hands get clammy on his desk top, and he felt uncomfortably hot. Jake smiled slightly at him. The remainder of the afternoon was an inner struggle for him.
>
> At the end of the school day he approached Ms. Gold, nearly in tears, but he felt he had to tell her that he had looked at the test. He felt guilty, as if he had let himself down. But he was also concerned about not snitching on Jake and felt scared Ms. Gold might get that information out of him.
>
> He walked back into the classroom where Ms. Gold was watering the classroom's carnivorous plants. "Ms. Gold, I saw your test out in the yard. I didn't look at it very long, but it was the spelling

test." Ms. Gold responded, "You know, Alex, looking at that test was cheating." Alex felt terrible but looked directly at Ms. Gold, and said glumly, "I know, that's why I'm here. I knew it was wrong. You should just give me an F on the test." Ms. Gold replied, "Yes, I should, but I would like to know who took the test?"

Alex squirmed but had made up his mind not to snitch; he said resignedly, "I know who did it, but I can't tell you, because that would be snitching. Snitching is like cheating in a way, and I've already done that once. I'm really sorry that I cheated, and I'm really sorry that I can't tell you who did it." Ms. Gold looked away, lost in thought. "Alex, I understand your choice. I am going to give you an F on that spelling test, but I am also going to give the whole class another test, one that I hope you will study for and do well on."

Alex left the room feeling relieved and curiously proud. He had stood up for what he had thought was right: admitting the bad thing he had done and also not tattling on Jake. He vowed to study for the next test and decided Jake was really a loser.

Takeo played baseball with a passion. He was a member of a team that had won many games. Now his team was scheduled to play a really good team, one that beat them last year. Everybody was excited and tense at the same time. The coach barked at them to get ready to go out on the field.

The game went badly. They were a couple of points behind, and Takeo came up to bat. He struck, struck again, and finally felt the ball hit the wood; it went straight up and then straight down into the pitcher's glove. Takeo was out. The coach looked coldly at him and then looked away. His teammates frowned and also looked away. Takeo flushed and grimaced; he walked dejectedly back to the bench.

The game ended shortly thereafter, with the other team winning once again. As they boarded the bus to go back home, the boys talked quietly among themselves. Aki said to Takeo, "We have won many games and we play well; that team is really good and we should learn how they do it."

Takeo felt that his team members were like a family. He sunk down in his seat, comforting himself with thoughts of future practice together and hoped he'd become better and never hit a fly-ball again.

These two vignettes illustrate shame, but they differ in social consequences. For Alex the experience of shame is painful and goads him to considering his action; as he contemplates his cheating and that he had a choice not to, his shame shifts into feeling guilty, and with remorse he strives to admit his wrong and "take his medicine." Afterwards he feels relief and also chooses to distance himself from Jake. However, it should be noted that throughout his ordeal, he is essentially alone. In contrast, Takeo's shame is shared with a larger group: It is the team that lost the game, even though individual actions led to losing. But their sense of belonging to a team, even one that has lost, remains strong and they collectively vow to strive harder. Both boys are keenly aware of standards, and their moral stance shows itself in Alex's case by admitting to a wrong with a willingness to take the consequences, and for Takeo it is in his commitment to work harder and to learn along with his teammates from the defeating team's prowess. Both boys demonstrate emotional competence even as they experience aversive self-conscious emotions; the outcomes for both boys demonstrate efficacy relative to their respective goals and cultural contexts.

"TYRANNY OF THE SHOULDS"

Horney's (1950) work presaged much of this thinking on the development of the self-conscious emotions, in my opinion, and her descriptions of the "tyranny of the shoulds" are rich in suggesting how the normal cognitive appraisals involved in determining the standards, rules, and goals that matter to us become distorted in harsh, punitive, and rejecting families. Horney thought that self-hatred and neurotic pride were somewhat like the two sides of the same coin; both are responses to an internalized coercive system of demands on the self to be that which it is not. In self-hatred, Horney saw a kind of self-flagellation going on that included self-accusations, self-contempt, self-frustration, self-torment, and self-destruction. But because these are so anguish filled, the self-hating individual goes to some bother to distract him- or herself from experiencing these self-condemnatory feelings. Classic distractions are addictions: binge eating, compulsive shopping, gambling oneself into debt, chemical dependency, and so forth. More subtle ways to conceal our self-loathing are found in relationships characterized by violence or exploitation (e.g., Feiring, Taska, & Lewis, 1996; Koss et al., 1994).

Horney concluded that duplicity and self-deception were the tools of defense cultivated by the neurotically prideful individual as well as by those defending against self-hatred. Both maladaptive patterns would appear to require a falsification of objective self-awareness and must therefore use a subjective self that is involved in constantly monitoring cues or seeking out "affordances" to stay in emotionally safe interactions (i.e., Neisser's *ecological self*). For such individuals, Neisser's *extended self* would probably be constricted in both past and future perspectives and limited to including only nonthreatening information; their *evaluative self* would be particularly vulnerability producing and therefore would also tend to be short-circuited when comparisons and evaluations signaled the possibility of falsified self-definitions being destabilized.

Horney's thinking about self-loathing in adults seems most congruent with Barrett's hypotheses when we look at those families in which disparagement of children is frequent and taken to extremes. In such families children are often the targets of scorn and harsh criticism, and if not offset by adequate love and affection, such children may have difficulties in developing emotional competence. My reasoning about why these children have problems in acquiring emotional competence is that, first, they are likely to have an impaired sense of self-efficacy (Barrett's sense of inadequacy) and, second, they frequently experience negative emotions that are not under their control. This combination of futility and feeling as though one is under siege by intense negative feelings contributes to a defeated self. In short, these children are likely to have problematic or deficient self-systems that put them at risk for incomplete or distorted acquisition of the skills of emotional competence as they proceed through childhood and adolescence. (I return to this topic in Chapter 12.)

CONCLUSION

If the self is the coordinator and mediator in our goal-striving transactions with an environment, then the multifaceted self described in this chapter can undertake such coordination and mediation in a branching, networking, and intersecting fashion. Multiple goals and multiple feelings are possible with a multifaceted self, and our emotional experience becomes more complex and nuanced as a result. Self-efficacy may be served by meeting most goals but not necessarily all our goals; greater frustration tolerance, coping, and resilience in the face of stress are all possible outcomes and will serve our emotional competence in future encounters with a provoking environment (usually ones that include other people). A self that can reflect on itself is also more likely to be able to expand its self-confidence in future as yet untested encounters, for self-knowledge allows for greater planful functioning. Awareness of the self's myriad facets also means that self-conscious emotional experience can become more complex: We can laugh at our moments of embarrassment or turn our shame into guilt that allows for repair, as in Alex's case.

We can better understand the development of adaptive and healthy self-conscious emotions such as those illustrated by Alex and Takeo by comparing them with their distorted counterparts, so aptly described by Horney. Her discussion of how shame can turn into self-hatred and pride into arrogance is exceptional and is a resource for deepening our theoretical thinking about emotional development in general and self-conscious emotions in particular. The combination of Horney's clinical work and Lewis's and Barrett's empirical–developmental work allows us to glimpse how self-construction proceeds with development and yet can diverge along paths of relative emotional competence or relative incompetence. Next we look at how families and peers contribute to emotional development and thus provide the "crucible" in which emotional competence is first forged.

Chapter 3

How We Become Emotionally Competent

*E*motional competence is embedded in cultural context. The particular society into which we are born provides us with a system of beliefs, which facilitates how we make sense of emotional experience. I illustrate how we become emotionally competent by presenting three extended descriptions of emotion *learning* in three cultural settings. The first is drawn from Mel Konner's (1972) work with the Zhun/twasi !Kung bushmen in northwestern Botswana; the second gives us an interesting comparison with the socialization of anger and aggression in a South Baltimore subculture (Miller & Sperry, 1987); the last is based on a Japanese sample (Conroy, Hess, Azuma, & Kashiwagi, 1980).

Konner (1972) described the !Kung child-rearing style as one that was permissive, attentive, affectionate, and extremely rich in stimulation and opportunities for exploration. I was especially intrigued by his description of tantrums and their relation to aggression in !Kung 2- to 5-year-olds:

> Unlike the passive tantrums we are familiar with, a Zhun/twa tantrum is often characterized by beating, object beating and throwing of objects, all directed at the mother, in addition to frowning, grimacing and

crying. Mothers are quite serene as the tantrum progresses, often laughing and talking to other adults while they ward off the tiny blows. They do not respond with the immediate anger characteristic of Western mothers hit by their children, but usually allow the episode to run its course. . . . If aggression *is* something that can be *displaced* or *redirected,* then this difference in the acceptability of real aggression against parents may help to account for the relative lack of fighting among young children in Zhun/twa society. (p. 301)

Konner also described the children as chasing and hitting animals such as dogs and cows that belonged to the village and even killing small animals; this aggression toward animals was also acceptable, for it was viewed as appropriate imitation of adult activities that would be undertaken in hunting. Peer aggression rarely occurred, and I can imagine that this sort of amicable atmosphere among !Kung children provided the foundation for the development of amicable adult relations, which would be adaptively necessary for a nomadic society with a hunter–gatherer economy.

In contrast to how aggression is channeled in Zhun/twa society, Miller and Sperry (1987) studied a South Baltimore community made up of working-class descendants from early immigrant Polish, Irish, Italian, and Appalachian laborers, in which mothers appeared to promote interpersonal aggression among young children. Mothers used teasing provocations to elicit mock aggressive reactions from their children; they reinforced their child's retaliation toward other children for presumed injuries or threats, and they modeled in both their discourse and their behavior the significance of aggressive interaction. As one mother put it quite vividly:

Oh, Peggy, she made me so mad one day I thought I'd take her by the neck and just strangle her, that's how mad I got with her. She kept throwin' a fit, wanted to get down [off the counter]. . . . She wants to go play the machines like those [bigger] kids do. . . . So she couldn't have her way. She couldn't get down so she threw a fit. And she almost, she scared me, she almost fell off the counter. I beat her. Oh, I was so mad. I think it, I was scared more than anything. (p. 11)

And another example:

Now she likes to wrestle with me. I'll take her upstairs and we go on the bed and start wrestling. And I'll say, "Take your fist and hit me." 'Cause I try to teach her in case somebody else is doin' it. 'Cause some kids do take their fist and hit you hard. [laughs] I let her punch me. Sometimes she sneaks a good one in on me. (p. 17)

Miller and Sperry's richly descriptive ethnographic study certainly presents us with a contrast to the gentle !Kung: Tantrums were met with violence and yet, vaguely similar to the !Kung mother, aggression toward the mother was tolerated (even encouraged), as long as it was conducted in an apparently playful context. The young 2½-year-old girls who were the objects of Miller and Sperry's investigation learned to become emotionally competent in *their cultural context* where self-defense and retaliation were necessary aspects for girls' and women's survival (physical violence toward women by men was commonplace in this community). Similarly, the !Kung children became emotionally competent *in their cultural context* but did so by learning just the opposite pattern from the South Baltimore children: They learned to get along with their peers in a friendly and cooperative fashion and channeled their aggression toward animals as part of rehearsal for hunting.

The Japanese sample of children was part of a cross-cultural comparison undertaken by Conroy et al. (1980). They questioned both American and Japanese mothers of 3- to 4-year-old firstborn children about a variety of hypothetical situations that were likely to occur in the home and which reflected noncompliance on the part of preschoolers. The results of their survey indicated that Japanese mothers were more likely than American mothers to appeal to *feelings* in order to gain their preschoolers' compliance. Conroy et al. (1980) give the following example of a Japanese mother's response: "It is not Mommy alone who is shopping. Other people are also here to shop, and the store owners have neatly lined things up so that the customers will buy them. Therefore, it will be annoying to them if you behave this way" (p. 168). American mothers were more likely to grab their child's arm firmly and order the child to stay close. Japanese mothers were also found to use gentle persuasion to elicit compliance from the child: "You drew very well. You can draw even better if you use paper instead of the wall" (p. 169). American mothers were more likely to demand an immediate cessation of the drawing on the wall and a command to clean up the mess. In other words, overt coercion was more often used by American mothers with noncompliant preschoolers, frequently leading to a battle of wills, whereas the Japanese mother appealed to her child's sense of wanting to please and cooperate, leading to strong emotional connection or *amae* (see also C. Lewis's [1986] analysis of Japanese parental control as reflecting their emphasis on cooperation). The willfulness of American preschoolers is congruent with American socialization values of independence and self-assertion; the responsiveness to others so noticeable in Japanese preschoolers is consistent with the Japanese socialization values of sympathy and social conscientiousness (Shigaki, 1983).

THE SOCIALIZATION OF EMOTION

Cross-cultural research on emotion socialization suggests that "emotions can be seen as both the medium and the message of socialization. Their uniqueness, and their crucial importance for understanding development, lies in this dual and encompassing role" (Lutz, 1983, p. 60). Certainly the examples of three different cultural contexts presented here illustrate how the parents' emotional responses to their children constitute both modality and meaning in the socialization of anger and aggression. Thus, even as we may observe emotional development *in the child*, those who interact with the child are communicating their own emotions *to the child*, often elicited by their evaluation of the child's emotional behavior. In addition to parents and other family members who are engaged in this reciprocal emotion-socializing process with children, the larger world of peers, media, and other adult figures such as teachers are also part of the social context. Thus, children acquire both emotion–laden beliefs and emotional-expressive behaviors that reflect these different influences. At the same time, their cultural beliefs about feelings and how they have learned to express their emotions converge toward (sub)cultural norms; in short, children become culturally predictable. Not that the adults in one's subculture necessarily approve of all aspects of children's and adolescents' predictable emotional behavior; rather they resignedly come to expect and tolerate to some degree, for example, "childish" crankiness, preadolescent irritability, or adolescent moodiness.

Folk Theories of Emotion

In the first chapter I briefly mentioned folk theories of emotion as cultural beliefs about what emotions are and how they function. The convergence toward cultural predictability in a child's developing emotional experience noted above reflects the child's learning his or her particular subculture's (folk) theory of emotion. We tacitly acquire such folk theories, not only about emotion but also about social relations, the self, and even the nature of thought, as we mature and are socialized within a particular cultural context. Such naive or folk theories of emotion function as internal guides or "working models" for both understanding *and* facilitating social exchanges that are mediated by emotion processes. A meta-level understanding of emotion that is embedded within a "working model" or folk theory of emotion may be important for children to comprehend more complex emotional transactions between people, such as when we witness another's chagrin, preemptive aggression, or ironic smiling upon receiving bad news. I list here, somewhat facetiously, some of my metaphors for assorted North American folk theories of emotion:

- The volcano theory ("If you don't vent your emotions, you'll explode," already mentioned in Chapter 1).
- The tidal wave theory ("Don't lose control or your feelings will build up until they overwhelm you").
- The out-of-sight/out-of-mind theory ("If you don't think about your feelings, they'll go away").
- The Vulcan theory from the *Star Trek* television series ("Your emotions are irrational and illogical, surely they get in the way of solving problems").

Apart from my attempts at parody, what is also noteworthy about these metaphors is that they are guides for how to cope. If emotions are the "products" of our goal-striving encounters with the environment, then some of the time we will not get what we want, and we will experience assorted negative feelings. What we then *do* with those aversive feelings and with the distressing circumstances represents our attempts to cope, and the coping strategies we pursue have much to do with emotion socialization. As these metaphors suggest, common coping strategies in North American culture include distancing oneself from one's feelings to appear "calm, cool, and collected" and, in seeming contradiction, expressing one's feelings—as in releasing pressure—to avoid a more intense emotional reaction. In Chapter 9 I return to discuss coping strategies at length.

My views about folk theories of emotion have been much influenced by anthropologist Catherine Lutz. She presented a view of folk theories of emotion that emphasizes social roles and relationships as integral to emotional experience (Lutz, 1987). Her term, "ethnotheories of emotion," refers to implicit and pragmatic guidelines and beliefs held by individuals for facilitating and understanding ordinary social–emotional transactions. She also emphasizes that ethnotheories of emotion are open-ended and subject to change. This feature is a key one, for as children mature, their naive theory for how emotion "works" and what to expect emotionally changes as well. As an illustration, Lewis (1989) found that a majority of preschool children thought they would feel *sad* if lost in a store, whereas a majority of adults expected children of that age group to feel *afraid* if lost in a large store. While it could be that there was some degree of misunderstanding of emotion labels by the child respondents, it does not seem likely, given the exhaustive work of Dunn, Bretherton, and Munn (1987) and Bretherton, Fritz, Zahn-Waxler, and Ridgeway (1986), among others, who have analyzed young children's discourse on emotions and found them to be impressively sophisticated by 3 to 4 years of age in our culture's emotion lexicon. What seems to account for the difference in expected emotional reaction is that different normative expectations exist for different age groups relative to what sort of emotion is likely to be felt in particular situations.

Lutz also takes into account in her discussion of ethnotheories of emotion that such theories typically include two different kinds of goals: (1) *action tendency goals* refer to the motivating value of an emotion for the individual to undertake some sort of action (e.g., to run away if afraid) and (2) *disclosure or attribution goals* refer to the degree of social acceptability surrounding an emotional experience that one has. For example, in the United States it is often more socially acceptable for a woman to report somewhat ambiguously to others that she felt *upset* rather than to say she felt *angry*; the reverse may hold true for men, and, indeed, investigators have found that boys report that they would be unlikely to disclose that they felt sad (Fuchs & Thelen, 1988) or fearful (Meerum Terwogt & Olthof, 1989).

Research on children's understanding that certain emotions tend to go hand-in-hand with particular motives and behavioral sequelae has been undertaken by Gnepp (1989a, 1989b), Stein and Trabasso (1989), among others. Saarni (1979a, 1979b, 1988, 1989a) has examined children's awareness of the social acceptability of certain emotional experiences and expressive behavior in terms of what they reported as socially appropriate expressions of emotion, which included not expressing any emotion at all under some circumstances (the Star Trek theory, perhaps). Zeman and Garber (1996) also examined grade-school children's expectations for appropriateness of emotional–expressive behavior and found that children generally thought it would be a "bad idea" to express vulnerable emotions such as fear or sadness with one's peers. Thus, Lutz's disclosure rules surrounding emotional–expressive behavior vary, at least in Western societies, with who witnesses one's emotional display.

Parenthetically, the "new" folk theory of emotion for the "high-tech information age" may be the set of assumptions assembled under the general rubric of "emotional intelligence" (Goleman, 1995; Salovey & Sluyter, 1997). Given my perspective on the significance of folk theories of emotion in how we come to construe what is emotionally meaningful, I have pondered whether emotional intelligence represents our society's folk theory about emotional functioning. Goleman (1997) suggests that emotional intelligence is what is needed "to learn to flourish in life," although I think an environment that provides educational, economic, and social opportunities is important for "learning to flourish" as well. Mayer and Salovey (1997) define emotional intelligence as follows:

> Emotional intelligence involves the ability to perceive accurately, appraise, and express emotion; the ability to access and/or generate feelings when they facilitate thought; the ability to understand emotion and emotional knowledge; and the ability to regulate emotions to promote emotional and intellectual growth. (p. 10)

I welcome the idea of emotional intelligence as a much needed addition to our thinking about intelligent and resourceful problem solving; however, I notice the absence of empathy, interpersonal focus, and moral character in the above conceptualization. My approach to emotional competence clearly also shares much with this definition as well as reflecting the influence of folk theories of emotion. Where emotional competence and emotional intelligence may differ is in emphasis: I consistently focus on emotions in social contexts and with regard to the individual's self-efficacy and moral sense. I return now to how we might think about emotion socialization in a more analytical sense.

COMPONENTS OF EMOTION

One way to look at the socialization of emotion is to think of emotion as consisting of components and from there to examine how each component is influenced by socialization processes. I especially like the components approach taken by Lewis and Michalson (1983), who proposed that our English language folk theory of emotion suggested five basic components:

Emotional Elicitors

These are the circumstances or context in which we experience an emotion, and they clearly reflect considerable social influence in that our culture determines to a great extent what are viewed as "typical" causes for particular categories of emotion (see, e.g., Russell, 1991, for a review of culture and emotion categorization). Thus, gustatory pleasure at the prospect of eating a lizard does not seem especially plausible for me, but in some other parts of the world, I might be quite pleased at the invitation to dine on such a delicacy. Even within a given culture, there may be considerable variability in what is viewed as a situational elicitor of an emotional response, and, for that matter, there appears to be variability due to one's age group that also interfaces with the social construction of causes for emotions (e.g., Lewis, 1989).

Emotional Receptors

These are hypothesized structures that allow us to react to the environment. I think of them as the *affordances* described in the preceding chapter: We are endowed with a rich biology for interacting with our environment, and this biology provides us with both sensory and cognitive information. I think that temperament might also be considered part of this biological affordance system for interacting with our environment, as in arousability and reactivity to stimuli, and individual differences in temperament may well be related to differences in emotional responsiveness (e.g., Derryberry & Rothbart, 1988; Rothbart & Bates, 1997). A possible clinical example of emotional receptors might be how the administration of Ritalin (methylphenidate) to children assessed as having attention-deficit disorder with hyperactivity changes the dynamic affordances of the environment for such children. It certainly changes how their teachers and parents view their behavior and thus alters the emotional tone of these children's social relationships.

Emotional States

Emotional states refer to the bodily changes that co-occur with emotional responding, including biochemical, neurological, and physiological activity associated with emotional arousal (e.g., Levenson, Ekman, & Friesen, 1990). I suspect that somatic activity associated with emotional states can be directly influenced by parents when they give their upset and irritable children snacks, candy, or a bottle of milk to calm them down.

Sugar, carbohydrates, and the distracting activity of eating may indeed alter the biochemical emotional state. It is likely that we learn to "self-medicate" our aversive emotional states by eating and drinking, which can be thought of as an outcome of emotion socialization and influenced by family, peers, and media. Caregivers may also try to influence the external manifestation of emotion-related somatic activity; for example, when a parent notices the pallor or hyperventilation of a badly frightened child, he or she offers coping suggestions, reassurance, or a reframing of the emotion-eliciting situation (e.g., "Try to breathe slowly and deeply so you'll feel better; it just looks dangerous when the roller coaster goes down the hill fast, but you're safely strapped in").

Emotional Expression

Socialization influences emotional expression in significant ways: In all cultures children learn rules or guidelines for where and when to express what emotion with which people. When children alter their external expression of their feelings, they are often attempting to bring their expressive behavior into accordance with cultural or subcultural beliefs about what is appropriate or socially desirable under certain circumstances. These beliefs about which expressions of emotions are socially desirable or appropriate are referred to as *display rules* in that there is considerable social consensus or predictability about what sort of facial expression is displayed. In Chapter 8 I go into considerable detail about emotional displays and their relationship to emotional competence. At this point I simply want to emphasize that emotional–expressive behavior is deeply embedded in the dynamics of social relationships, exemplified in the vignette in the first chapter about the twins Ned and Jack, who artfully arranged their revenge on the bully Steve.

Emotional Experience

Lewis and Michalson (1983) view this last component of emotion as the most cognitive one: It requires access to a language of and about emotion. This component takes into account knowledge about emotion and assumes increasing insight into one's emotional processes as one matures. Thus, reflection on the self's affective experience is implied as well as being able to infer emotional responses in others (see Saarni & Harris, 1989, for relevant reviews of children's understanding of emotion).

Understanding one's emotional experience reflects the influence of socialization in that inherent in the construction of emotional experience are cultural meaning systems (Lutz, 1983). Lutz argues that cultural values are embedded in the socialization of beliefs about emotional experience, and the transmission of these cultural values constitutes parental goals insofar as parents attempt to socialize and guide their children toward culturally desirable ways of feeling and behaving. To illustrate, Lutz, an anthropologist, lived with the Ifaluk people on a Micronesian island and had an opportunity to observe parents' teaching their children when they should feel *metagu,* a feeling evoked when an elder is justifiably angry with the child. Parents were most concerned that their children learn to experience *metagu,* for if they did not display *metagu* when another adult was justifiably angry with them (beginning at about 5 to 6 years old), then the judgment made about the children's deficient behavior was that *their parents* had failed to responsibly teach them. Although Lutz does not directly comment on this, I also see in her example the interconnecting web of influence that community and families traverse in the socialization of emotion in the young. This is one way in which cultural meaning systems are "enforced," namely, parents are encouraged to socialize their children according to consensually agreed on beliefs about desirable and appropriate emotional behavior, and if they do not, then the parents themselves become targets of negative social opinion and judgment.

Ethnographers and observers in natural settings have often collected information about how socializing agents (parents, teachers) use an emotional lexicon to interpret emotional experience to children. Pollack and Thoits (1989) found that explicit verbal linkages between situational cause and resulting emotion characterized the most frequently mentioned emotion statements used by teachers in a therapeutic school. Miller and Sperry (1987) found mothers using emotion language to specify the greater legitimacy (or acceptability) of some emotional responses over others relative to social context (e.g., retaliatory anger was encouraged toward provoking peers but severely discouraged toward adults, even if the adults had behaved in a provoking fashion). Russell's (1991) comprehensive cross-cultural comparison of emotion language categories provides one of the most thorough analyses of how emotion concepts can be viewed as systems of representational scripts. Such a script system implies that the meaning of any one emotion concept is related to a network of concepts with which it is integrated; for example, one's beliefs about anger may be influenced by one's beliefs about one's sex role (see Chapter 6 for an illustration of this anger/sex-role script network). Thus, the component emotional experience reflects this acquired network of concepts, which provides the growing child with scripts for representing his or her own emotional responses within a multidimensional matrix of causes, goals, values, social relations, and beliefs about emotion management (including both internal emotional regulation and expressive control). It is especially impressive that by 6 to 8 years of age (and likely earlier but less accessible to verbal articulation), many children have well-defined scripts that reveal such a "multidimensional matrix" (recall the story of Rachel with her grandfather in Chapter 1). Chapter 6 further addresses Russell's work, among others, on scripts and emotion concepts.

Summary

Children are exposed to emotion-eliciting circumstances, learn about the emotions involved, and subsequently incorporate that learning into their own emotional "map" of when to feel, what to feel, how to express feelings, and whom to express them to. In short, those aspects of emotion that are the clearest targets of socializing influence appear to be emotional elicitors, emotional expression, and emotional experience. Certainly these last two components of emotion have the most developmental research associated with them. These last two components also provide for the greatest communicative access to one another's emotional processes, namely, emotional–expressive behavior is meaningful and informative to one's interactants, and emotional experience permits the verbal description and exchange of emotional processes to others. The influence of socialization on emotional receptors and states is more ambiguous and awaits further research. Finally, readers are also referred to Gottman, Katz, and Hooven (1997), Garber and Dodge (1991), Halberstadt (1991), Lewis and Saarni (1985), Ratner and Stettner (1991), Saarni (1985, 1993), Saarni and von Salisch (1993), and Thompson (1990), among others, for additional consideration of what may be involved in the socialization of emotion. Comprehensive literature reviews on socialization processes more generally considered may be found in Bugental and Goodnow (1998) and Parke and Buriel (1998).

PROCESSES OF EMOTION SOCIALIZATION

Families are most often studied by social scientists as the locus of emotion socialization processes. Certainly the younger the child, the more likely it is the caregivers who make significant choices that influence the child's emotion socialization. With increasing maturity, the larger world of peers becomes the more salient context for emotion socialization. In this section I first address the family context of emotion socialization and then linkages between the family and peers for emotional competence.

Traditionally, socialization in families has been studied from the standpoint of (1) parents' modeling behavior that their children subsequently imitate, (2) parents' reinforcing (positively or negatively) their children's behavior, and (3) children's internalizing aspects of their parents' beliefs, feelings, and behaviors through unconscious processes of identification. However, we find that socialization is a two-way street: Children influence their parents' behavior toward them as well, and to complicate things further, children's developmental level affects greatly what they imitate or identify with and how effectively reinforcement functions (an absurd example should suffice: taking away telephone privileges from a preschooler for throwing a tantrum in a restaurant is not an effective use of negative reinforcement). Parents probably are most aware of trying to didactically teach their children about desired emotional–expressive behavior, but whether it is all that successful in modifying their children's behavior is debatable. Examples include the following: "You can't scream in church, Judy" [Judy begins to cry instead]; "You have to smile for Grandma when she wants to take a picture" [Joey looks cross-eyed while grinning demonically]; and "Look, you're just going to have to control yourself when Bob comes over tonight" [Bob being Mom's recently acquired boyfriend; Debbie proceeds to whine energetically all evening].

There is a considerable body of research on individual differences that are thought to affect emotional–expressive behavior and which may be viewed as mediating the socialization of emotion in children. Most often investigated have been gender differences (e.g., Eisenberg & Lennon, 1983; Fuchs & Thelen, 1988), temperament and/or personality differences (e.g., Goldsmith & Campos, 1982; Fox, Sobel, Calkins, & Cole, 1996; Rothbart & Bates, 1998; Rothbart, Ziaie, & O'Boyle, 1992), cultural differences (e.g., Gordon, 1989; Harkness & Super, 1985; Lutz, 1983, 1985), and those differences stemming from pathology-inducing circumstances (e.g., Allessandri & Lewis, 1996; Camras, Grow, & Ribordy, 1983; Camras, Sachs-Alter, & Ribordy, 1996; Casey, 1996; Cicchetti & Carlson, 1989; During & McMahon, 1991; Feldman, Philippot, & Custrini, 1991; Lewis & Miller, 1990; Zabel, 1979).

More subtle differences, such as the degree to which parents are controlling or accepting of children's emotional–expressive behavior and the degree to which they talk about emotion in the family, have been less easily and less consistently determined as having a *direct* effect on children's subsequent emotional behavior or emotional understanding (e.g., Cassidy, Parke, Butkowsky, & Braungart, 1992; Dunn, Brown, & Beardsall, 1991; Eisenberg, Fabes, Schaller, Carlo, & Miller, 1991; Eisenberg, Fabes, Carlo, & Karbon, 1992; Saarni, 1989a). It appears that relative to these parenting differences, other variables (e.g., family structure, presence of siblings, and level of maternal education, in addition to temperament, gender role, dysfunctional circumstances, etc.) mediate or influence how parenting differences translate into observable outcomes in children's emotional socialization. Thus, the sources of more subtle individual differences in emotional socialization are likely to be difficult to unravel because of their embeddedness in unique developmental histories and unique contexts.

The more significant socializing influences on children's emotional experience may stem from some of the choices that parents make about contexts their children experience, that is, when they act as "filters" or as "conduits" relative to what the child is exposed to (see also Ladd & LeSieur, 1995). Parents act as emotional filters when they, for example, screen television programs or playmates for what they believe to be desirable exposure for their children. Choosing one route (or conduit) over another may significantly affect the emotional environments children experience. A common example is when working parents enroll their toddlers in day-care programs as opposed to having the child spend the day with a grandparent. The former option is rich with peer interaction and nonfamily adults who impose limits; the latter option is rich with intensive adult interaction where limits may be more subtly imposed. Parents also act as "coaches" or managers for their children's emotional experience, and this viewpoint led to some of the more fascinating research discussed next.

Parents as Managers

I assume that processes of emotion socialization are embedded in relationships; therefore, the emotional dynamics of these relationships mediate the form and quality of emotion socialization in the individual child. I use a metaphor to try to clarify this dynamic. Think of the parents' affective relationship with their children and, for that matter, with one another, as a melody; the lyrics that accompany the melody are the more overt parental coaching/managing behaviors and verbalizations that we can more readily identify in empirical research. Parenting advice books also address the latter, whereas the former, the "melody," appears more often in the domain of psychotherapy, particularly object relations–oriented therapy and attachment theory.

Intersubjectivity

A few researchers have tried to capture this complex interplay of melody and lyrics. Ratner and Stettner (1991) used the term "intersubjectivity" to describe how people in close relationships, in this case, parents and their children, mutually influence one another's emotional responses, in part because they have a shared history of emotion-laden interactions with one another. Based on their arguments, I would infer that when children experience an emotion (e.g., fear), prior interactions with their parents having to do with when they felt fear before are evoked as *representations* accompanying the present fear response. Thus, the parents' own expressive behavior (e.g., judgmentalness, reassurance, and personal distress) becomes incorporated into how children feel about their own feelings. A child whose fear is ridiculed is more apt to try to suppress his fear or feel shamed about it in contrast to the child whose parent explains the source of the fear rationally and sympathetically. The latter child may be more likely to use his feeling of fear as a meaningful cue to seek support if it is available or to explore the problem situation for alternatives that are less scary. At the beginning of this essay I quoted Catherine Lutz's comment about emotion being both the medium and the message in emotion socialization, and that viewpoint appears relevant to understanding what intersubjectivity is all about: The parents' feelings about the emotion in question are "packaged" together in their socializing efforts directed at their children's emotions.

Similar to Miller and Sperry's (1987) theoretical interpretation of their ethnographic research on the socialization of anger and aggression in a South Baltimore community, Ratner and Stettner also distinguish between socialization *instruction*—or what is presented by the parents and/or other cultural agents (e.g., schools and television) as the "message" or content of what is to be transmitted to the child—and socialization *acquisition*, which is what the child actually internalizes and subsequently performs behaviorally. To return to our metaphor, the melody and lyrics of emotion-laden relationships that children "hear" may not always be the same as what the other family members think they are playing as the "music." And yet there may be a convergence over time as suggested by some early research by Chapman (1981). He found that mothers used discipline methods with their children based on their *anticipations* of what they thought their children would do. He argued that in the short run, parental expectations will affect children's behavior, but in the long run it was the children's behavior that affected the parents, for the expectations they developed were based on their children's past behavior. In a parallel fashion, Steinberg and Laird (1989) found that mothers who used primarily situational information for determining what they thought children were feeling tended to have children who also relied more on situational information for figuring out what they were feeling. Mothers who relied more on children's expressive behavior for inferring their emotions had children who similarly were more responsive to their expressive behavior. We cannot tell from this study who influenced whom given Chapman's perspective, but perhaps what is salient is the mutuality of interaction. Finally, Dix (1991) proposed a model of parenting that explicitly identifies emotional processes *in parents* that affect the parent–child relationship significantly. Specifically, he argued that analyzing which emotions are activated in parents, how they are managed, and how they influence parenting behavior toward children are critical issues for understanding children's emotional development. As we shall see later, these same sorts of concerns are reflected in Gottman et al.'s (1997) research on parents' emotions and their impact on their children.

Discipline Tactics

A significant body of research is emerging that further consolidates the notion that parents function as managers or coaches of their children's emotion socialization. Denham and her associates (e.g., Denham & Grout, 1993; Denham, Mitchell-Copeland, Strandberg, Auerbach, & Blair, 1997; Denham, Zoller, & Couchoud, 1994) conducted a number of studies with preschool-age children and their parents, typically their mothers. The overall pattern they found is that mothers who talked about emotions with their young children, expressed predominantly positive emotions, responded to their children's emotion calmly and reassuringly, and used emotion-laden explanations in their discipline tactics tended to have children whose emotional–expressive behavior was better regulated and socially more competent with peers. In short, such mothers had children who were both happier and more self-confident.

In a similar vein, Gottman et al. (1997) proposed that when parents interact with their children in ways that are warm, praising, facilitative of emotion understanding (as in Denham's work), and nonderogating, and they provide a supportive "scaffold" with which they encourage their children's development, their children learn to engage "with the world cognitively or affectively by self-soothing, inhibiting negative affect and focusing attention" (p. 105). Their use of the term "emotion coaching" entails that the parents (1) are aware of their child's emotion, (2) see their child's emotional experience as a learning opportunity, (3) help their child to label or verbalize his or her feelings, (4) empathize and validate their child's emotions, and (5) assist their child in dealing with the distressing circumstances. In their research, they followed a group of two-parent families for about 3 years, starting when the target child was about age 5. When the child was about age 8, the families were recontacted and an extensive battery of measures was again administered. Their data yielded exceptionally rich information and ideas about how parents set the stage for their children's emotional regulation in the preschool years and then how the children subsequently ventured forth into peer groups and classroom settings.

Meta-Emotion

One of the strategies used by Gottman et al. (1997) was to analyze interview data with parents to determine the parents' implicit beliefs and feelings about their own, their spouses', and their children's emotions. They used the term "meta-emotion" to denote the idea of our having emotions about emotions, similar to the terms "meta-communication" or "meta-cognition." (From my standpoint, their use of meta-emotion is similar to what I view as folk or naive theories of emotion.) They were able to predict 3 years later which children would be functioning well socially and academically, based on their careful examination of the parents' meta-emotion system. This meta-emotion system was embedded in how the parents used (not necessarily consciously) a complex network of beliefs and feelings about how emotions "worked" for them, especially anger and sadness. Their findings were complex, but one of their more robust (and expected) outcomes was that parental derogation and insufficient scaffolding/praising in the preschool years tended to be associated with less adequate academic and social functioning in their school-age children.

Gottman et al. (1997) acknowledge the limitations to the conclusions they drew. Ethnic diversity, serious economic stress, single parenthood, diagnosed psychiatric disturbance, and the like were not evident in their sample of families. They approached their families as research subjects rather than participants in complex contextual systems whereby such systems might well require adoption of multiple roles and possibly even style switching among different meta-emotion perspectives. However, in spite of these limitations, they *listened* to the parents with a sensitivity to their emotional processes that will likely have a profound influence on future research on parent–child or family interaction.

I next turn to a brief discussion of linkages between family socialization of emotion and their children's peer relationships. In this context I also consider how peers socialize the emotional–expressive behavior of one another, a topic that is more implicit in research on peer relations rather than explicitly investigated.

Linkages between Families and Peers in Emotion Socialization

Learning to Regulate Emotional Arousal with Peers

As Gottman et al. (1997) point out, families may model with their young children open and vulnerable emotional expressiveness and responsiveness; however, this is just how 8-year-old children typically do *not* act in our culture when they try to join a group of other children for play. Thus, children do not simply copy their family models for emotional behavior with their peers; something else occurs that links what children learn in the home and what they demonstrate with their friends. Gottman et al. believe that children in emotionally responsive families learn to regulate their feelings in sufficient measure so that they are able to attend to the other children and appropriately join in rather than becoming overly excited, aggressive, reactive, or withdrawn. Parke, Cassidy, Burks, Carson, and Boyum (1992) reviewed research on the links between parent–child interaction and children's social competence. They, too, proposed that it is emotional regulatory processes that are primary in mediating family-based emotion socialization and peer social contexts. Their review also concurs with the general patterns found by Denham and her colleagues as cited earlier: Socially popular children (typically between 3 and 6 years of age) tend to have parents who are warm, are responsively engaged with their children, and use inductive discipline methods rather than coercive and punitive ones. Parke et al. (1992) also reported that parents who play longer with their young children and who used indirect interactive styles during the play (asking questions, letting the child take the lead, etc.) had children who approached their peers similarly. Such children were generally more engaged for longer play periods with their peers and were less controlling. Rejected children tended to be coercive with their peers, an interactional style they had also experienced at home with their parents where they tended to respond with noncompliance to the barrage of parental directives. More recently Carson and Parke (1996) confirmed and extended these findings. They found that it was *fathers'* negative emotional expressiveness toward their children while they played with them that was associated with poor peer relationships.

Expressive Behavior and Peer Relations

Parke et al. (1992) reviewed the impact of parental emotional expressiveness on their children's social competence. They note that gender of parent and gender of child may interact but how the parents expressed emotions toward their children when the children were upset and distressed is more important. Moderate parental expressiveness combined with appropriate problem solving appeared to be the combination that was linked with children's learning to manage their social relationships more competently (see also Roberts & Strayer, 1987). Across a number of studies Parke et al. (1992) also note that fathers' negative emotional expressive behavior, including disgust, anger, and anxiety, was most consistently associated with their children being more likely rejected by their peers. Parallel to the idea that children learn controlling (and thus less flexible or adaptive) interactive strategies from parents who interact with them in this fashion, may be the outcome that children who experience frequent and intense bouts of negative emotional–expressive behavior from their parents also learn to display similar expressive behavior with their peers.

Parke et al. (1992) also reviewed a number of studies that suggested that children who have greater emotion knowledge were more likely to be socially accepted and sought out by other children. Emotion knowledge is obviously a broad concept, but for young children it is typically defined as the ability to identify facial expressions of common emotions, to describe eliciting circumstances, and to connect emotional experience with expressive display. Insofar as parents facilitate children's learning about various aspects about emotion, they help their children in peer contexts, for the children are better equipped to be able to figure out what others are feeling and why. They can then more adaptively adjust their own behavior to the potentially emotionally charged social interaction.

Parental Socializing Style and Children's Peer Interaction

Parke et al. (1992) raise many significant issues about the linkages between family emotion socialization and their children's subsequent peer interaction that are worthy of research. Intriguing to me was how the linkages might change with the child's development. The majority of the studies they reviewed focus on a relatively narrow age range, 3 to 6 years old. The fact that a number of studies suggest that learning to regulate one's emotional arousal is what children take from their family interaction into the world of peers may in part be a function of this particular age group. What would children in middle childhood or young adolescents take from their families' emotion socializing style into their peer relationships? A great many studies have been done on parental disciplinary styles and older children, and consistent with the above review, harsh and domineering discipline is usually associated with children experiencing peer difficulties (further reviewed in Ladd, 1992). At least one study suggested that this type of disciplinary style short-circuits children's interpersonal problem-solving skills and thus disrupts their ability to have more satisfactory peer relationships (Pettit, Harrist, Bates, & Dodge, 1991). Hart, Ladd, and Burleson (1990) also found that parents who used power-assertive discipline techniques—emphasizing compliance as opposed to trying to work with their children to understand psychological motives and feelings—had children (9 years of age) who displayed controlling and self-centered instrumental behaviors with their peers and, as a result, tended to be rejected. Combining the above studies with the work of Gottman et al. (1997), I would infer that this sort of harsh, power-assertive disciplinary style on the part of parents is accompanied by expressions of contempt, anger, and hostility toward the child being disciplined in such a fashion. A humiliated, resentful child would seem ill-equipped indeed to negotiate peer relationships satisfactorily.

Finally, Cooper and Cooper (1992) reviewed empirical and theoretical links between adolescents' relationships, both with their parents and with peers. Most relevant to emotion socialization and emotional competence was their own work with adolescents that yielded results similar to the findings of Pettit et al. (1991) and Hart et al. (1990) with younger children. Specifically, adolescents who had collaborative negotiation styles with their parents also had adaptive and collaborative interpersonal negotiation skills with their friends. Adolescents who regularly experienced family interaction characterized by more contentious disagreements and unilateral conflict negotiation strategies tended to have more conflicted and argumentative friendships (Cooper & Carlson, 1989).

Speculation about Peers' Socializing One Another's Emotion

I have been most influenced by research by Asher and his colleagues in terms of thinking about how peers may mutually socialize the emotional–expressive behavior of one another (e.g., Asher & Coie, 1990; Asher & Rose, 1997; Asher, Parker, & Walker, 1996). They examined close friendships among school-age children (as opposed to whether the children were simply rated as "popular" or accepted by others) for the sorts of emotional tensions and conflicts that are unique to close relationships between peers. Asher and Rose (1997) determined that there are five primary nodes around which children at times experience emotional dilemmas with their friends; in the following list I have included quotes taken from their chapter (p. 203) that illustrate these five nodes particularly well:

1. Respecting the need for equity and reciprocity:
   "He is my very best friend because he tells me things and I tell him things. He shows me a basketball move and I show him, too, and he never makes me sad."
2. Providing help, even when it might be inconvenient or have a cost to it:
   "My friend is really nice. Once my nose was bleeding about a gallon every thirty minutes and he helped me."
3. Being trustworthy and reliable, even when it might be in conflict with other desires:
   "Jessica has problems at home and with her religion and when something happens she always comes to me and talks about it. We've been through a lot together."

4. Managing disputes and conflicts (as opposed to terminating the friendship or escalating the conflict into aggression):

> "Angie is very special to me. If we get in a fight we always say we are sorry. And if she says she would play with me, she plays with me."

5. Recognizing that friendships are part of larger dynamic networks such as classrooms or neighborhoods (sometimes one's friend wants to spend time with others and sulking about it is both useless and potentially threatening to the friendship):

> "Tammy is really forgiving. She understands when I pick partners other than her."

As is evident from these quotes, children relish and value their friendships. From friendships they gain companionship, alliance, support, and validation, and given that they highly prize these interpersonal goals, children must learn to modify their behavior, including their emotional responses, to maintain these interpersonal rewards. What is it then that children influence in one another so they can do this? Asher and Rose's research provide some idea as to what children do to resolve friendship conflicts. First, they found that children who nominated retaliating strategies as ways to solve problems with friends were, not surprisingly, less likely to have any! Second, they also found that children who used verbally aggressive and/or friendship-terminating strategies also had fewer friendships. Third, children who proposed compromising strategies had more best friends than those who did not use this strategy. Fourth, in terms of the quality of the friendships that children did report, the most conflicted ones were associated with retaliating, controlling, terminating, and aggressive goals. Those children who espoused relationship goals ("I would try to stay friends") had the least conflict in their friendships, and associated with such a goal were presumably behaviors that were compromising, supportive, validating, and forgiving. In short, children with close friends appear to be able to cope with conflict and tension, show empathy and understanding of both their own and others' feelings, recognize that their emotional–expressive behavior affects others, desire emotional closeness, and have a moral sense of "doing the right thing" with their friends. This surely sounds like emotional competence, as manifested in close relationships, in that such children are demonstrating self-efficacy in emotion-eliciting social transactions.

I suspect that children's involvement in close friendships is a significant vehicle for promoting the skills of emotional competence in ways that extend them beyond what the immediate nuclear family may be able to do. The eight skills of emotional competence described in this volume are all relevant to close friendships, and I speculate that children reinforce one another's growing mastery of each skill as a way of sustaining and nurturing highly valued friendships. Extremely lonely children and children who are frequently rejected by others have difficulties managing their emotional responses to others (e.g., Parkhurst & Asher, 1992) and may be at considerable risk later in life for psychological disorders (e.g., Parker & Asher, 1987). Such children are neither emotionally competent nor socially competent, for deficits in either emotional or social domains will reciprocally affect the other deleteriously (see also Casey, 1996).

I conclude this chapter with a brief discussion of how children are also important constructors of their own emotional experience. This view derives from cognitive developmental theory and research, and specific studies are cited in the subsequent chapters when I consider developmental factors relevant to each skill of emotional competence.

COGNITIVE MEDIATION OF EMOTIONS

One of the more prominent aspects of Western culture's views of how emotion "works" is the emphasis on cognitive mediation of emotion or appraisal (e.g., Lazarus, 1991). What do we know about children's acquisition of this belief, namely, that emotion results from one's own cognition (as opposed to from one's kinship system, from dream spirits or ghosts, or from bodily illness)? I would argue that one of the corollaries to this Western folk theory belief about emotions as stemming from one's thoughts, images, and the like is our culture's emphasis on emotion as an *internal,* individual experience in contrast to the emphasis in a number of other cultures' on emotion as an *interactive* experience (see Kitayama & Markus, 1994, for extensive discussion of this topic). However, given that we are focusing on the socialization of emotion in children reared in Western cultures, let us look at how children acquire this specific facet of Western folk theory of emotion.

Understanding of Mental States

I have found the cognitively oriented work undertaken by Harris and his colleagues to be especially descriptive and useful for examining children's developing belief that emotions are connected to how and what one thinks. In a series of studies, Harris and his collaborators investigated how children (both English and Dutch) made sense of their own and others' emotional experience (e.g., Harris, 1985, 1989; Harris & Gross, 1988; Harris & Lipian, 1989; Harris & Olthof, 1982; Harris, Olthof, & Meerum

Terwogt, 1981). Their most recent data suggest that in the preschool years, children are already able to conceptualize emotional experience as stemming from "mental" causes. That is, they demonstrate in their understanding of others' experience that the perspective or belief held by the other is significantly involved in determining how the other feels (i.e., that emotional elicitors are *constructed*). As they move through middle childhood, children begin to invoke mental factors as well for how *to change* emotional experience. For example, Harris and Lipian (1989) interviewed children in boarding schools to find out how the children thought they could alleviate negative feelings such as homesickness and sadness. Older children (age 10) were much more likely to cite such strategies as distraction, focusing on something positive, reinterpreting the situation, and so forth. Younger children (age 6) tended to restrict their strategies to suggestions about how to change the situation rather than looking inward to seeing whether and how one might alter one's internal experience. This greater reliance by the older children on internal, mental states as part of the "emotional package" (i.e., one's folk theory of emotion) has an impact on several critical features of emotion, among them the cues used to identify emotions reliably, how emotional–expressive behavior is regulated, whether emotion moderates other psychological domains such as memory and beliefs, and, importantly, how to cope with negative emotions.

Stein and Trabasso (1989) emphasized the role of goals in children's appraisals of what gives rise to emotions and feelings (see also Wellman & Banerjee, 1991, discussed in Chapter 4, and Levine, 1995, discussed in Chapter 5). Liking or wanting something or the opposite, not liking or not wanting something, were prominent anchors in how preschool children determined how they or others were likely to feel. Such a goal orientation allows the young child to develop expectations for emotional experience and beliefs about "the right way" to feel. Socializing agents, whether they are parents, peers, or the media, influence what is liked or not liked and thus affect children's beliefs about how to feel when they do or do not get what they want. Stein and Trabasso's work also fits well with the social constructivist position described in the first chapter: As children's cognitive capabilities become more complex, they are able to construct a more sophisticated understanding of expectations for emotional experience, in themselves as well as in others.

Developmental Models

To account for children's progressive acquisition of this mental mediation of emotional experience, Harris and Olthof (1982) in an early theoretical paper suggested three developmental models, which are thought to operate integratively. The first was the *solipsistic model*, which proposed that children observe that their own emotional responses are more reliably identified by examining their own mental state than by relying on any particular situation they may be in. To illustrate, by school entry a child normally knows that children are usually happy at their own birthday celebrations. However, it can occur that children also experience a disappointment in the course of a birthday party and are no longer happy in that situation (e.g., they did not get what they wanted or their divorced father/mother did not show up as the child had hoped). Such children report that they are unhappy, despite it being their birthday celebration; that is, such children's mental states are more reliable for determining how they feel than looking to the customary situational elicitor for ascertaining what they feel.

What goes hand in hand with this solipsistic model is the idea that children become aware of their own mental state as consciousness. Harris (1995) suggested that this ability to represent consciousness also has a developmental trajectory which influences how children come to think about their own feelings. His research and theorizing led me to propose the following metaphors: The young preschooler tends to think of consciousness like a faucet; it can be turned on and off. The child of age 5 to 6 thinks of consciousness as a bit like a wild river; it is an uncontrollable flow. Finally, by about age 8 or 9, children think of consciousness as a managed water course: One can dike it, dam it, build a bridge over it, or turn away and not look at it. Applying my metaphors to how children think about their own feelings, 3- to 4-year-olds might view their emotions as coming and going, one at a time. Five- to 6-year-olds might say that they cannot control or change their feelings once they experience them, that is, they could not direct their appraisal at a different feature of the emotion-laden situation and thus modify their emotional response. However, 8- to 9-year-olds would believe that they could redirect their conscious attention to something else and thus alter how they were feeling.

The second model proposed by Harris and Olthof (1982) was a *behavioral* one, which emphasized that children draw their data for determining where emotions come from by observing others rather than themselves. Children undoubtedly notice that certain situations and people's reactions to them have some degree of correspondence. However, as they mature, children may also observe that not all people react the same way to a given situation and that a given reaction can occur in a seemingly noneliciting situation. The child might then come to attribute the emotional reaction to an internal mental state that a person has rather than to an external situation. A common example is found in children's comparison of food preferences: My daughter happens to love tempura-batter-fried octopus rings, but when she has told other children that she likes to eat octopus, she is immediately greeted with horrible retching noises. (She still likes octopus.)

The third developmental model was the *sociocentric model,* which suggested that the verbal community was the impetus for children to increasingly orient themselves to a more mentalistic view of emotional experience. The child's linguistic community presumably can direct the child's attention to the covert, internal aspects of emotional experience in the absence of immediate situational and/or behavioral contexts. As a result of this verbal "instruction," the child acquires the belief that emotions have both their source in and can be modified by the self's cognitive constructions (evaluations, beliefs, reinterpretations, intentional distractions, etc.). Several investigators have studied preschool children's exposure to and involvement in conversations about emotional experiences; the general result has been that given the redundant cues provided by both verbal and nonverbal emotional communication, young children tacitly acquire a great many "rules" by which emotions are linked to eliciting circumstances and coordinated with social transactions (e.g., Beeghly, Bretherton, & Mervis, 1986; Brown & Dunn, 1991; Dunn et al., 1991). I return to this topic in Chapter 6. In summary, these three developmental models operate in mutually influencing ways and allow us to look at how children's cognitive development interfaces with context. That interface yields the "tools" with which children engage with others in emotion-laden interaction, which in turn further expands children's emotional, social, and cognitive development.

CONCLUSION

The socialization of children's emotions is obviously intertwined with their history of relationships within the family, with the contexts to which they have been exposed, and with the kinds of peers with whom they have associated. The culture (or subculture) also influences profoundly how children's emotional experience is socialized, as does their developmental level. Where does this leave emotional competence? Given a healthy central nervous system and normal cognitive development, it seems fairly likely that favorable family, community, peer, and subcultural contexts foster the individual's likelihood of acquiring emotional competence. However, can one be exposed to an inadequate family, a harsh community, uncharitable peers, and rigidly held subcultural beliefs and still become emotionally competent? Conceivably yes, according to Lewis (1997) if the individual is subsequently immersed in an entirely different sort of social structure that facilitates emotional competence. Such radical contextual shifts do occur, but too many children from harsh family and community circumstances do not escape the limited range of personal choices and opportunities that might otherwise have helped them to alter their social structure in a profound way. Indeed, Lewis argues that rather than thinking in terms of "*cures,*" we should develop social policies that *care* and appropriately provide ongoing support to families and communities so that their children will thrive and become emotionally competent.

This emphasis on context is important to bear in mind as I move on in the subsequent chapters to discuss the different skills of emotional competence. Each skill develops in an interactive fashion; for example, learning about others' emotions is interfaced with the developing awareness of one's own emotional experience, and both are integrated with a growing verbal and conceptual knowledge about emotion as mediated by the individual's culture. Thus, separating out the different skills of emotional competence is an analytical strategy that lends itself to the following separate chapters for each skill, but we must keep in mind that these emotional competence skills are emerging, developing, and generalizing within an integrated and dynamic system, namely, the individual-within-context.

In the subsequent chapters I present what I see as the most significant skills and abilities for developing emotional competence. I include vignettes and case studies as well as selected relevant research. For those who desire more detailed sources, I include references to recent reviews. Given the current chapter's focus on socialization, I also address the cultural context surrounding the development of emotional competence as well as the tremendous variation among individuals in how these different facets of emotional competence are expressed.

✒ Chapter 4

Skill 1: Awareness of One's Own Emotions

*A*wareness *of one's emotional state, including the possibility that one is experiencing multiple emotions, and at even more mature levels, awareness that one might also not be consciously aware of one's feelings due to unconscious dynamics or selective inattention.*

This first skill of emotional competence is perhaps the most basic: Recognition of what we are feeling means that we acknowledge the significance of some event, which may also be an interpersonal transaction. Our emotional response provides us with crucial information: The event is rendered *meaningful* by our emotional reaction. We learn that our feelings have a distinctive pattern to them, which includes emotional state, expression, associated causes (elicitors), and our subjective experience of emotion. As we mature, we recognize that not only can we be aware of emotion *A* (e.g., sadness) but we can also feel emotion *B* (e.g., guilt) and even emotion *C* (e.g., anxiety) about the very same situation or about the same person. Thus, we become aware of the possibility of multiple emotions experienced virtually simultaneously or in rapid oscillation as we consider different aspects of the person or situation.

I elaborate further on the topic of multiple emotions later in this chapter. However, I want to note at the outset that the complex appraisals made by an individual about a multifaceted situation or relationship when more than one emotion is experienced are integral to mature emotional competence. Recognition of the different features that often interact with one another in a social situation allows for a richly faceted appraisal, and one's emotional experience is similarly more complex. An example is captured in English when we use the term "bittersweet" to describe a relationship. If one's memory of the relationship were strictly "bitter" or strictly "sweet," it would be a less elaborated and less complex memory about the relationship. By reflecting on a "bittersweet" relationship in the past, we summon up more nuance, subtlety, and texture in our reminiscence; we might even reexperience haunting mixed feelings.

We may also become aware that at times we are "unaware" of some of our feelings. This is most evident when we reflect on some really ridiculous thing we did and wonder what in the world was going on inside us that we acted this way. We may then infer that we must have been feeling X which influenced us to behave in this fashion, even though we may be reluctant to admit to ourselves our petty emotional reaction. Passive–aggressive behavior, fueled by less than aware angry feelings, is a commonly encountered example. Perhaps the feeling of anger was subverted because it was too risky to acknowledge or express, and only a sense of simmering discontent remained. On reflection, we might become aware of our *resentment* and realize that it was this feeling that prompted passive–aggressive behavior. Mature emotional competence lies in recognizing that at times we may need to look at the possibility that we can be unaware of or are selectively *in*attentive to some of our feelings. By acknowledging this possibility, we open up the range of cues we can use to resolve a problematic relationship or vexing situation.

Before I return to the topics of multiple feelings and awareness that we may be unaware of our feelings, I first want to present some material on how we acquire awareness of our own emotional states. There is much that is speculative here with regard to preverbal infants' awareness of their emotions, and the issue of how we know what we feel raises questions once again about the role of the self in emotional experience.

DEVELOPMENT OF EMOTIONAL AWARENESS

The Self in Emotional Awareness

For awareness of our emotional response to occur, we must have developed a sense of self: The young child must be able to cognitively apprehend that it is he or she who is feeling something. As mentioned in

Chapter 2, a young infant (perhaps under 6 months) would *have* emotional states but does not experience a conscious *awareness* of the emotional state. Lewis and Brooks (1978) stipulate that the infant must first develop a subjective self (self as agent) and then a self as object to have the capacity to know that he or she is experiencing an emotion. I do not consider young infants' emotional contagion responses as instances of awareness of their own emotional response. When 10-week-old infants appear to respond differentially to their mothers' emotion-laden facial expressions with facial expressions of their own (e.g., Haviland & Lelwicka, 1987), they may indeed be responding emotionally, but they lack the necessary cognitive representational skills for knowing that it is *they* who feel something distinctive and in relationship to something salient in their environment. However, I think that there may be some sort of "proto-awareness" by the middle of the first year, for we find that preverbal infants demonstrate something like a pragmatic awareness of their emotional experience when they show reliable intentional behaviors to sustain or reinitiate events (many of which are social transactions) that produce pleasurable emotional states. They also appear to be able to distinguish between positive and negative vocal tones with appropriate matching expressive responses, even when the words spoken were not from the same language as their caregivers and no other emotional–expressive information was available except the voice (Fernald, 1993). Thus, they can discriminate hedonic tone fairly well in others by the middle of the second year, but it is not clear that infants *know* what it is they are feeling, even though they are able to produce appropriate expressive signals in response to someone's positive or negative expressive behavior.

Lewis (1993b) has also argued that for us to have awareness of our emotional experience, we would need to know that the bodily *state* changes we feel when we are emotional are uniquely different from other bodily changes we might experience (e.g., the butterflies-in-our-stomach accompanying fear is not the same as hunger). A second cognitive process is the evaluation of context; for example, did something occur that was scary as opposed to anger provoking. For both of these processes, some degree of exposure and learning is necessary, as is the development of *agency*, namely, who or what is the cause of some event or change that is internal to oneself (see also Lewis, 1991). Knowing that the cause of the change in our bodily state was our own emotional response leads to acknowledgment of our emotional experience, which is the most basic of the emotional competency skills.

Social Referencing

Our inference of infants' emerging awareness of their own emotional responses is on firmer ground when we observe infants evaluate events and persons present prior to their expressing a distinct emotion. Social referencing is a good example of this, and infants as young as 10 to 12 months demonstrate such strategies as looking to their parents' emotional–expressive behavior when faced with a stranger (or some other emotionally ambiguous situation) as a guide to their own emotional reaction (Feinman & Lewis, 1983; Mumme, Fernald, & Herrera, 1996; Sorce et al., 1985). In her review of social referencing and emotion regulation, Walden (1991) suggests that infants of about 1 year of age may already have some functional notion of what is an appropriate response to a situation, because they are less likely to use their mothers' *in*appropriate emotional expressions as a guide for their behavior when her reaction does not fit the eliciting situation (see also Feinman, 1985). Sorce et al. (1985) examined this pragmatic awareness of feeling states by having the babies' mothers look sad (as opposed to the more fitting expression of anxiousness or fear) as the infants approached a drop-off (the "visual cliff"). Infants were more likely to look puzzled at their "sad" mothers. In a more recent review of social referencing with atypical children, Walden and Knieps (1996) found that for developmentally delayed infants, mothers tended to use social signals to "push" their infants to respond; they appeared to try to get their delayed infant to respond to a stimulus by sending out many expressive gestures, even though these infants' own social–emotional signals were assessed as difficult to understand. Thus, individual differences affect how toddlers acquire a practical awareness of their own emotional state, and it is also likely that different research methods, adapted to the unique features of different groups of atypical children, would yield more information as to those processes by which we all acquire awareness of emotional experience.

By age 2, many normally developing toddlers are able to verbalize simple feeling states and can describe anticipatory affective states such as liking or wanting something, and as "terrible 2's," they are especially adept at articulating what they do *not* want to do. Walden notes that by this time they often "negotiate" with their parents around "what to feel" in different situations and may choose not to use their parents' emotional expression as a guide to how to behave in some situation. (Try taking a toddler to a restaurant and you will see this "negotiation" in action. Parents' stern or wary looks go completely unheeded as their 2-year-old insists on getting out of her chair and walking around the restaurant or playing with her food.) On the other hand, in a genuinely new and uncertainty-filled situation, a 2-year-old still looks to others to see how to make sense of the situation emotionally. These "others" need not be the child's immediate caregivers, for by this age siblings and peers increasingly become a source of social–emotional information. To illustrate, I was with a 22-month old niece who had never been in an elevator before. Going up was OK, but during the descent she began to look a bit wary; at that point two older children started jumping up and down gleefully in the elevator trying to be "in the air" when the elevator landed. The little girl started jumping too and a smile appeared on her face as well to match the older children's emotional response to the elevator descent. I did find out from the child's mother that when they were in the same elevator about 3 weeks later, her daughter started to jump up and down, looking quite pleased with herself.

Understanding Contexts and Emotional Response

As children mature, they report a greater variety of emotions. Their exposure to different contexts for experiencing emotions broadens their conceptual awareness of the nature of emotion-eliciting events as well as their personal emotional response to such events (Gordon, 1989). Simultaneously, their linguistic skills are increasing, and thus it is not surprising that they report more emotionally varied experiences. A personal vignette illustrates this growth in awareness of personal emotional response when a child is exposed to novel contexts and is elaborating his linguistic skills:

> Four-year-old Andrew had never gone camping before; however, he was a child who had considerable exposure to adult interaction and had a very impressive vocabulary for his age. Among his favorite words for describing his emotional appraisal of negative events, objects, and people were "grotesque" and "scrofulous." The outhouses we encountered during our camping in national forests were indeed properly described as scrofulous, but when he explored the blackened cavern burned into the roots and base of a *Sequoia gigantea* and called it grotesque (which was not altogether inaccurate), I heard him correct himself, "No, it's not that, it's magnificent!" He then commanded his mom to take his picture in front of the "magnificent" tree.

Young Andrew expanded both his knowledge base about emotion-eliciting contexts (including outhouses and old trees) and how to label his personal response more appropriately (changing his verbal declaration to "magnificent" to describe the old sequoia). Thus, children embed their awareness of their emotional state within contexts, that is, the circumstances in which their feelings arise.

Harris (1995) has focused on the impact of children's cognitive skills on their awareness of emotions relative to contexts. He makes an important distinction in children's understanding of *intentional targets* of emotions versus *causes* of emotions. He contends that children primarily anchor their emotions in appraisal of the object, person, or event at which the emotion is directed (e.g., mad *at you,* scared *of spiders,* happy *about going to the amusement park*) as opposed to the causal or precipitating event (e.g., a squabble between siblings that leads to anger, finding a big spider in one's bed, and being told that the family is going to "Fun World"). Wellman, Harris, Banerjee, and Sinclair (1995) confirmed this finding for 2-, 3-, and 4-year-old children; however, they also found that this sort of construal did not hold for how children viewed physical pain. Children understood pain in terms of the eliciting or causal event rather than pain being directed at an intentional target (e.g., children would feel pain upon being pricked by a pin, but they would typically not feel pain *about* pins, although they could develop a generalized phobic reaction to pins or needles, in which case they have a *fear of* pins because pins can prick and cause pain).

The significance of this idea of intentional targets of emotions as a contextual anchor for children's understanding of their subjective emotional experience is important theoretically, for it points to the transactional encounter between person and environment; that is, children construe their emotions as directed at something. Functionalist and relational views of emotion as described in the first chapter emphasize this goal-oriented nature of emotion as opposed to other theoretical positions which emphasize the biological causes of emotions (e.g., Ekman, 1984). As I elaborate on in Chapter 9, children also tend to view their experience of negative emotions as tacitly tied to how to cope with aversive emotions and distressing circumstances (e.g., Saarni, 1997). When we are aware of our emotional response, we do not have a segmented linear emotional experience that unfolds in time as first an appraisal of a cause, then a physiological response, then some directly linked facial expression, and finally an "aha!" reaction of "I must be feeling *X.*" Instead, we more often see a child smack another child with a shovel in the sandbox with no particularly distinctive expression on her face (she might even look mildly interested), but upon being scolded, she says Sam squashed her sand castle, and she was *mad at him,* so she hit him. She may be using her feelings as cues for why she behaved aggressively, or just as plausibly, she used her aggressive behavior as a cue for how she might have been feeling. In any event, on being socially confronted, she is faced with having to *explain* the circumstances, and then she competently (and prudently) produces a self-justifying sequence of causal provocation, emotional response, and targeted reciprocal action.

To sum up, we construct a meaningful sequence for our emotional experience in terms of how we become aware of our feelings and subsequently act on them, and it is this meaningful construction that also allows for emotional communication with others. The fact that the sequence is "meaningful" is based on the child's learning her subculture's folk theories regarding what emotions are and what to do when one feels them. For example, consider a 4-year-old who comes home after nursery school and announces to his father, "Today I had six mads." A likely response from his father would be, "You had what?" The boy's statement is not culturally meaningful, because Western models of emotion assume that emotions are mass nouns and not count nouns (D'Andrade, 1987). The father might then correct his son by saying, "Oh, you mean you felt mad six times today." He might go on to query his son as to what was he mad about or whom he was mad at. These everyday sorts of emotion-related communicative exchanges further anchor for the young child that his or her feelings are part of a whole scenario of events, behaviors, and other people. In short, emotional experience is contextualized. Deconstructing this contextualization might be analytically interesting, but it would no longer be descriptive of how people make sense of their subjective emotional experience.

Wishes and Beliefs in Understanding Emotions

Research by Wellman and associates (Wellman & Wooley, 1990; Wellman et al., 1995) found that children as young as 2 to 3 years old could understand that emotion was connected with what they wanted or did not want. The notorious "terrible 2's" mentioned earlier also provide ample anecdotal evidence that young children can readily threaten an emotional reaction to a family member if they do not get their way. Liking, not liking, wanting, and not wanting are pivotal goal-related factors in young children's appraisals, which they are readily able to communicate to others (Stein & Trabasso, 1989).

At slightly older ages (4 to 5 years old), children begin more reliably to show in their understanding of emotional experience that beliefs and expectations are also important in predicting what they will feel. The considerable literature on the development of mind is rich with examples of preschoolers competently predicting that someone will be surprised, upset, saddened, angered, and so forth if an expectation for how an event "should" turn out does not take place (e.g., Harris, Johnson, Hutton, Cooke, & Andrews, 1991; Wellman & Banerjee, 1991). By middle childhood, children readily comprehend that their mental state (appraisal) is central to what they feel about a given target and that others with different views may experience different feelings about the same target (e.g., Harris, 1989). Interestingly, our informal conversations still reflect the concrete and seemingly external "causal" features found in younger children's thinking (e.g., "You make me mad!"). Upon probing, older children are able to say, "It was what she did that I really hated, and that was why I got mad at her." The preschooler, when asked why she got so mad at Sam, emphasizes Sam's destruction of her sand castle, not her thoughts about wanting her castle to endure forever in the sandbox and that Sam's behavior was terribly destructive to her goal of castle preservation.

Access to a rich vocabulary may also facilitate children's understanding of their emotional experience. Carroll and Steward (1984) examined two age groups, 4- to 5-year-olds and 8- to 9-year-olds, for their understanding of their own emotions relative to their verbal IQ (as measured by the Peabody Picture Vocabulary Test) and performance on several Piagetian tasks. They probed children's understanding of their emotional experience by asking them several questions: "Show me how you feel happy (or sad, mad, and afraid)." "How do *you* know when you are feeling happy" (or sad, mad, afraid)? "How would *I* [the interviewer] know that you were feeling happy" (or sad, mad, afraid)? Their results indicated that older children were more likely to describe their emotions as internally based (e.g., "I feel hurt inside, and then I get sad about it") whereas the younger children described their emotional experience in concrete situational terms (e.g., "I got mad at my brother when he turned the TV off and I was watching Ninja Turtles"). Interestingly, among the younger children, if they obtained higher IQ scores (despite demonstrating preopertional thinking on the Piagetian classification and conservation tasks), they were more likely to describe their emotional experience in ways that were more sophisticated and similar to the older children. Thus, access to a more elaborate verbal system permits *communication* of what is going on emotionally inside oneself and facilitates others' responding to those verbal cues. Carroll and Steward concluded their study by mentioning one 4-year-old girl who was the daughter of a psychotherapist. This child was apparently unusually mature for her age in understanding her own emotional experience in that she was able to verbalize how another would know what she was feeling. Carroll and Steward (1984) surmise that she had been exposed to a more enriched environment wherein emotional communication and sensitivity were enhanced beyond the more ordinary home environments of most preschoolers.

Besides developing (and even cultivating) an awareness of *what* we are feeling, we also acquire facility with *dimensions* of emotional experience. Degree of intensity and length of time an emotional episode lasts are two dimensions that are critical to coping with distressing emotions. I turn to this topic next.

Awareness of Emotional Intensity and Duration of Emotion

Regrettably few studies have directly examined children's awareness of emotional intensity or their evaluation of how long emotions last. Consider the following cases:

> Jorge, age 11, arrived home with a chipped front tooth and a bloodied nose. He had been in a fight after school with Charlie, a notorious bully. Jorge's father asked him, "You know what kind of a kid Charlie is, what in the world made you think you should fight it out with him!?" Jorge responded, "Dad, he just kept coming after me in front of the other kids, saying how stupid I was, how stupid our family was, and when he said he was going to hurt Selinda [Jorge's 8-year-old sister] and that I was too stupid to even notice it, then I was madder than ever and I knew I was so mad that I would be stronger than ever. And I was!"

> Teresa, age 10, tossed fitfully in her bed. It was hard to go to sleep not knowing what was going to happen to her family now that her parents were getting divorced. She knew they had been fighting a lot together; maybe if they had sort of like an intermission from one another and didn't see each other so much, they'd get less angry and start to feel better again. Teresa wondered how long that would take, and she guessed for grownups who'd been very mad at each other, it would probably take a month. She and her friend Maria had a real bad fight, and it took a week before they made up. But she figured her parents had been fighting more than she and Maria had, so it would probably take more time for them to get over it.

In the first vignette Jorge rated his anger along the "yardstick" of strength. He recognized the intensity of his anger, and in his description of his anger to his father he construed his anger as having energized or enhanced his physical strength. We can also infer that he believed the intensity of his anger was fueled by the onslaught of insult and provocation perpetrated by the bully, Charlie. In the second vignette, Maria estimated the duration of angry feelings between her parents and contrasted that with the time needed to overcome the negative feelings between herself and her friend after a quarrel. She assumed that a higher frequency of quarreling and a greater intensity of negative feeling require more time for dissipating the aversive emotion associated with marital conflict.

Both Jorge and Maria indicated in their understanding of emotional experience our culture's beliefs that emotions can be viewed as varying along an intensity continuum (or dimension) and a duration continuum. Maria's understanding suggested that she saw the duration of emotion as linked to frequency and intensity of its occurrence in a relationship. Another variable linked to intensity of emotion is its felt sense of controllability. In our culture, more intense emotions are assumed to be less often under one's control; that is, it is assumed that it is harder to suppress the expression of very intense feelings and more difficult to distract oneself from the aversiveness of very intense negative emotions. I do not discuss this aspect of emotional intensity here further but return to it in Chapter 9.

Later in this chapter, when I return to the topic of multiple emotions, I discuss one of the few empirical studies on children's awareness of emotion intensity and duration (Wintre & Vallance, 1994). Relevant here as well is research undertaken by Harris, Guz, Lipian, and Man-Shu (1985). The latter investigators examined the dissipation of emotion in children ages 6 to 11 years. Using stories featuring both positive and negative emotion-eliciting situations (e.g., getting a much-wanted pet dog vs. the dog's dying), they interviewed the children using open-ended questions. All the children believed that immediately after the incident, emotion would be intense and then gradually would diminish in intensity. They made the same attribution about their own emotional experience. Interestingly (and this also presages Chapter 6), the children also believed that if they did not think about the emotion-eliciting situation (especially a negative one), they would more readily feel *less* emotional. Harris, Guz, and Lipian (1985) interpreted children's beliefs about the waning of emotional intensity over time as associated with decreased thinking about the precipitating event as indicative of children's capacity to reflect on their own subjective experience. In other words, they learn this relationship between duration and intensity of emotion by looking inward at their own mental processes, which is essentially the solipsistic model described in the preceding chapter and proposed by Harris and Olthof (1982).

Children's Views of Emotion in Themselves versus in Others

A few studies have compared how children make sense of emotions in themselves versus in others (e.g., Karniol & Koren, 1987; Saarni, 1989a; Strayer, 1986). I comment on two of them here, for they suggest that there may be some degree of a positivity bias in children's assumptions of how they think they personally would feel. The qualification to these studies is that they use interview strategies and thus ask children to verbalize their anticipation of how they would feel if in the same situation as some story protagonist or to describe how they emotionally responded in the past in some situation similar to a story protagonist. In other words, these studies may be eliciting more children's knowledge of our culture's folk theory of emotion rather than their own spontaneously occurring emotional experience. The assumption here, of course, is that one is socialized according to the general tenets of one's cultural folk theory of emotion, and that as a consequence, one's spontaneous emotional behavior presumably has some congruence with the cultural consensus of what would be the predicted emotional experience for a given situation. In fact, children as young as 4 years of age have been found to understand many connections between situational causes and emotions in a fashion similar to adults (e.g., Barden, Zelko, Duncan, & Masters, 1980; Strayer, 1986), but clearly there are many subtleties that still elude them at this young age.

One study that compared children's expectations for how they would feel in contrast to what other children would feel was undertaken by Karniol and Koren (1987). They presented a series of brief scenarios to 6-year-olds and asked the children what they would feel if this happened to them or how the boy/girl in the scenario would feel. They were also asked to justify their responses. Karniol and Koren's data suggest (at least in this age group) that children make different inferences about their own anticipated emotional experience than they do about others'. Specifically, the children predicted more negative feelings for others but *not* for themselves. They also spontaneously gave more coping suggestions for how to transform the negative situations into more positive contexts when they were asked to infer how they would personally feel. Finally, when evaluating their own emotional response as opposed to others' emotional reactions, the children were more focused on the consequences of the story situation for themselves. It is interesting here theoretically that children do not appear to be simply "reading off" some sort of prototypical script for how they are likely to feel in some situation. If they did, there would be little difference between what children thought they themselves would feel versus what others would feel. Karniol and Koren argue that children use unique information available about the self as a way to flesh out their inferences for how they would feel in some situation. For predicting vague others' reactions, they probably do use more common social stereotypical scripts, but for themselves some element of anticipated coping with the emotion-eliciting event is built into their inferred reaction.

The expectation that one's own feelings would be more positive in tone than what others experience has parallels that appear in the literature on self-esteem (e.g., Harter, 1990; Taylor & Brown, 1988). Glasberg and Aboud (1982) also found that 5-year-olds were much less likely than 7-year-olds to describe themselves as sad. Thus, there may be a developmental transition here that speaks to how children can both conceptualize their own emotional experience and anticipate their ability to cope with distressing feelings (i.e., young children may not want to think about themselves in emotionally aversive situations as they fear they might begin to feel that way and subsequently anticipate feeling overwhelmed; see also Harter & Buddin, 1987).

The second study I briefly describe is one that I undertook with school-age children (Saarni, 1987, 1989a). I was interested in comparing adults' and school-age children's expectations about parental reactions to children's emotional–expressive behavior in situations that varied according to (1) whether expressing genuine emotion would contribute to *someone else* getting their feelings hurt or (2) whether the genuine emotional display would make the child more vulnerable and distressed. Examples of the former are expressing disgust toward Grandma's food being served at the table, staring at a physically scarred person, giggling at a funeral, and showing obvious disappointment upon receiving an undesirable gift. Examples of the latter are distress about getting an injection, sadness about having made a mistake during a solo performance, and fear about a bully's threats. These seven scenarios were used in interviews with children, and after answering several questions about the story protagonist, at the end of each story the children were asked what they personally would do if they were in the situation. Even though the children often described the story protagonists as concealing or somehow dissembling their genuine feelings to avoid making themselves even more vulnerable (e.g., "If she shows that she's scared of shots, then when she gets it, it'll hurt more"), for themselves they anticipated that they would indeed express their genuine feelings, either because they anticipated parental support for doing so or because they felt their feelings would be quite intense and therefore could not be dissembled. On the other hand, if they believed that expressing their real feelings would hurt the feelings of someone else, they anticipated that both their own as well as the story protagonists' emotional–expressive behavior would be managed to avoid that predicament (e.g., "Well, even if you don't like what your Grandpa got you for your birthday, you should try to smile and say thank you").

My data and Karniol and Koren's may be similar in that the children appear to scan the situations for how they would cope if they were in that situation. Then they respond with anticipated emotional reactions that already have embedded in them their expectations as to how they think they will be able to cope with the demands of the situation. Thus, if a child's real feelings give him a sense of fragility or vulnerability but his parents are nearby to comfort and support him, expressing his genuine feelings is acceptable, and effective coping lies in being with those who provide an "emotional safety net." Interestingly, other data collected with different methods and in another region of the country (Midwest) found a sex difference in children's expectations about whether they would reveal their negative feelings to their parents. Fuchs and Thelen (1988) found that boys were less likely than girls to communicate *sadness* (a vulnerability-inducing emotion) to their parents, but, if they were to do so, they would be more likely to reveal their sadness to their mothers. Such boys apparently would minimize or otherwise modify the expression of their vulnerable emotions—such as sadness—with their fathers; adopting an emotional front or dissembling the expression of one's feelings then becomes the more adaptive coping response for such school-age boys if they do not anticipate a supportive interpersonal context for the display of genuine emotions.

AWARENESS OF MULTIPLE EMOTIONS

Awareness of experiencing multiple emotions or conflicting emotions (as in ambivalence) is a development that may appear as early as 5 to 6 years of age (Stein & Trabasso, 1989; Wintre & Vallance, 1994) or not until late childhood (Donaldson & Westerman, 1986; Harter & Whitesell, 1989), depending on one's criteria and methods of eliciting such understanding from children. Stein and Trabasso interviewed 5- to 6-year-olds, using open-ended questions, and determined that at this age children could readily describe situations in which they felt good *and* bad or people whom they liked *and* did not like. For example, the children described feeling badly when a goal was blocked ("My mom said I couldn't go outside and play . . . ") but feeling good when an alternative goal presented itself instead ("But my brother said he was going to give me a present") (p. 64). Family conflicts were cited about 80% of the time when the children both disliked and liked a person ("I fight with my brother all the time, . . . but I still love him") (p. 65). However, Stein and Trabasso caution that this does not mean that children *simultaneously* feel conflicting feelings: Rather they first focus on one situation to which they attach values and attributions, respond emotionally to its impact on them (e.g., "I don't like her, because she took my Halloween candy"), and then focus on another situation with its accompanying values and attributions and respond emotionally to its impact (e.g., "But I like her when she plays with me"). Thus, ambivalence for Stein and Trabasso (1989) is a *sequential* process with different appraisals attached to the different or polarized emotional responses, and they suggest that this process is the same for adults, just much more rapid.

Studies conducted by Harter and Whitesell (1989) and Donaldson and Westerman (1986) are similarly concerned with children's cognitive construction of their own emotional experience, particularly when multiple emotions are involved. Harter and Whitesell (1989) focus on the cognitive developmental prerequisites for understanding the simultaneity of multiple emotions embedded in a situation or relationship (see also Harter, 1986a). Not until the child has access to "representational mappings," that is, the ability to consider *at the same time* one set of ideas that is at odds with another set of ideas, would the child be able to integrate opposite valence emotions (happy and sad) about *different targets* that co-occur in a *situation* (e.g., "I'm glad I get to live with my dad, but I'm sad about not being able to live with mom too"). An older child (now probably a preadolescent) can integrate simultaneously opposite valence emotions about the *same target* (e.g., "I love my dad, even though I'm mad at him right now for not following through on his promise"). Harter and Whitesell acknowledge that what may occur as we cognitively integrate contrasting emotions about the same target is a rapid oscillation between the multiple emotion-eliciting aspects of a relationship or situation.

Harter and Buddin (1987) also point out that it is not known whether children might experience simultaneously two (or even more) emotions but can only cognitively construct an explanation about the experience that focuses on one emotion. They also note that children may in some situations experience only one overwhelming emotion (e.g., fear), but as they seek to cope with the scary situation or have to communicate about it to someone else, they begin to cognitively construct a more complex system of appraisals about the emotion-eliciting situation or relationship.

Donaldson and Westerman (1986) used methodology that allowed them to probe whether children recognized that contradictory feelings toward the same target could influence or interact with one another. Specifically, they used two stories, one about a child who lost her kitten and then is given another one and a second one about a much-loved puppy who destroys her owner's favorite toy. Their interview strategy included many open-ended questions which sought to determine how the children made sense of contradictory feelings and whether they experienced ambivalence toward the kitten or puppy. They found that not until age 10 to 11 did children understand that contradictory feelings could interact with one another such that negative feelings might be ameliorated by more positive ones and vice versa. Older children were also more likely to explain how current feelings change as partially dependent on memories of other feelings (e.g., a child can dispel angry feelings toward his "naughty" puppy by remembering how much he really loves his pet and then forgiving the young dog for its misbehavior). Another common example of ambivalence occurs when children of divorced parents admit to reluctance about seeing the noncustodial parent: On the one hand they reexperience their memory of painful loss and anger at their parents for breaking up the family, but on the other hand they experience their love for the absent parent as well. They may end up coping with the emotional conflict by withdrawing from it and may be quite aware of doing so. From an 11-year-old: "Well, I'd just get upset seeing him, so it was easier just not to, but then I feel guilty sometimes that I don't want to visit him."

Wintre and Vallance (1994) introduced a methodological variation whereby school-age children rated the intensities of multiple emotional responses for a given situation. For example, relative to being home alone, children could say they might feel *a little bit happy* about being home alone but also *sort of sad* and also *very much scared.* They also had the children answer only with regard to predicting their own feelings and not a hypothetical protagonist, and for each emotion-eliciting scenario the children were systematically asked how much they would feel angry, sad, happy, scared, or loving by placing a mark on an "emotion intensity thermometer." Because of the format for eliciting their responses, the children did not need to verbally elaborate or justify their expectations for multiple emotions and their respective intensities, and thus their comprehension appeared more sophisticated than that of children in the Harter and Buddin study. Their results showed that by age 8, children could coordinate from two to four separate emotions for the same situation and combine these different emotions with variable intensities (as in the example about being home alone). They also found that girls exceeded boys in being able to combine more separate emotions, which is consistent with other research that girls acquire greater skill at talking about their feelings than boys (e.g., Golombok & Fivush, 1994).

Finally, Harris (1995), in a review of children's awareness of their own emotions, theorized that younger children (preschoolers to about age 7) scan a situation for its emotional meaning and when they find one, stop scanning. Older children do not exhaust the search, so to speak, for further possible appraisals that might yield multiple emotional responses. Harris and his associates (Peng, Johnson, Pollack, Glasspool, & Harris, 1992) undertook a training study to try to teach children ages 4 to 7 how to scan an emotion-eliciting situation for multiple emotions. They found that in comparison with a control group, the 6- to 7-year-olds acquired the cognitive scanning "persistence" needed to produce multiple emotion appraisals, whereas the training for the 4- to 5-year-olds did not yield any increase in their scanning skills.

The final feature of this skill of emotional competence is recognition of the possibility that we are not always aware of our feelings due to unconscious dynamics or due to selective inattention. I turn to this topic next.

AWARENESS THAT ONE MAY NOT BE AWARE OF ONE'S EMOTIONS

No empirical study of children systematically examines whether they know that the self may not be consciously aware of some emotion—except for the earlier cited work by Harris, Guz, Lipian, and Man-Shu (1985) on children's beliefs that emotion intensity wanes as one thinks about other things. The typical defense mechanisms of childhood, namely, regression, repression, and denial, all presumably function to defend the self against awareness of painful negative feelings, but clinicians using such constructs do not usually encounter young children who spontaneously announce that they are aware that they were not admitting to themselves their real feelings. What is more likely to appear to the clinician is that the young child displaces the painful negative feeling onto something or someone else. In play therapy the puppets or human figures throw one another out the dollhouse window and otherwise abuse one another. The clay figures get regularly smashed to bits, and the watercolors get splashed and slathered on top of one another on the paper—hiding, changing, or elaborating what first was drawn there. Clinical anecdote also suggests that acting-out behavior in children and adolescents may "mask" a depression; for example, the loss of something terribly important, such as trust in a parent or belief that one is both loved and lovable, may underlie the obnoxious aggressive behavior of an externalizing youngster.

A vague malaise may be consciously evident and experienced by an individual, but it may be hard to pinpoint more specific emotions. Zeroing in on what those specific feelings are also means evaluating the emotion-eliciting events and one's own involvement in bringing those emotion-laden situations about. Doing the latter may result in consequences that in turn are likely to evoke still more negative emotions.

Think of the young teen who finds herself pregnant: She feels despondent, unsure, and worried. She may be aware that she would be wise to make a decision before the birth as to whether or not to keep the baby and then to plan accordingly. However, she pushes from awareness her neediness for affection and feelings of shame and avoids any decision making—maybe her boyfriend will come around and marry her after all, maybe welfare will take care of her and her baby, and maybe even her father will let her live with him, especially after he sees how cute the baby is. She avoids confronting the full range of her feelings about the predicament she is in, including her anger at and despair about rejection from her boyfriend. Then it becomes too late to opt for an abortion, and passively she awaits the birth.

Social workers and counselors who work with foster families and families who adopt older children are likely to encounter children whose flat expressive behavior and somewhat depressed mood quality suggest malaise. Such children may be coping with their sad circumstances by pushing from awareness their feelings of rejection and abandonment on the part of their parents and/or other preceding foster parents (for excellent discussions of attachment disorders, see Bretherton, 1995; James, 1994). An illustrative case from one of my counseling students concretizes these sad circumstances:

> Eight-year-old Andy had been referred to the counseling intern, Toni, because he was apparently falling asleep in class a lot, but when asked about what time he went to bed, he had said about 8 or 9 o'clock, which was confirmed by a phone call to his mother.
>
> During the first meeting together, Toni asked Andy whether he would like to draw a picture of his family. Andy announced, "I have no family; I'm adopted and my parents are getting divorced," but he proceeded to draw a picture. His picture had a sun in one corner, a house of sorts, and a brown blob that he said was his dog. Toni said, "This looks like a nice picture, but where are you?" In response, Andy drew a stick figure without any facial features. Toni asked, "Is there anyone else with you and your dog?" Andy replied, "No, I'm by myself." Toni probed further, "How do you feel being by yourself in this picture?" Andy picked up the blue crayon and obliterated the human stick figure. He then turned to Toni, and said matter-of-factly, "I might as well be dead or never born at all." Toni was concerned: His expression was neutral, but the weight of his words did not match his demeanor; he might as well have been describing his homework.

Andy was a child overwhelmed by the enormity of his adoptive parents' pending divorce. His vulnerability was obvious, yet his way of dealing with the upcoming divorce was to suppress his feelings by tuning out (sleeping) and splitting off his emotion from his thoughts (the matter-of-fact announcement that he might as well be dead). When Toni inquired, Andy's parents said that they thought he was dealing with the situation quite well; they said he was compliant and not causing any trouble during their difficult separation. In fact, Andy would have probably been better off had he caused some disturbance to the parents and communicated to them his distress and great fear about the upcoming family disruption. He desperately needed their reassurance and support to cope with the divorce, yet they naively did not adequately or explicitly enough provide it to him, because his "emotional signals" were ambiguous and flat in quality.

In Chapter 9 I return to the topic of coping with aversive emotions and circumstances. However, for the purpose of this chapter on awareness of emotions and the realization that we may at times have been unaware of our feelings, I wish to stress that avoidance or suppression of one's feelings is likely to impoverish one's ability to cope and solve problems. In some situations in which we have little control over the circumstances, it may make sense to blunt or limit how much information we take in, and at times it may be appropriate to ignore our emotional state (as in urgent situations or emergencies). But most interpersonal situations or chronic social transactions are best dealt with by being aware of our feelings. When we are aware of our emotions, we can seek support (as was needed in Andy's case) or use our feelings as cues to help make a difficult decision vis-à-vis a relationship. Certainly in terms of a felt sense of self-efficacy, awareness of how we feel generally facilitates effective problem solving. I think intrinsic to acknowledging how we feel and seeing it as part of a complex interaction of ourselves with others means that we are using our feelings as valid cues to a problem to be solved. As a result, we have more complete information for use in generating solutions to problems.

Other clinical examples of selective inattention to emotions, yet accompanied by an awareness that we are avoiding something, may occur in the precipitating anxiety that precedes bulimic excesses or drug abuse (e.g., Attie, Brooks-Gunn, & Petersen, 1990; Dryfoos, 1990; Holderness, Brooks-Gunn, & Warren, 1994). Socialization of emotional coping within the family likely contributes to the development of such emotion-avoidant patterns and the use of emotion-numbing coping methods such as chemical dependency. Indeed, we see occurring across generations addictive behaviors (Ackerman, 1983), as well as patterns of family violence that suggest selective emotion avoidance, which are also often accompanied by substance abuse (Saunders, Lynch, Grayson, & Linz, 1987).

INDIVIDUAL DIFFERENCES AND CULTURAL INFLUENCE

People obviously differ in their competence in various activities. Consider how individuals might differ in emotional competence: We could look at individual differences for each of the skills and components of emotional competence that are described in this volume and relate that to how such differences affect self-efficacy in emotion-eliciting interpersonal transactions—this being the overall definition of emotional competence used here. Thus, looking at individual differences just in this first skill of emotional competence (i.e., our awareness of our own emotional experience) means that we would want to examine how differences in awareness of emotional experience manifest themselves in self-efficacy in interpersonal transactions.

There is a growing body of research on the contribution of individual differences to differences in awareness of one's own emotional experience, apart from age differences and emotion vocabulary differences (see the research by Carroll and Steward, 1984, described earlier). Traditionally, developmentally oriented researchers have explored the influence of age differences and gender differences and to a much lesser extent, the influence of culture, family structure, and what I call *social maturity* (obviously relative to one's age group and cultural context). Under this general notion of "social maturity" I include variables indicative of mental health, adequacy of social performance (i.e., social competence), and behavioral adjustment. It is in this area that the greatest strides have been made in recent years in investigating the influence of individual differences on awareness of one's emotional experience. In a review on children's social competence and emotional experience, Hubbard and Coie (1994) suggested that although children who can more accurately "read" the emotions of *others* enjoy higher social status, little research has been done on whether more sophisticated or incisive awareness of one's *own* emotional experience is in fact correlated with more adept social functioning with peers.

Because I have already discussed how awareness of emotional experience develops, I do not consider age differences any further here. However, there are some interesting data on gender differences and a few studies on cultural influence and "social maturity" differences in awareness of emotional experience that warrant our attention. I consider primarily research that takes a developmental perspective, but I include some material based on adults that seems related to how we develop this particular skill of emotional competence.

Gender Differences

One way to look at awareness of emotional state is to consider whether individuals are able to express an emotional state with their face, particularly if they are asked to adopt or pose an emotional facial expression. To undertake such a task, we need to know how to move our facial muscles to match a consensually agreed on belief as to what, for example, an angry facial expression looks like. A number of studies exist that have used judges to rate whether the posing subject has indeed *encoded* the facial expression that typically goes with the requested emotion. Relative to gender differences, some have found that girls (and women) do better than boys (and men) in encoding emotional facial expressions (e.g., Buck, Miller, & Caul, 1974; Hall, 1984; Zuckerman & Przewuzman, 1979), probably because girls in our culture are allowed or encouraged to be emotionally more expressive compared to boys. The result is that girls may learn to produce emotional expressions more readily on request; they simply have more practice than boys do in using their expressive behavior. As we see in Chapter 8, girls do indeed appear to have an advantage over boys in some situations in which it is strategic to manipulate emotional–expressive behavior (e.g., looking agreeable when they do not feel that way on the inside). On the other hand, boys get lots of experience at inhibiting their expressive behavior, especially that which would otherwise render them vulnerable (e.g., masking sadness, fear, anxiety, and distress), and they learn to adopt a stoic expression across a variety of emotion-eliciting situations (e.g., Fuchs & Thelen, 1988; Pittman, 1993).

In a similar vein, Casey (1993) also found sex differences in a study of 7- and 12-year-olds in which the children played a game and then received either positive or negative feedback from a televised peer, who was allegedly in the adjacent room and could see them. Girls were more expressive of both positive and negative emotions, regardless of the nature of the social feedback, whereas boys tended to be rather stoicly negative in both positive and negative feedback conditions. (Perhaps "churlish" is the descriptive word to use for the boys.) In the subsequent interview, girls were also more accurate in describing what they believed their facial expressions looked like than the boys were. But both boys' and girls' reports of their internal emotional experience were influenced by whether the feedback they received was negative or positive, and this response did not vary across the two age groups. Casey's data appear to suggest that for these school-age children, the boys and girls did not differ in knowing how they felt when they received either negative or positive feedback; rather, they differed in knowing how and what they expressed on their faces as they heard the feedback. In that regard, the girls were superior to the boys in being aware of what they expressed facially during the feedback experience. Casey interpreted the difference in terms of socialization values: Girls learn to regulate the social parameters of their emotion and thus become more aware of their facial displays.

It is simply not known whether over the long term, our awareness of our emotions is compromised by chronic inhibition or adoption of emotional fronts. I would argue that over time our awareness of our own emotional experience might be dampened or "bleached," because we would have a reduced amount of *social* feedback about our emotional experience. In other words, if people do not know what someone is really feeling, there are few or only inadequate expressive cues for them to reciprocally respond to, which in turn would reduce opportunities for validation or confirmation of the individual's own emotional experience. Andy's experience, cited earlier, could represent the sort of developmental history such an individual might have. Certainly women's popular magazines are full of articles on "How to Get Your Guy to Communicate" or "What You Can Do to Enhance the Marital Dialogue" and letters to the experts inquiring about how to get husbands and boyfriends to open up and be more emotionally intimate. Emotional intimacy is, in many respects, the capacity for genuine emotional expressiveness with specific individuals (see also Chapter 10, in this volume; Saarni & von Salisch, 1993).

Data regarding whether there are sex differences in awareness of emotional state when relying on felt internal physiological cues are contradictory. Shields (1984) suggested that women may be more attentive to their physiological changes when experiencing emotion. However, Roberts and Pennebaker (1993) suggested that men more accurately detect changes in physiological functioning than do women. They argued that women use both internal physiological cues and external social–situational cues to make sense of emotional experience. This is not to say that men do not; rather, men can more readily detect physiological changes, even in the absence of social–situational cues. Intriguing here would be to find out whether men then make attributions about those physiological changes that they detect as reflecting *emotional experience.* Perhaps men can indeed detect changes in pulse and respiration more readily than do women, but what meaningfulness do they attribute to these changes? Similar research also needs to be undertaken with children.

The research literature on school-age children's *understanding* of multiple or contradictory emotions has generally not revealed sex differences with the exception of Wintre and Vallance's (1994) research described previously. An age group that in my opinion has been underresearched is the transition from preadolescence into adolescence, approximately 11 to 14 years. It may well be that we would find some gender differences emerging in how emotion awareness is understood and experienced, because there do seem to be some gender differences occurring in this age group in frequency of affect disorder, namely, more adolescent girls are diagnosed as depressed compared to adolescent boys; yet no consistent sex differences have been found in incidence of depression in childhood (e.g., Rutter, Izard, & Read, 1986).

Social Maturity Differences

Several studies suggest that the ability to encode or display emotional facial expressions may be greater in children who are more popular, extroverted, and more socially competent (for a comprehensive review, see Feldman et al., 1991). Interestingly, Custrini and Feldman (1989) found that in the age group 9 to 12, gender had a pronounced effect on whether social competence and accuracy at encoding and decoding emotion were linked. For boys, level of social competence (assessed by parental responses to the Social Competence scale of the Achenbach Child Behavior Checklist; Achenbach & Edelbrock, 1982) was unrelated to accuracy of emotion encoding and decoding. However, for girls there was a rather large difference between those girls ranked below average in social competence as compared to those ranked above average in social competence. Custrini and Feldman (1989) suggest that this interaction of gender and social competence in accuracy of emotion encoding and decoding may be related to the differential value accorded to "emotionality" for girls as opposed to boys. If girls are socialized to use emotional communication more than boys, then deficits in emotion communication (i.e., encoding and decoding of emotion expressions) may well contribute to deficits in social adequacy as well. Of course, the causal sequence may also operate in reverse: Deficits in social adequacy lead to deficits in emotion communication. One caveat to mention here is that having parents rate their children's social competence may constrain what we can infer about the children's social competence with people outside the family and away from parental observation (e.g., social competence with peers).

An intriguing study conducted by Hubbard (1995) used peer ratings of social acceptance versus rejection and related such peer nominations to emotional expression, emotional awareness, and goal orientation (instrumental or task focus vs. social engagement). Her subjects were African American boys and girls, ages 7 to 8 years. Children who were rejected by their peers on the sociometric rating task tended to express both more positive and negative emotion compared to the nonrejected children in a "rigged" game with a confederate child with whom they subsequently lost the game and a prize. Interestingly, rejected girls reported experiencing the most negative emotion compared to any of the other subgroups of children, whereas the nonrejected girls reported the least negative emotion in this situation.

Finally, rejected children (no sex differences here) were more likely to say that they were more concerned with winning the game than with being liked by the game partner (the confederate). Hubbard hypothesized that these differences might derive from rejected children's being less motivated to engage socially with an unfamiliar peer, and in the case of the rejected girls who reacted the most negatively, it would seem unlikely that they were especially interested in making any social overtures. Nonrejected children appeared to be less concerned about winning or losing the game and balanced their desire to win with some interest in getting to know the other child; as a result, losing did not make them feel so badly.

Little research has been undertaken that links social competence or maturity with understanding multiple feelings. However, a Dutch study compared emotionally disturbed children with normally adjusted children (Meerum Terwogt, 1989) relative to their understanding multiple emotions. Both groups were of normal intelligence; the emotionally disturbed group was characterized as 60% anxiety- or affect-disordered and about 20% as conduct-disordered. The age groups sampled were 6 to 7 years and 10 to 11 years. Meerum Terwogt (1989) found that the normal and disturbed children did not differ in understanding multiple emotions, but where they did differ was that the emotionally disturbed children more often dichotomized their responses: Either they responded to the stories as not at all emotional or they ascribed all negative emotions to the stories. They also tended to judge the emotions in the stories as more intense than the non-disturbed children. Meerum Terwogt (1989) interpreted his results as suggesting that emotionally disturbed children of normal intelligence were capable of undistorted emotion understanding, but their maladaptive functioning was revealed in the way they embedded inadequate coping strategies into their judgments. Thus, some situations were judged as overwhelmingly emotionally intense, others as having no emotional salience at all, and still others as having only negative emotional meaning. A rigidity of perception seems evident in such all-or-nothing judgments and coping would be commensurately impaired. Their findings are also reminiscent of Harris's (1995) theorizing about preschool children's tendency to stop scanning a situation for possible other emotions after they have found one meaningful emotion-eliciting appraisal. The maladjusted children in Meerum Terwogt's sample appeared to perseverate in an immature form how they represented to themselves emotion-eliciting circumstances.

Finally, Greenberg, Kusche, Cook, and Quamma (1995) undertook a large-scale affective education program with second- and third-grade children in metropolitan Seattle (PATHS: Promoting Alternative

THinking Strategies). Their curriculum emphasized vocabulary for feelings, appraisal of basic emotions in oneself and others, and how to manage one's emotions. Their sample included regular classrooms as well as children in special education classrooms, many of whom were likely at risk for emotional maladjustment. Their posttest analyses suggested that all children increased their verbal fluency in labeling and discussing their emotions and the children in the special education classes may have made proportionately greater gains than the regular education children in learning how to manage their emotions. Greenberg et al. (1995) argued that the gains achieved by the children in meta-emotional knowledge as a result of the intervention program also helped them to develop further interpersonal problem-solving skills and behavioral self-control because of enhanced awareness of their own emotion processes and ability to think about them (see also Greenberg & Kusche, 1993).

Cultural Influences on Awareness of Emotional Experience

Mesquita and Frijda (1992) exhaustively reviewed cross-cultural data on many different aspects of emotion, including how situations are appraised, how physiological cues are used (or ignored), how emotions prompt subsequent action, how emotional expression and related behaviors function, and how emotions are regulated. Their review is extraordinarily rich in detail, and I shall not repeat their analysis and description here. However, their conclusions do warrant some attention. First, they conclude that global statements are inappropriate about either the universality of emotion or the other extreme, that all emotion is uniquely culturally constituted.

Second, if we use abstract levels of description, we tend to find cross-cultural similarity, while the more micro or specific level of description tends to yield cross-cultural differences. To illustrate, the generic and abstract idea of participating in a celebratory feast tends to elicit more cross-cultural similarity in people's expectations that such an event would be associated with happiness or pleasure. However, a *particular* emotion-eliciting situation may differ across cultures; for example, eating a barbecued lizard at some celebratory feast does not elicit pleasure for me, but it might for others in another culture.

Third, on one hand, a major source of cultural differences lies in what we might call emotion control or regulation strategies. The chapters in this book on coping, self-presentation, and emotional dissemblance all constitute topics around which considerable cultural variation exists. On the other hand, what is common to most cultures is the existence of some emotional expression control strategies; that is, we do not always show what we really feel, but how we go about doing this, with whom, and in which settings, is highly culturally variable.

Fourth, Mesquita and Frijda (1992) believe that there may be some emotion-eliciting events that have nearly universal meaning in stimulating similar emotional reactions across different cultures. They suggest that loss of a person with whom one has a close relationship, rejection by one's primary group, and threats by one's rivals to one's security may be typical of such universal emotion-arousing events. However, how such emotion-arousing events are specifically coped with and made sense of is culturally variable. For that matter, there is a range of individual variability even within a given culture or subculture in terms of how causes are assigned to such events and how one deals with the situation and one's emotional experience. For example, consider how two people might make sense of as well as cope with rejection by their primary group of friends. In both cases the two people might well feel sad or even devastated, but suppose person A constructed the causes of the rejection as stemming from irreconcilable differences in beliefs (e.g., she was pro-choice but they were not), whereas person B viewed the rejection as entirely his fault because he was allegedly insensitive to the viewpoints of his friends (e.g., he "should have known better" than to air his pro-choice views with these particular people who had just volunteered for Operation Rescue). Person A would probably cope by beginning to find new friends who shared her political outlook, whereas person B might withdraw from social situations for a period of time.

Fifth, Mesquita and Frijda (1992) point out that trying to determine how cultures differ or are similar in emotional experience is beset with methodological problems, among them lack of comparable translation of emotion terms, lack of comparable samples or "informants," and lack of comparable social environments in which emotional experience can be observed.

Do cultures influence degree of emotional competence? I would argue that this is the wrong question to ask, for emotional competence is part and parcel of culture. Our culture (or subculture) gives us meaning systems, and those meaning systems are very much applied to what is appraised as emotion eliciting. Anthropologist Brad Shore (1996) calls these fundamental meaning systems the "master narratives" of a culture, implying that the way that we go about constructing our stories about our emotional experience is imbued with the values and beliefs that constitute our cultural heritage. Rimé (1995) would probably add to this view that because people are apparently motivated to share with others their emotional experience, they must be able to describe it according to culturally meaningful forms. If they could not access mutually comprehensible terms with which to describe their feelings, then at the very least interpersonal confusion results, and at worst outright rejection or avoidance occurs. The loneliness felt by many newly arrived immigrants and foreign students may be due in part to this inability to share one's emotional experience meaningfully.

Lazarus's (1991) encompassing approach to emotions as indicating an adaptational "goodness-of-fit" between the individual and his or her environment is also very appropriate here. He would argue that culture defines what are meaningful goals (i.e., how we appraise events as emotion eliciting) and what constitutes personal well-being (i.e., how we cope with emotional experience). These two broad variables yield a complex matrix of transactions between individuals and their multifaceted environments that include not only the nature of emotional experience but also how individuals cope and regulate their emotions, their cognition, and their behavior. Not surprisingly, this begins to sound like our general definition of emotional competence, namely, the degree to which one is self-efficacious (i.e., effective at promoting one's well-being) in interpersonal emotion-eliciting transactions. It is these emotion-eliciting transactions that are embedded in cultural meaning, and thus our emotional competence is inextricably intertwined with our cultural context.

I think it is also important to note that neither Lazarus nor I would say that experiencing a negative emotion is undesirable or is somehow not related to promoting one's self-efficacy. Indeed, just the opposite: Awareness of our negative emotions provides us with important information about our social and physical environment. In addition, negative emotions can also be culturally prescribed and can function to promote social bonds and elicit support, for example, receiving sympathy while grieving a loss. Think also of the children cited in my research who felt that if they were in the context of a supportive interpersonal "safety net," they would indeed express their vulnerable distressed feelings. It is how we cope with emotional arousal that is the key here to emotional competence and ultimately to Lazarus's notion of adaptation within a cultural context.

CONCLUSION

Awareness of one's emotions facilitates problem solving, and it is a capability central to emotional competence. Knowing that we feel scared instead of sad yields different avenues for figuring out what to do; in the former circumstance it might be a good idea to run away, but if we are sad, seeking support might be the most adaptive action to take.

Awareness of experiencing multiple emotions about an event or a relationship also promotes effective adaptation: One can take into account the pros and cons of a situation and act accordingly or make a decision that weighs the advantages and disadvantages of an outcome. And, finally, awareness that we are not always aware of our feelings may serve to intensify our self-reflection when we are faced with a crucial choice. Knowing that some feelings render us acutely vulnerable is still significant information for solving thorny and resistant interpersonal problems.

It is also important to remind ourselves that our respective cultures define, for the most part, the details of emotional meaningfulness in our daily experience. However, even in cultures that have no equivalent term for "emotion," the *significance* of events, relationships, and experiences is noted, and subsequent behavior or interaction is influenced accordingly. Individuals who are impoverished in their awareness of their emotions (or of what is culturally defined as significant) would have parallel deficits in knowing how to respond adaptively to their environment, and concurrently, their self-efficacy in emotion-eliciting social transactions would be impaired.

Skill 2: The Ability to Discern and Understand Others' Emotions

Ability to discern and understand others' emotions, using situational and expressive cues that have some degree of cultural consensus as to their emotional meaning.

An edited excerpt from one of my cases illustrates a relatively mature level of this skill of emotional competence. The case also shows that the ability to understand what others are feeling develops in conjunction with awareness of our own feelings, with our ability to empathize, and with the ability to conceptualize causes of emotions and their behavioral consequences. In addition, the more we learn about how and why people act as they do, the more we can *infer* what is going on for them emotionally, even if it is not especially obvious or may even be counterintuitive. The case involved C, a sensitive and compassionate eighth-grader, who was approached by her school counselor, G, to become a peer counselor at the middle school for sixth- and seventh-graders. G noticed that C had a special talent for understanding other kids' feelings, without their actually saying in so many words what they felt. After C completed the peer counselor training, G approached her to videotape one of her sessions with a small group of students who had been referred for a variety of family transitions and crises.

J (*speaking in a blasé, pseudo-bored manner*): We had to go see my dad at Lompoc [a federal penitentiary] over the weekend. It was really weird and creepy; it was hard to relate to him like my Dad. And afterwards my mom was all crying and mad at us [J has two siblings] during the drive home. I'd just like to move out.

C: So going to Lompoc was sort of like being on an alien planet, but your Dad's there, and you felt, maybe, like he was sort of an alien too, not part of you anymore, but he's still your dad. And then your mom is all upset and takes it out on you guys. It seems nothing you do fits or works right: how to show you love your dad, how to help your mom, and yet your dad's in jail and you feel ashamed of your family.

J (*wiping away some unexpected tears*): It'd almost be better if he were dead; then it would be over with, and I wouldn't have to explain about my father. (*She covers her face with her hands, and C passes her the tissue box.*)

After watching the tape segment with C, G asked her how she knew that J felt ashamed and defeated ("nothing you do fits or works right"). C said she thought about how she would feel in J's situation with a father in jail; she thought she would feel embarrassed and uncomfortable talking about it. Yet she noticed that although J was acting as if it was no big deal, she said she wanted to move out, even though she was only 12. C elaborated, "When you just want to escape, get away from it all, because staying there is so awful, but you can't. Then I guess the person feels trapped, and the only way she can act in front of others so she still feels some pride is to act like it's no big deal, it's not important to her."

C's skillfulness at reading in between the lines of J's verbal and nonverbal messages allowed her to develop hunches about what sort of emotional experience J might be having. She used her own estimate of what she would feel like in a similar situation but modified it in light of unique information she noticed about J, for example, her acting as though it was no big deal but at the same time wanting to move out of her home. C took a greater inferential leap when she guessed that J might feel as though nothing she did "fit or worked right" and elaborated on this as a trapped feeling from which one would simply want to escape. The image of feeling trapped implied that C believed J felt as though she had little control over the circumstances facing her, and it

reflected C's use of a "causal search" that might underlie emotional reactions. We might surmise that C combined J's communication with
the fact that J had also been referred to this small support group by a
teacher or counselor, the implication being that J was probably revealing some difficulties in other areas of her life that were becoming noticeable at school. Indeed, J's grades had plummeted, and she had been
truant several times.

C's competence at discerning and understanding another person's
emotional experience is sophisticated but not uncommon for adolescents. I introduced this case to bring into focus how significant inferring and understanding others' feelings are for guiding our subsequent
social interaction with those individuals. Indeed, the whole complex
process of dyadic emotional communication is a weaving back and
forth of two individuals' reciprocal inferences about the emotions of
the other, which in turn are integrated with one's own emotional reactions (see also Chapters 8 and 10, in this volume, for further elabora-
tions of this theme). However, let us back up and consider some of the
developmental tasks that need to be mastered before arriving at this
mature stage.

DEVELOPMENT OF UNDERSTANDING OTHERS' EMOTIONS

At a rather young age children are able to act pragmatically vis-à-vis others' emotional–expressive behavior, which suggests that they both
discern others' emotions and can use others' emotional–expressive behaviors as reference points for guiding their own emotional response
(reviewed in Michalson & Lewis, 1985). For example, try smiling at the
next few young babies you see in the grocery store checkout line. If
they are between 4 and 9 months and within touch of their caregiver,
they will probably smile back. Now try frowning at a baby (preferably
not one of the same ones you just smiled at); he or she will probably
show a distressed face or turn away and reach for the caregiver. The
baby's behavior in response to an unfriendly facial expression is adaptive and appropriate; by turning away, reaching for the caregiver, or
expressing distress, the baby shows that he or she pragmatically understands the implication of your expression: This is not an exchange to
be pursued!

As discussed in Chapter 4, infants also learn to scan others' facial
expressions (especially their caregivers') in order to figure out the emotional meaning of an ambiguous situation (i.e., social referencing). In a
sense, learning "to read" others' emotional–expressive behavior precedes one's own emotional response to new and uncertain situations.

Social referencing provides infants and toddlers with a valuable strategy with which to learn their families' and subculture's meaning system for how situations and events are to be appraised in terms of their emotional significance.

However, let us move beyond social referencing to examine what children have to understand to generate *sophisticated* insight into another's emotional experience: (1) They need to be able to decode the usual meanings of emotional facial expressions; (2) they need to understand common situational elicitors of emotions; (3) they need to realize that others have minds, intentions, beliefs, or what has otherwise been referred to as "inner states;" (4) they need to take into account unique information about the other that might qualify or make comprehensible a nonstereotypical emotional response or a response that differs from how oneself would feel in the same situation; and (5) they need to be able to apply emotion labels to emotional experience so that they can verbally communicate with others about their feelings. I describe several studies that address these facets of how we come to understand others' emotions; however, I consider the last item about emotion labels in greater detail in the next chapter when I discuss the emotional competence skill of acquisition of an emotion lexicon.

Understanding Facial Expressions

A review by Gross and Ballif (1991) of research on children's understanding of emotions in others based on facial expression cues and situational elicitors of emotion concluded that, not surprisingly, as children matured, they became more accurate in their inferences about what others were feeling. The easiest emotions to figure out were positive ones: smiling faces and situations depicting pleasure and getting what one wants were readily comprehended as associated with happiness. Negative facial expressions depicting sadness, fear, or anger were more difficult for children to decode, but if paired with a detailed emotion-eliciting situational context, children were much more likely to infer the negative emotion in question. An example of a study illustrating these more general findings with quite young children is described next.

Variable Meanings

Michalson and Lewis (1985) conducted a study with 2-year-old middle-class children and found that they understood the verbal labels for most of the facial expressions of six basic emotions (happiness, surprise, anger, fear, sadness, and disgust) in that they could point to the photo of the appropriate posed facial expression (on the part of a 10-year-old girl) when asked to pick out the face that showed the emotion word (happy, surprised, angry, etc.). Happy and sad faces were accurately selected by about 86% of the children; disgusted and fearful faces received the lowest accurate matching rates (29% and 14%, respectively). None of the children could (or would) produce the verbal labels for the facial expressions themselves.

These same 2-year-olds also demonstrated a limited degree of understanding about which situation was likely to elicit which emotion (between 25% and 71% were able to choose the appropriate facial expression for the happy, sad, and surprised situations). However, as Michalson and Lewis pointed out, the meanings attributed to facial expressions and eliciting situations were variable, for already by age 2 family "rules" or customs may be in place that influence what sort of facial expression is likely to occur in what sort of situation. Adults, for example, may almost as often match a sad facial expression as an angry facial expression to a situation in which damage is intentionally done to one's achievement (i.e., for children, the situation for eliciting anger was having a sibling deliberately knock over one's tower of blocks).

Adults recognize that an expression may be a *social* response and not necessarily identical to their emotional response. One person may have learned that a sad expression upon having one's accomplishments damaged may elicit repair or compensation from the perpetrator; another person may have learned that by expressing anger, she can prevent the perpetrator from doing such damage again in the future. Both are legitimate instrumental expressive responses intended to influence the social exchange. For researchers to call one "accurate" and the other "inaccurate" is an oversimplification of emotion understanding. Indeed, as Lewis and Michalson (1985) have discussed elsewhere, facial expressions can have a dual function; they can be *signs*, in which case they bear a one-to-one correspondence to internal emotional state, or they can function as *symbols*, in which case they point to something else, for example, placating someone, deterring someone, or presenting oneself in a more favorable light (recall J's seemingly bored and disinterested behavior while discussing her father's imprisonment). The dissociation of facial expression from internal emotional experience will be taken up in detail in Chapter 8.

Bearing in mind my reservation mentioned earlier, by age 4 children can nominate the sorts of situations that "go together" with a simple set of emotions (Barden, Zelko, Duncan, & Masters, 1980). Their accuracy in decoding posed facial expressions of idealized basic emotions is quite good, with only a little lingering confusion over the negative emotions (e.g., sad, mad, and afraid expressions), and, indeed, by school entry at ages 5 to 6, children reliably distinguish among the negative facial expressions as well (reviewed in Camras, 1985). However, in reality, children must decode the meaning of facial expressions that are neither carefully posed nor presented as idealized static two-dimensional stimuli, as was done in the preceding research studies. More often than not, they also have some degree of familiarity with their interactants. Results based on experimental procedures may actually be quite limited in their generalizability to children's ordinary experience of having to make sense of others' emotional–expressive behavior and then using their interpretations to guide their subsequent social interaction. We need more research that uses observational strategies combined with controlled pseudo-naturalistic situations that allow us to examine just how children use their hunches about others' emotional experience to shape the ensuing interpersonal exchange (as an example of such a study, see Underwood, Hurley, Johanson, & Mosley, in press, described later in this chapter).

Bias in Attributing Meaning to Expressions

To address the issue of familiarity, Barth and Bastiani (1997) examined 4- and 5-year-olds' *biases* in labeling the expressions of their classmates' facial expression photos. First, they had the children produce five different emotional facial expressions, which were photographed. These then became the assortment of expressions each child was subsequently asked to label. Although the expressions were static, they were more ecologically valid in that they were based on familiar peers. Accuracy scores were based on congruence of the judged expression and which expression the classmate was intending to produce expressively. Bias scores were calculated as the proportionate number of times a child used a particular expression label (e.g., sad, happy, mad, surprised, or afraid) relative to the total number of classmate photos that were judged. The children made these ratings at the beginning of the school year and again 5 months later; a variety of other social data were also collected.

Their results indicated that it was the preferential bias for "seeing" some expressions more often than others that had greater stability over time than accuracy scores. In addition, bias scores were more strongly related than accuracy scores to children's peer acceptance (based on sociometric ratings) and children's social adjustment (teacher ratings). This pattern was especially noticeable if the bias was for "seeing" angry facial expressions, even if that was not what the familiar classmate was trying to produce expressively. Such children were found to have less satisfactory peer relations and their adjustment was more likely to be rated as hostile–dependent, which is consistent with research with older children who use a hostile attribution bias in their peer relationships (e.g., Crick & Dodge, 1994). Thus, some young children may already have well-established patterns of bias in what expressions they believe their peers are displaying; when their bias is toward perceiving angry expressions, they may engage in more socially distancing behaviors, resulting in less peer acceptance.

Understanding of Emotion-Eliciting Situations

As children mature, they combine both facial and situational cues as they attempt to discern and understand the emotional experience of others (e.g., Hoffner & Badzinski, 1989). Some researchers suggest that when there is a contradiction between a facial expression and the emotion-eliciting situation, school-age children are more likely to opt for whichever cue is more clearly presented (e.g., Wiggers & van Lieshout, 1985). Such a cue represents a "better bet" about what a person is feeling than relying on any particular category of cue alone. An example used by Wiggers and van Lieshout is a scenario depicting a boy with a weak smile about to get a fearsome injection. The situation, in this case, is more definitively portrayed than the boy's facial expression, and as a result, children conclude that the boy is anxious or afraid, despite the attempt at a smile. If the situation is also one familiar to children, they may use their own likely emotional response as a good bet for what the other child might also feel—even if the other child does not express the feeling behaviorally. Children also recognize that others might feel a mixture of feelings about a situation. As an illustration, Camras interviewed 5- to 6-year-old children using several different stories (e.g., "My friend came home from school one day and his mother told him that the family dog had just had puppies. My friend didn't even know his dog was going to have puppies."). The children were then asked to infer the story protagonist's feelings. Happiness and surprise were equally selected, but some children thought disgust might occur as well (personal communication, cited in Lewis & Michalson, 1985).

Strayer (1986) has documented that by age 5 to 6 years, children are able to provide reasonable determinants for emotions experienced both by the self and by others. She elicited this information by asking the children open-ended questions about their experience (e.g., "Tell me what would make you feel happy"). She next examined several thematic shifts in situational determinants of emotion such as impersonal versus interpersonal attributions, achievement themes, the role of fantasy, and degree of agency or control. Older children (7 to 8 years) made more use of interpersonal and achievement themes relative to the younger children (5 to 6 years), and, interestingly, there were no significant differences in explanations given for whether the emotion was experienced by the child or by somebody else. However, her methods for obtaining this understanding from children did not include the sort of stimuli that elicited the positivity bias toward the self that was mentioned in the last chapter (e.g., "I'd feel fine, but the other guy would probably not").

Understanding Others' Inner States

Relations with Pretend Play

As mentioned earlier, children may try to put themselves in another's place and thus try to figure out how someone else is feeling. Paul Harris (1989) argues that the emerging capacity of young preschool children (i.e., age 2½ to 3 years) to carry out more elaborate imaginative games of pretend is indicative of their ability to comprehend that others have wishes, beliefs, and feelings much as they have themselves. What is significant about pretend play is the distinction between "this is someone else" and "this is me." The 3-year-old child is able to portray herself as "Cat Woman" chasing around after her playmate who is "Batman," and a mere 10 minutes later may be imagining herself as the preschool teacher ordering the other children to sit at the table because it is time for lunch (a make-believe lunch, that is). In other words, the young child begins to recognize that others might have wishes, beliefs, or feelings that *differ* from what the child experiences as her own. Recall 4-year-old Andrew from the preceding chapter with whom I went camping and who loved words such as "scrofulous" and "grotesque":

> Andrew brought along on the camping trip a shoebox filled with "GI Joe" figures, contraptions, weapons, and I don't know what all else. He located a boulder and with a small shovel began to excavate nearby a "pit" (his word). He arrayed his various characters around the pit's edge and proceeded to stage an intense battle. Some plastic dinosaurs also appeared on top of the boulder who leapt down and did awful things to the GI Joe guys, who, in turn perpetrated equally ghastly things onto the poor dinosaurs. This siege was accompanied by Andrew's passionate discourse on what everyone (dinosaurs included) was thinking, feeling, and especially what they were going to do next to avenge themselves. After about 20 minutes of this din, his mother looked up from her book and somewhat wistfully asked who was winning. Andrew replied in a calm voice, "No one. But I have to bury the dead ones now." And thus the pit was filled up with the carnage, the trowel coming into good use to smack down any recalcitrant creatures.

Apart from how we might worry about our culture's influence on young children in the way of contributing to violent imaginings, Andrew's play sequence contained multiple perspectives on who was feeling what and intending what. His vehement dialogue accompanying the fantasy characters' action was in distinct contrast to his response to his mother's question, suggesting that he knew when his voice was part of the imaginary battle and when his voice represented *him,* answering his mother.

On the other hand, imagination and reality have a dynamic relationship to one another, and it was Andrew smacking the "bad" dinosaurs with the trowel during their burial. Play therapists recognize this dynamic fluidity in young children's play; that is, sometimes what the child feels is projected onto the play character. But the point here is that this is not always the case. Preschoolers such as Andrew also know that what they feel, think, or want is *not* necessarily the same as for others; and sensitive play therapists are able to distinguish these different sorts of play sequences in their observation of the child (e.g., Slade, 1986, 1994).

Mistaken Beliefs

Harris and others have examined extensively young children's developing comprehension that others can be misled or mistaken in their beliefs and thus can have feelings about something the child knows to be untrue (e.g., Gross & Harris, 1988). Indeed, children by 3 years of age (and perhaps even younger) can lie to avoid punishment and can understand "tricking" others (e.g., Josephs, 1993a; Lewis, 1993a; Peskin, 1992; Sodian, Taylor, Harris, & Perner, 1991). In terms of emotional competence, the ability to appreciate that others have feelings that may differ from their own in the same situation—because the other has a different belief about the situation—is a major step in children's intellectual, social, and emotional differentiation. The considerable literature on the development of "theory of mind" repeatedly demonstrates that children can take into account the wishes, desires, and needs of another (e.g., Astington, Harris, & Olson, 1988; Harris et al., 1989). In short, children recognize that others also have beliefs about emotion-eliciting situations.

Taking into Account Unique Information about the Other

The whole topic of how children combine the *unique* information they possess about another individual with what they infer that other person is likely to feel is surprisingly underresearched. Related research, cited previously, on children's acquisition of a theory of mind literature typically emphasizes particular beliefs, wants, or mistaken perceptions as opposed to the personality or prior experience of the individual. Virtually the only studies for more fully describing this feature of emotional competence in understanding others' emotional experiences were conducted by Gnepp and Gould (1985) and Gnepp and Chilamkurti (1988) and theoretically elaborated on by Gnepp (1989).

Gnepp and Gould (1985) examined whether children (ages 5 to 10) could use information about a story character's past experience (e.g., being rejected by one's best friend) to predict how the character would feel in some new situation (e.g., subsequently meeting the best friend on the playground). Not unexpectedly, the youngest children were more likely to use the current situational information to infer what the character was feeling (e.g., she would be happy at seeing her best friend) and older children were more likely to infer the character's emotional state by taking into account the prior experience (e.g., she would feel sad upon seeing her best friend). An interaction also occurred between the hedonic tone (positive/negative) of the emotion and the use of personal information: If the story character experienced a negative *emotion* at time 1 but encountered a commonly assumed positive *situation* at time 2, children were more likely to use prior personal history information when inferring how the character would feel at time 2. Gnepp (1989) suggests that children must first recognize what a person's perspective was at time 1 and then must apply that inferred perspective from time 1 to time 2 to come up with the atypical emotional response. Her data confirm what we would expect from older children: They can better keep track of the transitions individuals might go through that would affect their subsequent emotional experience. In addition, they can link together experiences a person might have that would lead her or him to appraise a situation in a counter-conventional way such that they would respond with atypical emotions.

Personality Traits

In an analogous investigation, Gnepp and Chilamkurti (1988) presented stories to elementary school children and adults in which characters' personality traits were systematically described as either negative or positive or desirable (e.g., agreeable and likable) or undesirable traits (disagreeable and unlikable individuals). The story characters then had some experience befall them, and the children were to infer the emotional reaction of the character to this new experience. Older children and adults were more likely to take into account the prior trait information in inferring the emotional response of the character in the new situation. The younger children (6-year-olds) were less consistent in doing so, but a number were able to take personality trait information into account when inferring how someone might emotionally respond to an emotion-eliciting event, even when the emotional reaction might be atypical for the eliciting event.

These two investigations show us that by school entry, children are on their way to superimposing multiple frames of reference onto one another across time intervals to predict or infer other people's emotional responses. In her research, Gnepp did not distinguish between emotional state and emotional–expressive behavior; the assumption was that children would infer emotional state. Whether children could also infer what sort of expressive behavior would be displayed, and whether it would be congruent with an atypical internal emotional state or with the consensually defined "typical" emotion response to the situation, was not part of the focus of these studies. In terms of emotional competence, being able to take into account multiple frames of reference for making good guesses about how someone else is likely to react emotionally is strategic and functional. It is strategic because one can negotiate social transactions with considerably more finesse. It is functional because it promotes relationship bonds and facilitates "depth" of communication. Such depth is likely if one's communication is sufficiently insightful about an individual whose atypical emotional reaction can be understood as highly probable, *given the personal knowledge one has about that individual.*

I suspect that this ability is most evident in close relationships (e.g., between good friends, between intimates, and between parents and their children). It is fairly easy to recall instances in our own close relationships in which our knowledge of someone's personality trait or a past anguish-filled experience allowed us to appreciate his or her unusual or atypical emotional reaction and not judge the person as weird or "unbalanced." We may have wished that the person did not feel this way, but we can understand the basis on which he or she appraised an emotion-eliciting situation and thus responded to it quite differently than most people would. Several studies have examined emotional interactions experienced by children and youth in close versus casual relationships, and I turn next to a brief review of several of these investigations.

Understanding Emotions within the Context of a Relationship

It is probably a commentary on Western cultures that the emotion of anger has been most frequently studied by psychologists relative to children's dyadic interaction. Some of this concern is driven by the association of anger with aggression and its obvious disruptive effects on social exchange. Frequent bouts of anger, combined with hostility, also appear linked to poor health outcomes. The conclusion drawn by Lemerise and Dodge (1993) in their review is that highly aroused anger, expressed hostilely and aggressively, is associated with a wide variety of maladaptive outcomes, especially if it is chronic; anger that is expressed calmly and in socially constructive ways yields, by comparison, considerably more favorable outcomes.

Anger and Relationship Closeness

Some studies with children and youth have examined how anger is controlled within friendships (e.g., Fabes, Eisenberg, Smith, & Murphy, 1996; von Salisch, 1993), and other studies have varied closeness of relationship as a predictor for how anger is experienced (e.g., Whitesell & Harter, 1996). A review that included a comparison of anger between friends, casual acquaintances, and siblings (von Salisch, 1996a) noted that preadolescents rather quickly regulated their anger when it occurred with close friends, but with their siblings, even habitual and predictable quarreling was accompanied by frequent and overt anger. Von Salisch suggested that anger among siblings may have the function of helping children assert their "rights" as well as becoming more aware of their own attitudes and wishes as individuals within their families.

Observation of Emotion-Laden Exchanges

Research in this area is progressively moving toward more use of observational methods to probe the dynamics of emotional exchanges. I describe a recent ingenious study that warrants greater attention and demonstrates this methodological approach. Underwood et al. (in press) had a large sample of school-age children (8 to 12 years) participate in a pseudo-naturalistic situation whereby they individually met with a confederate child of their gender who was a trained actor. The children did not know each other. The pair of children played together a rigged computer game in which the subject child more often lost than won. During the game playing, the confederate child made mildly insulting remarks ("Are you sure you're really trying?"), boasted ("I could beat you at this game with my eyes closed!"), or invalidated the subject child's occasional win ("That's just beginner's luck"). The pair were videotaped throughout their game playing.

   Among the findings that emerged in the complex data set was that genuine expressions of anger were quite rare, despite 25% of the subject children terminating the game playing before the allocated 10 minutes were up. The children were somewhat more likely to express sadness, especially the girls, upon being teased and losing the game so often. Immediately after the actor child made a provocative statement, the subject children were most likely to remain silent, but when they did make negative remarks, the remarks were more often harsher when made by boys, and girls had a slight tendency to make more self-deprecating comments. Girls also responded more often with what appeared to be nervous laughter and giggling. However, overall, Underwood concluded that the boys and girls were more alike in their reactions to the confederate child's socially aversive behavior than they were different. She also found an age difference: Older children adopted more stoic or controlled expressions than did younger children. Underwood recognized that a variety of demand characteristics influenced her subject children's emotional–expressive behavior: They wanted to make a good impression; they were in an unfamiliar context with an unfamiliar peer.

Underwood (1997) also tracked the sociometric peer status of her subject children. Most interesting is that in this contrived interaction, there was no significant effect of peer status (popular vs. rejected) on reactions to the child actor's provocative statements. What was significant was that more of the rejected children were among the group who elected to stop the computer game altogether. Underwood suggested that it may well be that the negative reputational bias that develops within children's social groups determines an important part of the pattern of aggressive and/or withdrawn behavior demonstrated by "rejected" children (Hymel, Wagner, & Butler, 1990), and in this unfamiliar laboratory setting involving an unfamiliar peer, angry or aggressive reactions were not elicited. This study raises many fascinating questions, but it emphatically demonstrates the powerful effect of context on the interpersonal exchange of emotion. The argument raised by Lewis (1997) as presented in Chapter 3, on whether context is the more significant determinant of *present* emotional and social functioning than one's prior developmental history, is germane to these results. I turn next to a brief discussion of another theoretical approach associated with a social psychological view of how we discern and understand emotions in others.

ATTRIBUTION OF CAUSALITY AND INFERENCE OF EMOTION IN OTHERS

Weiner and Graham proposed that how we infer others' emotions, and, for that matter, reflect on our own, depends on what we believe to be the causes of these emotional experiences (see also Graham &

Weiner, 1986; Weiner, 1985; Weiner & Graham, 1984; also reviewed in Thompson, 1989). In particular, Weiner and Graham (1984) focused on several attributions that they argue shape the kinds of inferences we make. The first is the dimension of *stability*, which means to what extent will an event recur: Is it a completely random and rare situation that one finds oneself in (i.e., unstable) or is it one that we frankly realize is all too familiar (stable). Generally speaking, if we notice that a particular sort of emotional experience recurs quite repetitively for someone, we attribute something to the person's personality, disposition, or aptitude that contributes to the person's being in this frequently occurring emotion-eliciting situation. In other words, we assume that it is a feature of the person that is rather stable—although this may be inaccurate. For example, I tend to attribute hostility as a generalized personality trait to those who seem to be reacting angrily on a frequent basis or to what I view as trivial eliciting situations (e.g., instances of "road rage"), but, in fact, I may be in error, and it is the context (driving in traffic while under time pressure) that is "stable" in its reliable elicitation of "road rage" from otherwise not especially anger-prone people. Thus, attributions of a stable nature about the causes of human emotion do not have to lie only within the person(s); they can also be directed at cultural context. When we attribute causes of emotional experience to something within the individual, we are using an *internal locus*, according to Weiner and Graham. When our causal attribution is about the environment (e.g., the cultural context), the locus is *external*. Finally, the feature that contributes significantly to our perception of emotional causes is the perceived *controllability* of the eliciting event, of ourselves, and of the emotional experience itself. For example, depressed people do not typically perceive their emotional state of depression as personally controllable; they cannot turn it off and on at will.

Expectations and Excuses

When we combine these three aspects of attributions about causes of emotion, namely, stability (ranging from random/rare to high recurrence), locus (internal or external), and controllability (ranging from none to a lot), we gain considerable insight into how people *expect* themselves to feel in future situations as well as how they *explain* why they felt as they did in some situation. Often such explanations have a tone of making an excuse for our emotional reaction, and such excuse making has been examined by social psychologists as one of the more frequently used means of self-deception, as in "I just couldn't help myself, but I'm sure it won't happen again . . . " (e.g., Baumeister, 1993b;

Sigmon & Snyder, 1993). Weiner and Handel (1985) also investigated excuse making among school-age children and found that it was the dimension of controllability that was typically used to excuse their action; that is, they did not have control over the causal circumstances and therefore could not be held responsible. From a developmental standpoint, children just at the age of school entry can discriminate accidental events from controllable ones (Yirmiya & Weiner, 1986), but they do not reliably take this information into account when making attributions for specific emotions, especially anger, which typically presumes that the violation was intentional as opposed to accidental. By age 7, Yirmiya and Weiner (1986) found that children did take into account intentionality and controllability in their attributions of anger to others.

Developmental Critique

From a developmental standpoint, Thompson (1989) has argued that the attribution dimensions suggested by Weiner and Graham (1984) may not reliably characterize younger children's inferences about others' emotions. His critique suggested that we need to carefully rule out semantic constraints operating on children's understanding because they are typically asked to provide an emotion label for some hypothetical character's response. Do they really understand the label they are using? For example, younger children (4 to 7 years) generally do not discriminate between embarrassment and shame. Much of the attribution work with children uses situations involving achievement and the experience of success and failure, with causal ascriptions related to luck, ability, or effort. Thompson's own research revealed that younger children tended to attribute pride to *any* successful achievement, even if it did not require any effort but occurred as a result of "luck" alone. Failure experiences were also more likely to result in a search for causes than were successes. Thus, the use of an attributional search strategy appears related to what the outcome was, especially if it was an onerous one.

Attribution research needs to be broadened to include other kinds of emotion-eliciting situations, for children may demonstrate use of these dimensions in their causal search for understanding their emotional experience (e.g., interpersonal anger) but fail to use them in understanding their own or another's feelings in another situation (e.g., perhaps one involving anxiety). It is also possible that children do indeed use these attributions but may fail to verbalize them when they are interviewed. Devising methodological strategies that clarify children's use of attribution-based reasoning is much needed. An example that comes to mind is to present children with probable and *im*probable attributions and have them pick one and show how it "explains" the emotional response of some character. Using puppets to act out emotion-laden interaction might also be a good strategy for probing young children's causal searches.

Thompson (1989) also emphasized the need to consider individual differences in the use of such attributions; that is, what may be viewed as controllable by one subculture may not be so viewed by another. An example may be violence in the inner city: Such violence may be perceived as unpredictably repetitive (i.e., its recurrence is highly likely, but the where, when, and how are unpredictable), as having an external cause, and perhaps much of it is experienced as uncontrollable; the resulting feelings may range from despair to fear to anger. A youngster growing up in this context has a different set of attributions about his personal safety than one who grows up in suburbia.

Outcome as a Factor in Children's Emotion Inferences

Levine (1995) examined more thoroughly how younger children construed beliefs about the causes of anger and sadness. Her sample consisted of 5- to 6-year-olds, and she found that for anger they focused on the aversiveness of the outcome as well as espousing a "righteousness" toward the reinstatement of the protagonist's goal. For sadness the children more often mentioned the loss felt by the protagonist and that the goal was impossible to reinstate. Thus, it was the focus on outcome and goal reinstatement that determined what emotion the children believed would be felt, for, in fact, Levine used the same *event* for both anger and sadness stories, but she varied the attributions surrounding goal outcome. To illustrate, she used an episode involving a child who could not go out to play because of an injury. In one version the child has to stay inside and *does not want to* and in the other version he or she wants to play outside but *cannot*. The former elicited attributions of anger and the latter sadness. Thus, children appear to learn (in our culture at least) that their feelings can be explained by the status of their goals—whether they are met, violated, endangered, or lost.

In terms of emotional competence, children need to be able to *infer* others' emotional responses, as situations and expressive behavior are often ambiguous, indirect, or conflicting. Children use their inferences to guide their subsequent social interaction, and if those inferences are fairly accurate, appropriate and efficacious interpersonal transactions should result. For children whose inferences are biased (as in the Barth and Bastiani [1997] study described earlier), relatively less adaptive social outcomes result. I would also argue that being able to undertake a causal search about our own emotional experience facilitates future personal coping and ideally leads to maximizing our efficacy in such future situations. In emotional experiences that leave us with a diminished sense of self (e.g., shamed), it is important to apply such a causal search to our emotional experience so that we can either avoid the causal circumstances that lead to such situations in the future or *shape* them differently so that our self-efficacy is more likely to be fulfilled. This argument needs to be addressed empirically and clinically in research with children and youth (see also Reimer, 1996).

INDIVIDUAL DIFFERENCES AND CULTURAL INFLUENCE

Gender Differences

Boys and girls do not seem to differ very much in their capacity to *understand* others' emotional experiences. Sex-role socialization in conjunction with cultural and familial context appears to influence more our motivation to attend to others' emotional experience or how we cope with or control emotional experience and expression of emotions, but the ability *per se* to understand others' emotions has not typically been found to be gender linked among children (e.g., Meerum Terwogt & Olthof, 1989; Saarni, 1989b; Thompson, 1989). However, Custrini and Feldman (1989) report that among girls, but not among boys, degree of social competence greatly influenced their overall accuracy score in encoding *and* decoding others' emotions. Girls who were below-average in social competence scored well below boys, regardless of their social competence level, and the highest-scoring children were girls who were above average in social competence.

Another view of how gender might influence children's understanding of others' emotions may be found in the notion of *gender schemata* (e.g., Bem, 1981; Ruble & Martin, 1998). Gender schemata are hypothesized to be a framework of beliefs and associations that act something like a colored lens on how we process information. For example, if we hold traditional and stereotyped beliefs about how males and females "should" behave, we would be more apt "to see" an angry woman as upset rather than angry. Gender schemata may color or bias how we perceive others' emotions in that we may make systematic errors of misattribution about others' emotions, or we might simply not pay attention to emotion information that does not fit with our gender schema. This area is wide open for some fascinating developmental research. Gender schemata have been investigated with regard to toy preference, play activities, and other sex-role stereotyped behaviors (reviewed in Ruble & Martin, 1998), but I am not aware of any study that has systematically examined children's gender schemata in conjunction with understanding others' emotional experience. Perhaps an adaptation of the Barth and Bastiani (1997) study in terms of gender schema and biases in emotion understanding would yield an interesting outcome.

Social Maturity Differences

Social Competence and Discerning Others' Feelings

Do children who are exceptionally socially competent show an enhancement of understanding emotion and expression linkages? Custrini and Feldman (1989) suggest that they may, if we take gender into account. Other research undertaken by Walden and Field (1988) suggests that preschoolers who obtained high sociometric peer preferences as play partners were also those who tended to be better at discriminating among emotional facial displays and who tended to demonstrate high spontaneous expressivity (but they did not excel in posed expressions). Another study by Edwards, Manstead, and McDonald (1984) of somewhat older children demonstrated a similar relationship: Children's sociometric rating was positively related to their ability to recognize facial expressions of emotion.

Further support for a link between social effectiveness and emotion knowledge can be found in research undertaken by Denham, McKinley, Couchoud, and Holt (1990) and in a study on family-peer connections by Cassidy et al. (1992). In the Denham et al. (1990) study, preschoolers were followed for 9 months relative to their sociometric ratings (which were modified and subsequently referred to as their *likability* among their peers). Observations of naturally occurring emotion episodes in the preschool were also collected as were measures of children's understanding of emotion. Among the latter was a task that required the children to select a situationally appropriate facial expression from a felt board and place it on a puppet's otherwise neutral face such that the affixed expression properly matched the situation that had been enacted by the puppet. Their results showed that children who demonstrated greater knowledge of emotion in the puppet task (especially in understanding anger and fear) were perceived by their peers as more likable. Their results also indicated that prosocial behavior was positively related to likability, but emotion knowledge in the puppet task was unrelated to prosocial behavior.

In the Cassidy et al. (1992) study of kindergarten children, emotion understanding was measured by interviewing the children about identification of emotional facial expressions, how particular emotions were situationally elicited, and the social consequences to such emotions. They found that children who demonstrated more complex emotion understanding were more accepted by their peers. The investigators also looked at parental expressiveness and determined that mothers' expressiveness in the home was also positively related to their children's peer acceptance. The authors suggested that the children may have learned from their parents' expressiveness appropriate ways to negotiate relations with their peers.

Social Control and Witnessing Others' Emotions

Another source of individual difference that appears to be related to social adjustment is personal control. Bugental, Cortez, and Blue (1992) studied school-age children who differed in the degree to which they viewed themselves as having relatively more or less personal control over the outcomes of social interaction. In contrast to children who believed they had high personal control over outcomes, children who believed they had little control tended to be dependent on the expressive cues of others in their construction of what was going on and how to respond to it. (We might think of these children as using social referencing to a greater degree than their high-control peers.)

Bugental et al. (1992) were especially concerned with whether or not situations were construed as threatening by children who had developed "social scripts" that differed in the degree to which the self was viewed as a powerful agent. To determine whether children experienced themselves as having higher or lower social control, they used a picture-plus-story instrument in which children assigned causes to problems and solutions involving ordinary family interaction. The children's performance on this instrument yielded scores which were thought to be indicative of perceived social control (realistic attributions of causes and solutions were coded as showing personal control). Bugental et al. (1992) then monitored the children's heart rate while the children watched a videotape of a boy seemingly about to get an injection with an unusually long and ominous-looking needle in the course of a medical exam. Not surprisingly, the child on the videotape looked afraid.

Children with low perceived social control made more errors in recalling the videotaped situation than those with high perceived social control; for example, they thought the boy did get a shot, when in fact he did not. The high perceived social control children also sought out additional new information, whereas the low perceived social control children relied on conventional expectations about children getting shots or medical exams, despite these conventions being "violated" in the videotape (e.g., the videotape child received his "prize" before the exam, not afterwards, which is more customary in pediatric settings).

The research of Bugental et al. (1992) is significant for the concept of emotional competence in that it suggests once again the importance of how the self is constructed and experienced in emotional interaction. In a sense, the self is a filter or mediator for how we appraise situations and that appraisal contributes not only to our emotional response but also to how we cope with our emotion and with the complexity of the situation. If we witness someone else's negative emotional state (in this case, fear), or we find ourselves in a scary situation and react with *diminished* understanding, our ability to cope will be compromised by these deficits in accurate information.

I think of low perceived social control as entailing reductions in scanning and connecting: If we react solely based on the expressive cues of others (which is essentially social referencing), then we may have a short-term gain in that we do not have to do the work in trying to scan for diverse information and connect what we already know to integrate our emotions with our coping strategy and with the nuances of the immediate context. It is adaptive and appropriate for infants and young children to use social referencing in their making sense of what is going on emotionally or in their figuring out what to feel in an ambiguous and unknown situation. They do not have the cognitive depth to be able to scan and connect meaningfully, but to rely exclusively on this approach as we mature is to limit and rigidify both our emotional repertoire and our emotional competence in interpersonal transactions. This topic, too, is wide open for developmental as well as clinically oriented research.

Problematic Outcomes and Understanding Others' Feelings

Discerning and understanding others' feelings do not necessarily always contribute to our emotional competence. Paradoxically, in certain circumstances, some children would be better off tuning out others' emotional behavior. Children who are exposed to and involved in their parents' depressed feelings represent one group who are at risk for an aversive emotion socialization experience; another group consists of those children exposed to marital conflict accompanied by overt anger. Clearly, it is unrealistic to assume that children can tune out their parents' negative emotions, but the outcome for the children if such experiences are frequent, intense, and started early in life may be negative. Downey and Coyne (1990) and Zahn-Waxler and Kochanska (1990) reviewed investigations of how children of chronically depressed parents (for the most part, mothers) develop emotionally. Cummings, Ballard, and El-Sheikh (1991) reviewed research on children who witness interadult anger.

Zahn-Waxler and her associates noticed in their work with children of chronically depressed mothers that such young children appeared to be *overinvolved* and *overresponsible* in their interaction with their distressed mothers. Some of these children attributed the cause of their mothers' distress to themselves and developed a seemingly precocious repertoire of strategies for "repairing" their mothers' unhappiness (e.g., excessive solicitousness). Zahn-Waxler and her colleagues see in this behavior a contradictory blend of impotence and omnipotence, which contributed to the children's becoming vulnerable to inappropriate guilt when they failed to make their mothers happy. The seeds of depression were perhaps also planted in that inefficacy, or helplessness, was frequently experienced by such children; they could not reliably succeed in pleasing their mothers.

Zahn-Waxler and her colleagues found that when young children were involved with emotionally troubled parents, the children were constantly exposed to having to cope both with their parents' distress and with the demands that such negative emotional experiences placed on them. At the same time, these children were having to maintain and "nourish" their attachment to their parents (as opposed to the parent more appropriately nurturing the attachment with the child). These excessive emotional demands appear to contribute to an intergenerational transmission of maladaptive emotion socialization. Not surprisingly, depressed parents tend to have children who later also show depressive tendencies (e.g., Fendrich, Warner, & Weissman, 1990; Garber, Braafladt, & Zeman, 1991; Weissman et al., 1987).

Exposure to Anger and Conflict

Turning now to the research on children exposed to adults' anger and conflict, children as young as age 4 readily recognize such interactions as angry ones and respond to them with negative feelings of their own (Cummings, Vogel, Cummings, & El-Sheikh, 1989). Across a series of investigations on school-age children, Cummings and his colleagues found a pattern that suggested that boys in the age range of 6 to 9 years were more likely to respond to interadult anger and conflict with their own anger and aggression; girls were more likely to experience distress and anxiety. Children perceived angry conflict between adults that was also accompanied by physical aggression as the most reprehensible. Cummings, Ballard, and El-Sheikh (1991) investigated age changes in response to witnessed interadult anger in older children and adolescents. They found that the 9- to 11-year-olds had the strongest negative reaction to interadult anger and the oldest adolescents (17 to 19 years old) had the least. Interestingly, they found that the gender difference was reversed from that noted earlier with younger children. Adolescent girls reported more anger than boys, who, in turn, reported more sadness. Cummings, Ballard, and El-Sheikh (1991) speculate that this reversal of sex differences among adolescents may be a function of the boys' feeling sympathetic distress for the "couple" engaged in the mock conflict, whereas the girls may have felt aggravated at the couple having this ridiculous and petty conflict. What is unclear is the extent to which the adolescent felt self-involved as he or she responded to this staged argument between a couple.

What does stand out in these studies is that the youngest children were the most ardently involved in having an aversive reaction. Thus, we may infer that the younger the child, the greater the stress when the child is exposed to angry, hostile conflicts between adults. Given that this research was undertaken with mock conflicts between adults whom the children and youth did not know, we can only surmise how much more involving and upsetting it is for children exposed to their parents' anger and conflict. Indeed, clinically oriented research on such families shows that such youngsters are at risk for developing behavioral problems, for becoming victims and victimizers themselves, and thus for perpetuating the cycle of abuse (e.g., Egeland, Jacobvitz, & Sroufe, 1988; Emery, 1989; Grych & Fincham, 1990; McCloskey, Figueredo, & Koss, 1995).

Cultural Influence

Discerning and understanding others' feelings is obviously embedded in cultural context. Consider how interpreting the meaning of facial expressions as either signs of internal emotional state or symbols of social interaction requires us to take into account cultural context. Similarly, if we use unique information to which we have access in order to understand the atypical feelings of another, we must also be familiar with culturally defined personality traits and how personal meanings are attributed to events over time. We can readily appreciate how cultures and even the "subcultures" of families might influence children's developing this skill of emotional competence.

The management of emotions and feelings is relevant to all cultures, and thus it is adaptive for children to learn what people feel in terms related to the culture's meaning system. How children themselves go on to respond to what they see or infer as others' feelings is highly variable and includes the child's coping capacities and the nature of the relationship between the child and the other person. As we saw in the research with children exposed to interadult anger or those who grow up with depressed parents, children most definitely have emotional responses of their own to witnessing and understanding others' feelings. But, again, exactly what those responses would be depends on cultural context. Thus, in our culture children may feel angry or sad when they see adults angry at one another; in another culture children might feel fear or shame. In some cultures (including our own) children might cope with a chronically withdrawn and depressed parent by being able to find affection at a nearby relative's house, and the parent's depression may be explained as due to spirits or some other phenomenon (e.g., unemployment and marital desertion). In North American culture, extended families have become widely dispersed, and many children may not have the option "to escape" to a relative's home to receive compensatory and appropriate affection. Thus, some cultural contexts may more adequately support young children's coping efforts as they seek to understand others' emotions by having social structures or networks of relationships that are more responsive to young children's needs. A society (or subculture) stricken by poverty, famine, chronic disease, or war is itself under systematic siege, and under more benign conditions might have the capacity to shelter and foster its children's emotional development through its cultural institutions and social structures. But when survival is at stake, cushioning or facilitating children's emotional development tends to have low priority, and, indeed, children may be pushed toward emotional indifference and stoicism as a way to cope with overwhelming trauma (for further discussion, see Garbarino, Dubrow, Kostelny, & Pardo, 1992; Garmezy & Rutter, 1983).

One way to organize theoretically the relatively few studies that have looked at non-Western children's perception of emotions in others would be to take Hofstede's (1991) work-related dimensions of cultural variation and apply them to emotion understanding patterns. Hofstede's list of cultural dimensions consists of degree of individualism (as opposed to collectivism), power distance (the degree to which relationships should be structured according to rank or dominance), "masculinity" (the degree to which instrumental agency is valued more than communal caring), uncertainty avoidance (the degree to which social relations should be made more predictable by rules, norms, and laws), and the Confucian work orientation (the degree to which a long-term orientation in social relationships is valued). If these value dimensions occur in the realm of adult work relationships, it would seem that they might also shed light on how a given society socializes its children's orientation toward emotion, both in oneself and in how emotions are construed interpersonally. A systematic description of how these values might be linked with emotional socialization strategies in non-Western societies would be most beneficial.

As an illustration of the effect of values on emotion socialization, Cole and Tamang (1998) examined emotion beliefs in two subcultures in Nepal, the Tamang Buddhist majority and the Chhetri Brahmin (Hindu) minority. They found that Tamang mothers valued peaceful demeanor and believed that their children learned "right conduct" implicitly or automatically, whereas the Chhetri Brahmin mothers felt they had to teach their children more explicitly about good behavior and socially desirable conduct in settings away from home (e.g., school). The apparent effect of these two different parental emotion socializing beliefs was that the Tamang school children were more likely to report a generalized benign and calm emotional response to a variety of challenging situations with infrequent experience of negative feelings and no need to mask or conceal feelings. On the other hand, the Chhetri Brahmin children were more likely to report specific negative emotional reactions to some challenging situations which were then to be regulated by concealing one's feelings.

As the Cole and Tamang study reveals, if we are to understand better how children in societies quite different from our own acquire emotional–expressive communicative "styles," we need also to take into account the childrearing values espoused by the society at large and by the parents in particular. Chen, Dong, and Zhou (1997) examined the childrearing practices among parents in the People's Republic of China and found that rigid, unaffectionate, and authoritarian parenting practices were *negatively* related to their children's being perceived by their classmates as shy and sensitive, whereas for European North American children, authoritarian parenting has been *positively* associated with shyness and sensitivity in children. But when we take into account that Chinese society *values* expressive restraint, a tempered demeanor, and a degree of social inhibition, not only in its children but also more broadly as an indication of mature and socially appropriate behavior (e.g., Bond, 1993, 1996), this reversal of the North American socialization pattern makes sense. In fact, *authoritative* parenting was associated with socially competent children in this study, and these children were more shy and restrained than the less socially competent children, who were more likely to have parents subscribing to authoritarian practices.

CONCLUSION

How children make sense of others' emotions and the contexts in which they occur remains a rich area for further research. Some topics for future research have been alluded to in the text, but additional concerns include the following: First, much of the research in this area relies on how children *verbally* respond to hypothetical examples whereas observational data describe children's *behavioral* response to others' emotional displays. Second, in addition to expanding our methodological approaches, we must undertake further research on the developmental transition from childhood to adolescence. What shifts in interpretation of others' emotions occur in the years between 12 and 14? Recent research on young adolescents' experience of anger with close friends compared to casual acquaintances suggests that they can appreciate how the nature of the interpersonal relationship affects emotions and subsequent coping (Whitesell & Harter, 1996). However, we do not really know how emotionally competent understanding of others' feelings affects the formation of social networks and emerging self-constructions of identity during this important developmental transition. Third, given the significant cultural influence on this emotional competence skill, examination of individual differences from a cultural standpoint is much needed, taking into account childrearing beliefs and folk theories about emotion.

In the most general sense, we can conclude that this particular skill of emotional competence is initiated at a relatively early age and the degree of sophistication is influenced by the relative adequacy of social relationships experienced by any given child. By "adequacy" I mean here the perception of self-worth and being connected to others. Social competence is affected by the skill with which children and youth can understand others' emotional experience, and being able to negotiate the increasingly complex relationships that emerge in middle to late childhood is well-served by being able to infer and undertake "causal searches" about the other's emotional response. I also think that children's and youth's moral codes (fairness, "doing the right thing," moderation) become more explicitly integrated into their inferences about others' emotional experience at this time. They more readily make judgments about others' intentions, good or bad, about others' emotional styles as being like a loose cannon or the other extreme, sluglike, and about the likelihood of others' fairness and reciprocity. These judgments affect the target child's perception of emotion in the other, much as a bias might. Emotional competence, with its emphasis on self-efficacy in emotion-eliciting social transactions, is revealed when we can relatively accurately understand another's emotional experience even as we simultaneously bear in mind our own beliefs and values that give meaning to our personal emotional response in the interpersonal exchange.

Chapter 6

Skill 3: The Ability to Use the Vocabulary of Emotion and Expression

*A*bility *to use the vocabulary of emotion and expression terms commonly available in one's subculture and at more mature levels to acquire scripts that link emotion with social roles.*

THE PIVOTAL ROLE OF LANGUAGE

The ability to represent our emotional experience through words, imagery, and symbolism of varied sorts promotes two major accomplishments: (1) Behaviorally we can communicate our emotional experiences to others across time and space, whether by talking on the telephone about how we felt about what happened yesterday or painting a picture of a maelstrom to represent our inner turmoil; (2) conceptually, by having access to representations of our emotional experiences, we can further elaborate on them, integrate them across contexts, and compare them with others' representations about emotional experiences. Some of the developments in awareness of our own multiple feelings or in understanding others' atypical emotions described in earlier chapters would not occur if we did not have access to a language or representational system for symbolically encoding and communicating our emotional experiences.

Without a shared language of emotion, much of the research with children described in this volume would not be undertaken. As the anthropologist Geoffrey White (1994) states, "When people talk about emotion, they are not talking primarily about states inside the individual, nor are they talking about responses or events outside the person. Rather, they are talking about processes that *mediate* or link persons, actions, and events" (pp. 235–236). When we interview children about their expectancies about which emotions they are likely to feel in *X, Y,* or *Z* situations, we are asking them about linkages between feelings and contexts whose meanings are culturally based. Discourse theorists such as White and Wierzbicka (1992; 1994) emphasize how our language creates our social and emotional reality and that such a reality is highly *relational.* By this they mean that not only does our language give us the tools for efficiently representing our emotional experience, but the use of emotion language literally shapes social relations as well. Katherine Nelson (1996) also emphasized that the acquisition of language is more than a communication tool; its use dynamically changes and alters how we think. She contends that language becomes the symbolic medium in which children develop and try out different *scripts* or representations of event sequences. Thus they can rehearse and discard if necessary the tentative models with which they try to make sense of their experience. (I resume the discussion of scripts in some detail later in the chapter.)

Nelson reports that children as young as age 3 can provide an interviewer with general scripts about everyday events and routines such as "having dinner." Given that language is socially transmitted, the way that young children come to develop these scripts or working models is by definition socially mediated. What this means for emotions is that their meaningfulness is embedded in the process by which children acquire a lexicon to describe their own affective experience as well as to understand what others are saying about their feelings. The language we speak is inextricable from how we conceptualize what the words symbolize, and that has major consequences for our emotion-laden beliefs, expectancies, and attributions. For example, the word, *tiken* in Nepali–Tamang society (Cole & Tamang, 1998) has as its English equivalent, "feeling OK," but *tiken* means more than just "OK." Its *connotative* meaning includes the Tibetan Buddhist value of a centered calm, a state of balanced emotion without extremes, with overtones of peacefulness (Cole & Tamang, 1998). Tamang school children do not report experiencing strong negative emotions that must be masked in social settings or managed in some way, because for the most part they feel *tiken.* The cultural values implicit in their emotion socialization have stressed the spiritual desirability of this state of *tiken,* and thus their process of emotion regulation takes an altogether different path than children might experience in other societies. Tamang children do not expect to become upset, nor do they expect to be exuberantly happy or exultant, but they do believe in living in accordance with their Tibetan Buddhist philosophy.

White (1994) has argued further that negative emotions are more "finely conceptualized and lexicalized" (p. 226), because negative emotions draw our attention to the fact that some situation or relationship has significantly deviated from what we want or value. Thus, verbalizing our emotions, especially the aversive ones, is highly likely to have consequences for our interpersonal relations. To illustrate: If we tell someone that we are angry with him or her, the message serves at least two functions (1) it labels our emotional response, and (2) it communicates to the other that he or she caused or contributed to our emotional reaction, and by implication he or she had better change his or her behavior if our negative emotional reaction is to end. Some of the research reviewed later in this chapter on young children's early use of emotion-laden language with their siblings shows that they do intend to influence others' behavior with their use of emotion-descriptive words and phrases.

Nelson (1996) similarly contends that with the acquisition of language, young children not only learn the lexical forms of cultural meaning systems but that access to language itself gives children further tools for shaping and transforming those very meaning systems. How this "language-as-meaning-shaping tool" works for children in the realm of emotional experience is undoubtedly quite variable, but I suspect children use language as a symbolic way of giving their unique emotional "thumbprint" to the patterns that are emotionally salient for them. In addition, older children and youth frequently inhabit more than one social niche; with the strategic use of language forms, especially the ones that are emotion laden, they can indicate their membership in these different groups. Examples that come to mind are how young adolescents conveniently change their slang to fit their different peer groups (one set of words is used for the adult-approved social venues of scouts, Junior Rangers, etc. and the other for one's buddies in the locker room).

Alexithymia

Despite the rich and emotionally expressive discourse that we encounter among verbally inclined children and youth, some children rarely seem to speak about their own emotions or to refer to others' emotions. Clinicians refer to individuals with a *severe* deficit in ability to use emotionally descriptive language as alexithymic (e.g., Krystal, 1988). Not only are their relationships with others impoverished, but their own self-awareness of emotional experience is extremely limited. Krystal, among others, attributes this deficit to severe childhood trauma. Given the arguments of discourse theorists cited earlier, even individuals who do not have severe deficits but who minimize emotional experience would be expected to have less elaborated on, less reflected on, and perhaps even frequently repressed feelings (see also Fischer & Ayoub's [1993] discussion of affective splitting and dissociation, which may be related to why an individual has an impoverished emotion lexicon). Not surprisingly, such individuals may have relationships that seem superficial or full of misunderstanding, for without ready access to a language of emotion, we are unable to talk about our emotional experiences with others and vice versa.

EMOTION-RELATED IMAGERY AND SYMBOLISM

I do not wish to limit our ability to reflect on and communicate about our emotions to the narrow labels typically used by psychologists studying emotion. A rich world of linguistic imagery may also be tapped into by those who communicate about emotion. Writing about emotion without using any specific emotion labels would challenge us to come up with evocative images that suggest emotional experiences indirectly, and, indeed, this is just what poets do so well. For example, I recently came across a poem by Mei Yao Ch'en[1] (1965), whose sorrow over his wife's and son's deaths was richly evoked by phrases such as "My eyes are not allowed a dry season" and "I have / No one to turn to. Nothing, / Not even a shadow in a mirror." As for what children understand about the language and verbal imagery of emotion, at an early age they are immersed in storytelling that is rich, engaging, and reciprocal in that the child is both listener and narrator (e.g., Miller, Potts, Fung, Hoogstra, & Mintz, 1990; Sperry & Sperry, 1996). The flow of emotion is inherent in such narratives, and I thought to illustrate how children during their school-age years use emotional state and expression vocabulary as well as emotionally evocative imagery by reprinting excerpts from some stories I have collected over the years from my daughter. I present the excerpts first and comment on them later. The words are Heather's own; I have added some punctuation here and there and have abbreviated some of the material (indicated by ellipses [. . .]).

THIRD GRADE, AGE 8: "THE ANT AND THE ORANGE MOUNTAIN"

Once there was an ant and an orange mountain. The mountain was very spooky. There were orange swirling clouds overhead. . . . But this one little ant had no home. Wherever he went he was not wanted. . . . The ant stared down in wonder [from the mountain top]. "It is perfect!" he cried. "There is not another ant in sight. I can live here."

The ant made his way down the mountain. Suddenly the mountain boomed, "How dare you enter my valley?" The ant, taken by surprise, cried, "Oh, mountain, please let me stay! I shall do no harm!" "No!" shouted the mountain. The ant sat on his rear and cried. "No one wants me," he bawled. "Everyone hates me!" The mountain took pity on the ant. "Oh, alright! You can live here," the mountain finally agreed. The ant stopped crying. He looked up at the orange mountain and smiled. . . .

One day the mountain said, "I must tell you something. There is another ant in this valley. I'm sure you would like her." The ant walked away. Her? Her? There was a girl ant here? Suddenly the ant rushed out immediately to find the girl ant. The mountain watched him with interest.

The boy ant searched furiously. Then he saw a young ant. He went up to her. It was the girl ant. He strutted over and showed off for the girl ant. "Hello," she said pleasantly. . . . The mountain smiled. He could already see that he was going to have a lot of baby ants in his valley. . . .

The following excerpt is from a story about the survival of a young girl caught in a tidal wave caused by a massive earthquake off the California coast. She has just felt the massive earthquake and realizes that as a consequence a *tsunami* might develop. The story was written about a year after the destructive 1989 earthquake in the San Francisco Bay Area.

FIFTH GRADE, AGE 10: "STRANDED"

I looked out to sea, but the sun shone right in my eyes, making it impossible to see the horizon. I sat on a rock and waited for sunset. Soon I could see the ocean, and what I saw made my heart skip a few beats. A huge wave was silhouetted against the sky! . . . I lay down flat on the rocks on the opposite side of the island so the tidal wave would not hit me full force. I heard the enormous wave approaching. I glanced up. The tall wall of water was coming. Fear shot up my spine. No! No! No! I don't want to die! I clutched the rock more tightly. The sound was like a lion roaring in my ear. Suddenly the wave struck, and it was cold as ice and so strong. . . .

The following excerpt is from a story about a girl who flees her abusive foster parents and manages to survive by living in the attic of the local library. The social crises of child abuse and homelessness had affected the nation and were frequent topics of discussion.

SEVENTH GRADE, AGE 12: "HOMELESS"

In late July I decided to enroll in school. . . . The weather did not match my mood; it was a clear day, the sun bright, and summer showing everywhere. A foggy, gray, dismal day would have suited me much better. I reached Greenwood school and nervously entered the building through the wide double doors. A sign directed me to the office, and I saw a thin, withered lady behind the desk.

"May I help you, young lady?" she said in a tiny voice.

"I've come to sign up for seventh grade," I replied.

"Sorry dear, we need your parents here to sign some forms to let you attend school."

I was prepared, and said, "My mother is very sick and bed-ridden with a virus. She sent me, and I can surely bring her the papers to sign." I held my breath tensely in anticipation. The lady finally consented, handing me a pack of forms. . . .

This excerpt is probably self-explanatory.

EIGHTH GRADE, AGE 13: "THE STORY OF JULY: A GIRL WITH AIDS"

"Snap out of it, July," I told myself aloud. I walked along the beach, letting my bare feet get wet in the water. I waded in to my waist and stood still as the waves churned around me. My eyes filled with unexpected tears. I looked out at that deep, shimmering, blue sea that went on and on to the horizon. I was tempted to just dive in and forget everything else. I wanted to swim out into that wide, never-ending expanse of ocean until I could swim no more. Then I would just float along and be attached to absolutely nothing. I would be free from everything. Is that what being dead feels like?

In this excerpt the protagonist has just been taken to a cult community in the desert by her mother; the current real-world context at the time of her writing this story was that of the Waco, Texas, tragedy involving the Branch Davidian sect.

EIGHTH GRADE, AGE 13½: "CHILDREN OF THE CULT"

Clara was flabbergasted. This could not be happening. It was her first day, and already she was being tormented by this woman, who seemed intent on hating her and every child here. The kids all around her rose from sitting on their beds at the supervisor's command and lined up perfectly in order to go to the Dinner Hall. Clara sat miserably, her anger writhing in her stomach like snakes. She stared down at her hands

in her lap as the children filed out in complete silence. She vaguely
heard the heavy wooden door slam shut, and then she heard the springs
of a mattress squeak. Clara's head snapped around, and she saw the
bleak face of a girl who looked to be about her age.
    "Hey, what did you do?" Clara asked softly. . . .

The increasing sophistication in use of emotion language and emotion-evocative imagery as Heather matured is apparent in these excerpts. (Bear in mind that if children can demonstrate this sort of conceptual complexity in their written language, they are capable of comprehending and possibly producing this in oral language at a much younger age (e.g., Shweder et al., 1998.) At age 8 she has begun to use vocabulary to describe the *expressive aspects of emotional experience* (booming "voice" of the mountain, bawling, watching with interest, searching furiously, strutting and showing off, being pleasant, etc). By age 10 she uses images to describe the *physiological experience* of some emotions (heart skipping a few beats, fear shooting up her spine, sound like a roaring lion in her ears, etc.) and by age 13½, she uses more complex images to suggest how an emotion feels in the body (e.g., "anger writhing in her stomach like snakes"). By age 12 she has begun to incorporate more *complex images for mood states* (e.g., she would have preferred a foggy dismal day to match her mood), and by age 13 she uses physical imagery to suggest an *abstract emotional experience* (e.g., floating in the ocean, detached, as perhaps feeling like death). In the final excerpt, Heather distinguishes the protagonist's emotional experience by *juxtaposing it with others' contrasting emotional–expressive behavior*; for example, Clara is "flabbergasted" and "tormented" but the other children "lined up perfectly"; a moment later she sees the "bleak" face of another girl, but her voice is "soft" toward this other child. Her use of social juxtaposition allows for more dramatic portrayal of the ebb and flow of emotion in this narrative, creating tension and a state of dread for the protagonist.

Children's use of narrative structure is more than just tying together a string of scripts, although they do include script knowledge of event sequences. Narratives are stories, which means that they involve a goal or a problem to be solved (Nelson, 1996), and the previous excerpts capture this awareness of a "problem." The truncation of the excerpts prevents showing how goals were reached and problems solved in Heather's stories, but what is evident even in these brief excerpts is that emotions are the motivational dynamic behind the goals and problems. In addition, children's narratives reflect the varying emotional issues of both their day-to-day experience and more dramatic or intense events to which they may have been exposed (Shweder et al., 1998). Narratives have as their "grist for the mill," as it were, both the ordinary and the extraordinary experience of their creators. With the exception of the first story, all the others reflect the growing awareness of a young girl in our society of social issues (AIDS, cults, homelessness, abuse) or the impact of sudden natural disaster on humankind. I echo Shweder et al. (1998) in a plea for more descriptive research of how children's narratives, including those from different societies and subcultures, transform in the face of contextual change and individual development. I turn next to a discussion of a variety of studies on children's acquisition of an emotion-descriptive lexicon and its use in communication.

DEVELOPMENT OF EMOTION LANGUAGE AND LEXICON

On the one hand, emotional *development* is clearly evident in children's becoming able to access an emotion lexicon in ways that promote their insight into their own and others' emotional experience. Recall in Chapter 4 my description of Carroll and Steward's (1984) research on children's understanding of their own emotional experience; they found one exceptional 4-year-old child of a psychotherapist who demonstrated especially sophisticated emotion-related understanding, comparable to children twice her age; yet her performance was similar to the rest of her age group in that all performed at a preoperational level on Piagetian tasks. Thus, there seems to be a particular linkage between access to an emotion-related lexicon and exposure to adults who *talk* about emotion-laden events and a child's acquisition of more competent insight into emotional processes. I discuss research that confirms this view later in this chapter. On the other hand, *emotional competence* is evident in being able to use an emotion-descriptive lexicon in ways that more powerfully or creatively command social attention (perhaps by eliciting a shared emotional experience, through the use of emotionally evocative metaphors, etc.). In this sense, children who are emotionally competent with their emotion-related language may be even more socially efficacious than those children who demonstrate simply average expected emotion language development. The intriguing work of Gottman et al. (1997) suggests that this is indeed the case (see Chapter 3, for a discussion of their work).

Assuming an intact nervous system and an environment that is not overwhelmingly trauma-filled due to chronic or severe maltreatment (e.g., Cicchetti & Toth, 1993), children do show some commonalities in our culture in learning how to represent emotion. Harris

(1995) described the development of representation of emotion as children's learning to conceptualize consciousness, with *emotion being one aspect of consciousness.* He suggests that there may be three phases in children's understanding of consciousness: As preschoolers they believe consciousness to be completely under arbitrary control, perhaps a bit like a faucet. With the onset of concrete operations, children seem to view consciousness as having more continuity and perhaps not always under one's control (i.e., there is an involuntary quality to consciousness as well). Toward middle childhood children may recognize that consciousness has its limitations, and therefore it can be regulated; that is, one can change one's thoughts, one can distract oneself, one can strategically not attend to a disturbing thought or feeling. Tantalizing possibilities exist in this area for further research to address these three postulated phases of emotion as an integral facet of consciousness.

In addition to age-related differences in the normal acquisition of an emotion-descriptive lexicon (which also functions as a system for representing emotion), individual differences and cultural influence are again strong forces in the development of this skill of emotional competence. This is not surprising, as one of the critical functions of an emotion lexicon is to be able to communicate with others, which obviously entails reciprocal communication about emotion (or the relative lack thereof). We would expect socialization differences, family milieu, and culture-based meanings to affect not only *what* sort of emotion-related symbolic system is acquired but also *how* children develop their emotionally descriptive language. There has been a tremendous growth in research on children's representations of emotion, and I include here references to more detailed reviews for the interested reader. However, this area of emotional functioning continues to be "ripe" (if I may use an emotionally connotative word) with issues for further research.

EMOTION WORDS

Bretherton et al. (1986) reviewed the relevant literature on children's acquisition of emotion words, and what follows is substantially drawn from their material. They note that many toddlers can use emotion words toward the end of the second year, but as Smiley and Huttenlocher (1989) caution, what may be included as an emotion word, (e.g., crying) may simply be a behavioral action noted by the young child and conceivably is not used by the child to denote internal emotional state. By 3 years of age children can much more readily label the emotions of others in addition to their own feelings; they can refer to emotional experiences in the past and anticipate them in the future (try talking to a 2½-year-old about how he feels about injections). Increasingly, they can also verbally address the consequences of emotional states as well as the situational causes of emotions (e.g., "Grandma mad. I wrote on wall").

Children can also apply emotion terms to pretend play by age 2½, and, indeed, hearing a child talk while playing out a fantasy with her figurative toys (dolls, action figures, "little ponies," stuffed animals, etc.) is an excellent way to observe a young child's competence with emotion language, for she constructs both the causes of the figure's emotional response and the consequences of the emotion, including how the figure copes. One of my sisters related the following vignette to me, and it captures as well the narrative quality of children's fantasy play with goals to be reached or problems to be solved:

> Three-year-old Sanna had a long stuffed toy snake, named Sam, which she loved to wind and drape around her body. One day on a trip out in the countryside, her mother abruptly pulled the car over to the side of the road and with great distress announced that she thought she had just run over a "huge" snake. Of course, everyone was terribly curious, and it did turn out to be an impressive California Mountain Kingsnake; unfortunately, it continued to writhe while in its death throes, and Sanna's mother became quite distressed about its prolonged suffering and accidentally killing it. Sanna's older brother, John, wanted to take the body home and skin it for Show-and-Tell at his school; his mother successfully resisted this plan.
>
> On a number of occasions after the Kingsnake's death, Sanna acted out long, complicated fantasies with her toy snake, wherein chairs, strollers, and even doors were made to "crush" Sam-the-snake. Sanna then pretended to be Sam experiencing the pain with many moans, groans, and shrieks and cries of "help me, help me; I'm dying." Next Sanna "rescued" him, comforting him and telling him she would fix his hurt (she wrapped dishtowels around his "crushed" mid-section like a giant bandage). She told Sam, "Don't be scared," and sometimes "don't be sad." Then she began an elaborate hiding sequence of Sam so that her brother couldn't find him and "skin him." Nine-year-old John took great delight in teasing his sister about how he was going to skin Sam if he found him, causing Sanna to come unglued and to cry for her mom's intervention.

Researchers have also studied parents' reports of their children's understanding and use of emotion-descriptive words. Using parents' ratings on checklists of words indicating emotion states (e.g., "happy"), emotion traits (e.g., "good"), and physical states (e.g., "sleepy" and "clean"), Ridgeway, Waters, and Kuczaj (1985) tabulated the percentages of children at 6-month intervals (starting at 18 months and extending to 6 years of age) comprehending emotion words and also using them. The most frequently understood words at 18 months were "sleepy," "hungry," "good," "happy," "clean," "tired," and "sad" (50–83% comprehension). The toddlers' use of these words in their own verbal production was much lower; 50% used the word "good" whereas only 7% used the word "sad." By age 6, children comprehended such words as "nervous" (83%), "embarrassed" (77%), "jealous" (60%), and "miserable" (53%). Their corresponding production of these words was half to two thirds of the percentages for comprehension.

EMOTION DIALOGUES

Going beyond the description of frequency and range of feeling-state words, Dunn et al. (1987) investigated naturally occurring conversations in the home between young children and their mothers and siblings. They were particularly interested in determining the sorts of functions conversations about feelings had in the social exchange within the home and how children communicated causes of feelings in their exchanges with others. They followed the young children from age 18 months to 24 months and recorded the conversations as unobtrusively as possible. They found that the vast majority of feeling-state conversations were with the mother as opposed to the older sibling, although conversations involving all three occurred more often than those between just the two siblings. This finding suggests that access to an adult who is interested in their feelings may be pivotal to children's having opportunities to talk about emotions. Conversations about causes of feelings increased significantly in the 6 months they tracked the children. Mothers tended to use conversations about feelings as a functional way to guide or explain something to their children, whereas the children were more likely to use feeling-descriptive words simply to comment on their own reaction or observation of another. Thus, they were learning to communicate their own self-awareness of feeling states to their mothers, who in turn were likely to communicate *meaningfulness* to their children by using guiding, persuading, clarifying, or otherwise interpretive feeling-related language.

My reading of Dunn et al.'s research is that the mothers anchored for their young children *how* to make sense of what they were experiencing in themselves and occasionally about others. Interestingly,

Dunn et al. (1987) found a considerable decrease in mothers' responses to the children's use of distress-related feeling words as they matured from 18 to 24 months. This may be an example of mothers trying to deemphasize their children's attention to distress. Alternatively, by 24 months these children may be going through the "terrible twos" stage with their attendant bids for autonomy at all costs; they end up experiencing more distress because their mothers set limits (e.g., "No, you cannot put your toys in the toilet!" or "Don't play with the phone!") and therefore thwart them, causing a greater frequency of distress episodes which the mothers prudently ignore.

Dunn et al. (1991) continued their research on naturally occurring conversations about feelings in the home, but this time they extended their longitudinal study of children from 3 to 6 years of age. They again focused on children's and mothers' exchanges around causes and consequences of feelings and additionally tracked how disputes and conflicts in the home provided occasions for emotional growth in terms of how children were exposed to and had to use emotion-descriptive language to negotiate the conflict. They found a tremendous range in variability among the children in frequency of "feeling talk"—from 0 to 27 occasions per hour of observation. The mothers also showed a similar variability, ranging from 0 to 22 occasions of "feeling talk" per hour of observation. Unfortunately, Dunn et al. (1991) do not provide us with information as to whether the mother–child dyads were matched in their rates of "feeling talk." Given the findings of their earlier study where mothers were pivotal in providing opportunities for children to verbally communicate about their feelings, I would speculate that if a mother did not talk much about feelings and related inner states, it was likely that her child did not do so.

Relative to disputes, Dunn et al. (1991) found that an average of 22% of "feeling talk" concerned conflicts between child, mother, or sibling or among all three; the range was again considerable, varying from 0 to 75% across the households. When disputes were being negotiated, 67% of the conversations included reference to causes of feelings, whereas conversations that did not focus on conflicts referred to causes of feelings only 45% of the time.

Dunn et al. (1991) also examined the relationship between their various measures of "feeling talk" (taken at age 3) and a measure of social sensitivity at age 6. They assessed social sensitivity by using Rothenberg's (1970) audiotapes of a man and a woman in scenarios that depicted happiness, anger, anxiety, and sadness (note that we do not know the generalizability of their data based on this measure using adult models). The children were asked to describe the emotional transitions that occurred from beginning to the end of the tapes, and the adequacy of their commentary provided the rating for social sensitivity. The correlations between the Rothenberg measure and the "feeling talk" variables assessed at age 3 were impressive: The highest significant correlation was .47 with diversity of feeling themes present in mother–child conversations (themes as diverse as pain, disgust, distress, pleasure, etc.) and the lowest significant correlation was .34 for incidence of disputes. In between were conversations about causes of feelings and total number of "feeling talk" conversations between mothers and children. Although these correlations might not seem terribly large, when we take into account that these measures span 3 years, it is quite impressive to obtain that sort of continuity in children's understanding of and sensitivity to emotional cues at age 6 with their earlier conversations about feelings with their mother at age 3.

The special role played by conflict should also be reassuring to parents. As taxing as disputes with one's preschooler may be, disputes play an important role in children's learning to understand their own and others' feelings and to acquire the emotional lexicon to make themselves understood to others. As Dunn and Brown (1991) point out, when children are feeling badly, they are motivated to express, verbally and otherwise, their feelings to get their needs attended to. For them to attain that goal, they need to learn to communicate their feelings in ways that regulate not only their own behavior but that of others as well. Learning to express affection to a parent is also a highly effective way to elicit positive attention, and Dunn and Brown are emphatic in their contention that children desire pleasurable interaction, not just attention to their distress or pain.

Another study by Dunn and Brown (1994) shed further light on the effects of family emotional expression on children's acquisition of emotion-descriptive language. Again they found that occasions of negative feeling on the part of the child were when most emotion-related discourse occurred between mother and child. Quite intriguingly, this study also demonstrated that if families were characterized as high in frequency of anger and distress expression, the children were *less* likely to be engaged in discourse about feelings. But if the families were low in frequency of negative emotional expression, then when a negative emotional event did occur for the child, the likelihood of an emotion-related conversation to ensue between child and parent was greater. This research suggests that children's acquisition of emotion-descriptive language is anchored in relationship contexts: If everyone is angry or distressed a lot of the time, then an episode of distress on the part of a child may be viewed as trivial. What may be meta-communicated in such families is that a child's feelings are not very important. We can surmise how differences in the families' emotional milieus provide varying preparatory stages for their children's later emotional experiences in the world beyond the home (see, e.g., Davies & Cummings, 1994, for a review on marital conflict and child adjustment).

Finally, in research that looked at shared fantasy material, namely, storybooks, between young children and their mothers, Denham and Auerbach (1995) analyzed the emotional content of mothers' and preschoolers' dialogues while looking at picture books together (whose contents were emotion laden). They found that such an interaction was rich with adult–child exchanges that included affect labeling and causes and consequences of emotional experience. In addition, both mothers and children used their emotion-descriptive language in ways that suggested social influence of the other; for example, mothers who limited themselves to simple comments about the emotion-laden material in the picture books had children who asked more questions to engage their mothers more. However, those mothers who made use of verbal explanation to a great degree appeared to stimulate their children further to use more complex and elaborated emotion-descriptive language. These children tended to respond with more guiding and socializing language about the characters' emotional experience (e.g., "We don't hit cats with baseball bats," from the coding appendix). In a similar vein, Nelson (1996) reported on research that found that mothers who used narrative styles with their children while on outings to museums and the like also appeared to influence their children to use more frequently narrative structures in their own renditions of emotion-laden events.

STRUCTURAL ANALYSIS OF EMOTION-DESCRIPTIVE LANGUAGE

Moving on to older children, Russell and Ridgeway (1983) examined emotion-descriptive adjectives used by children in elementary school. They found that these words could be statistically analyzed using procedures (principal-components analyses and multidimensional scaling) that allow one to explore ways that word meanings can be grouped together. The result was that two bipolar axes (dimensions) were found that provided an organizational structure for the many emotion-related terms used by school children. These two dimensions were degree of pleasure or hedonic tone and degree of arousal, as in energizing quality. This structure can be visualized as a graph by placing the pleasure and arousal axes perpendicular to one another (i.e., make the vertical line the arousal axis and crossing it at midway is the pleasure axis). In the resulting four squares, such terms as "delighted" would be placed fairly high in the upper-right quadrant (relatively high pleasure and high arousal), whereas "droopy" would be in the diagonally opposite square, indicating that it is characterized by low energy or arousal and relatively low in pleasure or hedonic tone as well.

This dimensional analysis of emotion concepts is of interest for it suggests something about the way emotion is categorized and perhaps even organized as subjective experience. A number of cross-cultural comparisons have been made on emotion concepts used by adults in other languages (reviewed by Russell, 1991), and the pleasure/displeasure dimension has been reliably found in all the cultures studied. The arousal dimension has sometimes been mixed with degree of dominance/submissiveness. Perhaps in these cultures, as probably in our own, dominance is associated with high energy or arousal vis-à-vis others, whereas submissiveness is associated with low energy. Russell suggests that hedonic tone is relevant in all cultures in terms of how feeling states are differentiated (i.e., one's feelings can range from bad through neutral to good), but the English word "emotion" is not necessarily present in all languages, although an equivalent term is more the rule than the exception (exceptions appear to be the Tahitians, the Bimin-Kuskusmin of Papua New Guinea, the Gidjingali aborigines of Australia, the Ifalukians of Micronesia, the Chewong of Malaysia, and the Samoans; cited in Russell, 1991). In these few cultures where no term similar to emotion exists, feelings may be referred to as arising within certain body parts or organs; for example, the Chewong view the liver as the source of what for them might be called thoughts and feelings.

The significance of the virtually universal presence of the pleasure dimension in emotion-descriptive concepts may indicate that feelings get us ready for action. If something feels aversive, negative, and unpleasant, we are prepared to avoid it, flee or escape from it, or destroy it. Conversely, if something feels pleasurable, comforting, joyous, or fulfilling, we seek it out, we protect it, we want to prolong or repeat the experience. These have been referred to as *action tendencies* that are implied by most of our emotion terms (see Frijda, 1986, 1987, for further discussion). Having such feeling cues available to us clearly is an adaptive way for human beings to evolve in a collective sense, but it is also adaptive in the individual's own course of development. For the child learning emotion-descriptive concepts, a rapid shortcut now exists for figuring out what sorts of situations or interactions to avoid and what sorts to engage in. If parents tell a child that deep water is dangerous, scary, and something to be wary about (because he does not know how to swim yet and he is only 4 years old), and then they enroll him in swimming lessons the summer he turns 5 years old, no wonder he panics at the edge of the pool! This common occurrence can be looked at from how emotion language has been used with children by their care-givers to protect them from harm, that is, from actions that young children might undertake because they had no *negative* feelings about a situation or interaction. Thus, parents warn their children to stay away from certain situations, people, and events by using emotion-descriptive words that connote dire and terrible outcomes. Conversely, parents also cajole their children to act in certain ways or to engage in certain activities because of "how much fun it's going to be" or "you'll really like it after you learn how to do it." As an illustration, I suspect the majority of young children learning how to play a musical instrument hear such parental litanies, which are intended to encourage their perseverance in the face of all too frequent emotional defeat.

EMOTION SCRIPT LEARNING

Acquisition of emotion-descriptive concepts continues throughout childhood and into adolescence, but little research has examined these older age groups. I think that the way that emotion language develops further in the school-age child and adolescent is evidenced in their greater ability to add variety, subtlety, nuance, and complexity to their use of emotion-descriptive words with others. (For illustrations, see Heather's stories at the beginning of this chapter.) But also intriguing to me is that children's *scripts* for understanding social *and* emotional experience are reciprocally influenced by their growing access to increasing complexity of emotion concepts. A brief review of scripts in psychological research follows.

Definition of Scripts

Such theorists as White (1994) and Shweder (1993) have defined emotion scripts as interpretive *schemes* that provide a routine or plan for making sense of emotional experience in ways that are meaningful to the individual. However, we are still addressing an abstract construct that does not readily allow us to see how scripts are pragmatically used, especially in social interaction (cf. E. Goffman, 1967). The theoretical position taken by Abelson (1981) permits us to specify exactly how scripts might operate. He hypothesized that scripts provide us with a set of inferences about how certain situations "ought" to unfold. Scripts entail *sequential* expectancies and, as such, they allow us to access our beliefs about a *predictable event sequence* (Abelson, 1981). Abelson also emphasized that scripts require learning: One must learn that antecedent and consequent events are meaningfully linked, indeed, "enabled," to use Abelson's term. This means that when one of these antecedent events occurs, an expectancy is activated to embark on a course of action that follows the script. However, scripts are much more complex than simple habitual routines; they are fluid cognitive constructions that have built into them *variability that takes into account contextual features*. For example, we might have a script about anger that unfolds *generally* as follows:

1. An offense occurs that is perceived as intentional.
2. The offended person experiences intense negative emotion with accompanying physiological changes.
3. The offended person directs expression of negative emotion at the offender.
4. The offended person considers retribution.
5. The offended person undertakes reciprocal harm to the offender.

Let's concretize this sequence with an example.

1. Eleven-year-old Kate felt betrayed (offended) when Ellen blabbed all over the class the secret she had told her, namely, that her parents were getting divorced (Ellen's act was intentional and harmful to an innocent person).
2. While sitting at her desk, she felt herself getting hot and tense; she broke the tip of her pencil pressing down so hard on the paper (physical changes accompanying the negative emotion).
3. Kate glared at Ellen across the classroom (expression of negative emotion directed at the offender).
4. Kate knew that Ellen secretly liked a boy in the class named Tony; she imagined what she could do to Ellen to get back at her (retribution).
5. During the next recess Kate sneaked back into the classroom and put a note on Ellen's chair seat that said, "Tony says you are ugly and stupid." She added to the note a picture of a cross-eyed, stringy-haired face for good measure (reciprocal harm done to the offender).

Given that we learn variability as part of this anger script, that variability can influence each of the five subevents listed. The angered person may or may not require intentionality for some event to be perceived as offensive. The offended individual may not be aware of any accompanying physiological emotion-state change, and he or she might have limited awareness of feeling angry; perhaps he or she feels "irritation" or despondency instead. The expression of anger at the offender is highly variable: the risk of retribution from a more dominant individual or the violation of still other scripts may suppress this subevent. The offended person may consider retribution, but whether he or she actually undertakes it, simply imagines it, or flatly discounts it as appropriate behavior depends on contextual influence as well as on other scripts the individual may have that countermand the generic anger script. For example, a parent may be angry at her preadolescent, but she does not seek reciprocal harm because of her beliefs about appropriate parenting behavior.

My thinking about emotion scripts has also been much influenced by Russell (e.g., Russell, 1991), and he notes that even within the same culture, scripts for the same emotions may differ from person to person, for emotion scripts are linked to other belief networks, including scripts about the self and about the social roles we occupy. I take Russell's point here seriously. When we link a script for an emotion such as anger to a network of concepts we have about, for example, our sex role "adequacy," then the anger script may well have additional emphases or omissions if our machismo or our femininity is implicated in the anger episode. Consider, for example, the possible linkages between scripts for shame and scripts for gender role. The shame–rage cycle seen in male batterers and the frequent occurrence of shame–depression seen in women—also addressed by Lewis (1992b)—may illustrate intersecting scripts for emotion and gender role. I am also intrigued by the possible linkages between emotion scripts and scripts having to do with self-concept and self-attributions (see also Eder, 1994). Indeed, what we refer to as self-conscious emotions may in fact represent an interplay of scripts about standards for behavior and scripts about *how* the self plays a causal role in events.

Clearly scripts vary from culture to culture, and many social scientists have addressed the unfolding of emotion scenarios as predictable sequences. Just examining the many chapters in Russell et al.'s (1996) recent edited volume *Everyday Conceptions of Emotion* suggests how rich this area is for descriptive research. Recall the discussion of folk theories of emotion in Chapter 3: Such folk or naive theories are essentially a collection of scripts ascribed to by a given culturally defined group, and these naive theories may be tied together by an overarching dynamic or functional theme that was captured in the somewhat facetious metaphors I used to describe North American thinking about emotional functioning (the volcano theory, the tidal wave theory, etc.). Now consider some beliefs about emotion from a decidedly different culture: Wierzbicka (1994) provides the following examples from a longer list of *liver* images, used by the Australasian people Mangap-Mbula of New Guinea, for describing what we in English might call feelings:

Expression	English equivalent
kete- (I)malmal	angry (liver is fighting)
kete- (I)bayou	very angry (liver feels hot)
kete- pitpit	get excited too quickly (liver jumps)
kete- ikam ken	startled (liver does snapping)
kete- kutkut	anxious (liver beats)
kete- patnana	calm, unmoved, long-suffering (liver is rocklike)

Wierzbicka (1994) suggests that what diverse cultures have in common is the more generic term "feeling" and that the concept of *emotion,* if it is used to refer solely to internally experienced subjective states, may be limited to an Anglo-Saxon view. She concludes that "people all over the world . . . link feelings with notions of what people do and say and of *what they regard as good or bad*" (p. 155; emphasis added). It is this linkage of feelings with expectations of human action, which is more often social than not, and with evaluation of desirable or undesirable outcomes that yields discernible emotion scripts. To claim that one's liver is snapping does not qualify as a script per se; it needs to be linked with a predictable sequence of events. Perhaps the Mangap-Mbula script would take the form of "something quite unexpected happened, causing my liver to do some snapping, and it would be a good idea to find out what caused this unexpected event." But, perhaps their script would dictate instead that when someone's liver starts snapping, some spirits are sneaking about, and he or she must undertake appeasement rituals. In sum, we find cultural similarities if we stay with fairly general statements about human beings' propensities *to feel,* and we find diversity when we venture into specific cultural scripts that vary in the meanings attributed to antecedents of emotional experience, in what are viewed as desirable goals, and even in the concept of emotion itself.

Children's Use of Scripts

Children learn emotion scripts not as full-blown symbolic structures but cumulatively through such emotion-laden interactions as social referencing (Walden, 1991), narrative interaction with others (Miller & Sperry, 1987), exposure to emotional events (Gordon, 1989), significant others' socializing responses to emotional–expressive behavior (Saarni, 1993), and so forth. Not surprisingly, emotion scripts become more complex as cognition develops and the social domain expands. How might one examine emotion script *deployment* among children? At least four strategies are available for empirical purposes.

1. One strategy is to examine how children behave when a social expectation is violated. When this happens, the antecedent event within a script has occurred, but the predicted consequence has not, and children are pressed both to manage the unexpected social interaction and to regulate their own emotional experience in it.

2. Another method is to sample directly developmental differences in children's deployment of complex script understanding in social–emotional interaction, such as "How do you cheer someone up?" That is, one can take a particular emotion-laden social interaction and examine the developmental differences that occur in children's interactive behavior (e.g., interpersonal negotiation skills). These developmental differences should reflect differences in the children's cognitive complexity and social maturity such that their understanding of the script(s) surrounding the emotion-laden interaction influences how they respond in the interaction.

3. A third strategy is to elicit from children their expectancies about "good" and "bad" consequences as a result of some emotional experience. "Good" consequences are more likely to represent consensually defined and predicted script outcomes; "bad" outcomes are due to not following the socially prescribed script sequence.

4. Finally, a currently popular strategy is to collect narratives that are told to children, about children, or overheard by children such that children acquire verbally mediated representations about views of the world, attitudes toward others as well as toward the child, and beliefs about the self (e.g., Miller, 1994). Narratives embody multiple scripts, and narratives and scripts are structurally similar: Both are typically based on personally meaningful events, they are causally and temporally ordered, and they are oriented toward value-laden outcomes.

Justifications as Scripts

To illustrate what children's script usage might "sound" like in their own words, I refer to a social cognition study I undertook (Saarni, 1997) with children, ages 6 to 8 and 10 to 12 years, to investigate their expectancies for how to cope when feeling sad, angry, afraid, hurt, or ashamed. I designed five hypothetical vignettes, each featuring one of the preceding emotions. The controllability of outcome, intensity of emotion, and degree of affiliation between the peer protagonists were controlled. The children were provided with coping strategies, including problem-solving, support-seeking, distancing, internalizing, and externalizing options (these are further defined in Chapter 9). Children chose the "best" and "worst" coping strategies and justified their choices as well as responded to what they would do in a similar situation. Results indicated that there were no age or gender differences in which strategy was selected as best or worst for any of the emotion-linked vignettes; however, younger children tended to provide more simplistic justifications, as expected. Problem solving was most often cited as the best coping strategy when feeling shamed or angry, support seeking when feeling sad, and both problem solving and support seeking were equally nominated when fearful. Distancing was viewed as the best strategy when one's feelings were hurt. Children overwhelmingly chose the aggressive externalizing coping strategy as the worst option across all emotion stories, and both social and nonsocial consequences were cited as the justification for why it was the least desirable coping strategy (but see one of the rare exceptions among the examples shown next).

The justifications that children provided for their choices allow us to examine their script knowledge as well; namely, they are able to suggest a predictable event sequence with clear indication as to why the particular behavioral sequence yields desirable or undesirable consequences. Indeed, the children's scripts were well-anchored in context and socially shared meanings as illustrated in a few of the justifications they offered as to why a particular coping strategy was selected as best. Note how the younger children's justifications represent more concrete scripts about coping with upsetting emotions:

> Seven-year-old female, after choosing the distancing coping strategy when the protagonist felt hurt: "Maybe if she did that [walked away from the other kids teasing her about her new jacket], it wouldn't hurt her feelings, because she wouldn't hear what they are saying."

The schematic script knowledge here is that when one's feelings are hurt, one should leave the scene to avoid further hurt.

> Eight-year-old female, after choosing the problem-solving strategy when the protagonist felt afraid about a big growling dog: "It's better to be late and go the other way than get chewed up, because if you're chewed up, your arm would be really hurt."

The schematic script knowledge here is that some negative consequences are worse than others and one should weigh the relative risks of choosing between "the lesser of two evils."

> Eleven-year-old female, after choosing the problem-solving strategy of assertively explaining to a friend (who had irresponsibly damaged the protagonist's new toy and thus provoked her anger) the importance of restitution for neglectful damage: "Debbie [the one who damaged the toy] would probably get a new ball in the end [to replace the one she had neglectfully wrecked], and Allison and Debbie would still be friends."

The schematic script knowledge here is that between friends it is a good idea to speak one's mind and provide a solution to an interpersonal conflict that would otherwise threaten a relationship if left unresolved.

> Eleven-year-old male, after choosing the externalizing strategy when the protagonist felt shamed by the teasing received over his pants ripping open on the playground: "He'd get even with him [for teasing him about the ripped pants], but he'd feel kinda' gross because he forgot his underwear, and that's kinda' stupid."

This boy's response was rare in the sample; however, it demonstrates the variability of schematic script knowledge, which in this case appears to be that if one's status is diminished, one should seek to reciprocate the damage to the "offender." Additional script knowledge here suggests that the boy thought the protagonist *should* feel shamed because he acted stupidly in allegedly forgetting his underwear. Interestingly, in the story the protagonist ripped his pants and his underwear were showing, not absent, as this subject child interpreted the scene.

In summary, these children had learned very well by the early school years what the socially approved scripts for dealing with aversive feelings and circumstances were, including, for the last preadolescent boy cited, the "necessity" for maintaining one's status. Yet it is also readily apparent that knowing what is socially sanctioned as a coping strategy is not necessarily how children actually behave when they are feeling scared, angry, hurt, sad, or ashamed. A critical missing ingredient that links scripts and immediate, contextualized behavior is the self's perceived vulnerability, which the last boy's response suggests may be critical when children react aggressively to their peers' minor provocations. Scripts provide children with culturally meaningful emotional experience, *and* they provide plans of action for managing both one's feeling state and the circumstances surrounding the emotional experience. In this sense, scripts span a time frame that extends from emotion elicitation through emotion management and culminates in adaptive social–situational behavior. With development, children both acquire and further revise their emotion scripts such that subtlety and complexity become more accessible to them in their emotional experience and in their interpersonal negotiation skills. I turn next to a discussion of individual differences in children's use of an emotion-descriptive lexicon and scripts for emotional functioning.

INDIVIDUAL DIFFERENCES AND CULTURAL INFLUENCE

Gender Differences

Researchers have typically not found sex differences in children's use of emotion words per se at young ages, but at older ages girls appear to be more motivated to talk about feelings and thus gain more experience in doing so. Thus, by adolescence girls are likely to be more comfortable using an emotion-descriptive lexicon, but many girls may exhibit a less well-developed repertoire of emotional scripts to deal with some emotional experiences, such as anger (Golombok & Fivush, 1994) . However, the gender of the young child does appear to elicit different styles of talking about emotion from the children's caregivers. For example, Dunn et al. (1987) found, in their study of young British children who were learning to talk about feelings, that little girls *received* more comments and inquiries about feelings from their mothers and their older siblings than did little boys; however, the boys and girls themselves were similar in their initiation of conversations about feelings. In a later study, Dunn et al. (1991) also did not find gender differences in children's production of emotion-related language when using an older age group (3 to 6 years). Fivush (1991), in a study with mothers of 3-year-old boys and girls, also examined whether caregivers speak differently to children depending on their gender. She found that mothers tended to talk in a more elaborate fashion about sadness with their daughters and more about anger with their sons. She found that mothers tended to embed their discussions of feelings in social frameworks more with their daughters than with their sons. Relative to script notions, she also found that when anger was involved, mothers emphasized relationship repair with their daughters and were more accepting of retaliation by their angry sons. Using methodology that involved storytelling accompanied by props (a toy house and family figures), Cervantes and Callanan (1998) did find sex differences: Young preschool boys showed an age-related increase in their use of emotion terms whereas the little girls did not, because these little girls had a higher frequency to begin with in using emotion words. Finally, in terms of range and frequency of comprehension and production of emotion-descriptive vocabulary, Ridgeway et al. (1985) did not report finding sex differences, even though they took care to balance the number of pre-school boys and girls whose vocabulary was evaluated by their parents.

In research on elementary school children's verbalized under-standing of emotional experience, such as the studies described in Chapters 4 and 5, gender differences in use of emotion-related lan-guage are similarly uncommon. However, when we consider the idea of script knowledge, especially the idea of emotion scripts interacting with other social behavior scripts such as sex role, we would expect gender differences to appear in how emotion scripts are to be played out vis-à-vis social transactions with others. Fivush's (1991) research suggests that parents may indeed expose their young children to different scripts for some emotions. That adults appear to experience sex differ-ences in style of emotion communication is certainly borne out by the spate of popular books (e.g., Brown & Gilligan, 1992; Gilligan, 1982; Glass, 1992; Gray, 1992) that speak to men's and women's different styles and approaches to emotional communication. In Chapter 8 I re-turn to this idea of multiple scripts interacting with one another, for when children realize that they need not show how they really feel, they learn to manage their emotional–expressive behavior *in conjunction with* other social goals (e.g., how to save face, how to impress others, and how to spare the feelings of another). Indeed, when sex differences are found in children's emotional functioning, it is more often in their behavioral enactment and expression of emotion (e.g., Casey, 1993; Da-vis, 1995; Saarni, 1984; Terwogt & Olthof, 1989) rather than their ver-balized knowledge of emotion.

Social Maturity Differences: The Special Case of Deafness

Given this chapter's emphasis on the acquisition of an emotion-descriptive lexicon, I thought it would be interesting to look at how hearing-impaired children acquire emotion categories. Investigations of children's acquisition of an emotion symbolic system when sensori-motor impairments are present not only provide us with much needed information about how to serve the social and educational needs of these children but also shed light on how emotion symbolic systems function communicatively and conceptually to promote emotional competence. Within the parameters of the disability, deaf (or blind) children may be able to develop an emotion symbol system that is self-efficacious in their interactions with others (e.g., Greenberg & Kusché, 1993). Indeed, within "deaf culture," those who cannot sign are less emotionally competent than those who can when it comes to effective communication with similar peers (cf. Kusché, 1984).

The more I read in this area the more I began to realize that the methodology used in research on deaf children's understanding of emotion concepts was frequently poor and insensitive; often the interviewers did not even attempt to use the communication "language" (i.e., sign language) of the subjects. This would be analogous to asking a Spanish-speaking child who knew only a little English to respond to a variety of complex questions solely in English! As Manfredi (1993) notes, hearing experts reciprocally demonstrate their handicap in communication skills when they attempt to converse with deaf signing experts. Indeed, Manfredi reports in her own research that when deaf subjects were administered the Thematic Apperception Test in sign language by another trained deaf individual, their signed projective responses were more articulated and complex than when they responded to a hearing test administrator. In short, when using their own emotion symbol system, they readily demonstrated competence. Greenberg and Kusché (1993) also contend that differences between deaf and hearing children are reduced or become negligible when nonverbal tasks are used; however, they believe that deaf children will generally show socially immature attributions about emotion-eliciting situations because their verbal labeling of emotions tends to be underdeveloped relative to hearing children.

Deaf children's play seemed like an area in which their emotion symbol systems should be observable, given the prevalence of nonverbal play activity and the low performance demands. Spencer and Deyo's (1993) excellent review of young deaf children's play informed me that much of the research is difficult to interpret because most investigators did not consistently track whether the deaf children had deaf or hearing parents. This critical piece of information is related to how readily, quickly, and reciprocally signing is introduced to the deaf infant. Preschool-age deaf children with deaf parents are apparently not especially different from hearing children when it comes to the social and cognitive sophistication of their play, according to Spencer and Deyo. However, deaf children with hearing parents who do not learn to sign are at risk for social and cognitive delays. This finding tells us that exposure to emotional conversations, whether they are spoken or signed, is what is important for young children. With such early exposure they are more likely to acquire a system of symbols with which they can communicate meaningfully about emotional experience, whether their own or others'. A replication of the research of Dunn and her colleagues (Dunn et al., 1987, 1991) with deaf children and their signing parents would be very useful.

True, the deaf child is restricted to having someone in her visual field to both send and receive communications, but given the repetitiveness and redundancy in most emotion socialization encounters between child and parent, I would guess that deaf children acquire their families' messages about how to make sense of things from an emotional perspective in ways similar to hearing children and in a similar time frame (assuming the parents sign with their infant or toddler). A problem for the majority of deaf infants is that their deafness is not hereditary and is more often the result of fetal or maternal medical complications. This means that there may be other conditions surrounding such young infants' early lives that compromise development. In addition, hearing parents may not realize that their baby is hearing impaired and thus do not initiate the compensatory communicative strategies needed for nurturing a deaf infant (e.g., emphatic nonverbal communicative cues, increased touching, gesturing and signing). Although some research has found that deaf children have lower frustration thresholds, tend to be impulsive, and act immaturely (reviewed in Greenberg & Kusché, 1993), it may not be the deafness per se but rather the neurological impairment involved in the original cause of deafness, ongoing stress in the birth mothers' lives, or deficits in hearing parents' communication with their deaf infants that contribute to such a behavioral pattern. Finally, although it would not be surprising to find out that deaf children acquire emotion categories and concepts that have some qualitatively different features when compared to hearing children's emotion concepts, such differences do not mean deficiencies. This is clearly an area that is more than ready for investigations that are both sound in methodology and sensitive in their approach; interested readers are referred to Marschark (1993) for further review of relevant issues in investigating development in deaf children. Readers are also referred to Greenberg and Kusché (1993) for a discussion of the positive gains in emotion understanding found after using a yearlong school curriculum "package" with deaf children.

Cultural Influence

We can think of cultural influence on the acquisition of an emotional lexicon as related to how societies use language to regulate emotion within social interaction. Many societies emphasize some emotional responses over others by attaching special importance to certain emotion-descriptive words. In American culture, the word "love" is such an emotionally loaded word. In recent years, "shame" has also been found to be a similarly emotionally loaded word, perhaps so much so that people do not especially even want to talk about shame, probably because emotionally aversive reminiscence ensues. Thus, when we use the word "love" with someone, we want to evoke in our relationship with that person joyful, affectionate, and enduring feelings. In contrast, when we tell others that they ought to feel ashamed, we create for ourselves a controlling, put-down, judgmental stance toward the other, whom we expect to cease and desist from doing whatever it was that we righteously thought they should not be doing.

Many anthropologists have examined emotion-descriptive language (see Russell, 1991, for an excellent review of cultural similarities and differences in how emotions are categorized in different languages and cultures as well as Wierzbicka, 1992). Briefly, Russell argued that our emotion lexicon should be understood as scripts (see the earlier anger example). These scripts can vary in how narrow or general they are for assorted feelings; the result is that in some cultures an emotionally toned response may be represented in the lexicon with relatively little elaboration (it is generally defined) and in others it would have many descriptors attached to it. A good example is anger. In English, anger has many variants (irritation, annoyance, frustration, vexation, aggravation, etc.) whereas for the Buganda of Uganda, anger and sadness may be interchangeable (Orley, 1973) and appear to be appropriate to a rather broad range of events which an English speaker would differentiate (as cited in Russell, 1991). Russell contended that to understand another culture's emotion scripts, we also need to understand the larger folk theory of emotion in which individual scripts are embedded. As a result, we cannot simplistically make comparisons across cultures of whether one or another emotion concept or symbol is much the same or, for that matter, radically different, a view similarly echoed by Wierzbicka (1994).

The perspective on ethnotheories (or folk theories) of emotion, which were described in Chapter 3, has also been emphasized by Catherine Lutz (1987, 1988; Lutz & White, 1986) in her work on cultural meanings in an emotion lexicon. Lutz (1987) states, "Emotion concepts have embedded in themselves crucial cultural propositions and in turn are nested in larger networks of knowledge about persons, roles, and goals" (p. 307). I believe that the more that two societies differ from one another in these cultural propositions and in the larger networks, the more their emotion symbol systems also differ from one another (recall the earlier list of liver images, used by the Australasian people Mangap-Mbula of New Guinea, for describing what we in English might call feelings). In sum, we find cultural similarities if we stay with fairly general statements about human beings' propensities *to feel*, and we find diversity when we venture into specific cultural meanings, goals, and social systems, including the concept of emotion itself.

Before concluding this chapter, I thought it would be interesting to provide a couple of descriptions of how children develop skills in their society's emotion lexicon such that they become effective emotional communicators. The two societies I will describe clearly show the children becoming emotionally more competent and self-efficacious as they acquire these emotional lexicons.

Samoa

Elinor Ochs's (1986) review of Samoan children's acquisition of emotion-descriptive language provides us with a delightful contrast to English-speaking, Western-reared children's acquisition of emotion-related concepts. I begin with a quote from Ochs, which refers to how the "terrible 2's" are experienced in Samoa:

> Every Samoan parent we questioned said that their child's first word was *tae,* a term meaning "shit." The term is a curse, a reduced form of *'ai tae,* meaning "eat shit." This conventional interpretation of a child's first word reflects the Samoan view of small children as characteristically strong-willed, assertive, and cheeky. Indeed, at a very early point in their language development, children use the curse frequently and productively to disagree, reject, and refuse and to prevent or stop some action from being carried out. (pp. 264–265)

I had to laugh when I tried to imagine American parents hearing such expletives every time their 2-year-old intended to say "no!" Samoan children also learn very early to use sympathy-inducing markers in their speech when referring to themselves to increase the likelihood of getting something for themselves (attention, food, etc.). Thus, these 2- to 3-year-olds typically refer to themselves as "poor me" or "dear me," and I would guess that if they were not successful in getting what they wanted, they probably cried out, "Eat shit!" Only later do Samoan children apply such sympathy markers to others in their speech.

Early speech is clearly used for emotional communicative purposes, even though the Samoan language does not have an equivalent word to the English word "emotion." According to Ochs, emotion is encoded in Samoan grammar phonologically, morphologically, and syntactically. It is embedded in who speaks to whom and in what sequence, and of course, emotion is also conveyed by loudness, pitch, and intonation. It is almost as though affect and feelings are so omnipresent in Samoan speech, that a specific word designating emotion as an internal state is not necessary. Indeed, feelings are viewed more as reactions and actions in Samoan society rather than internal states. For example, Ochs describes parents warning their naughty children that they will not love them anymore. Because of how verbs of feeling (e.g., loving) are used with a morphological marker that renders the verb as *instrumental,* what this means is that withdrawal of love in Samoan is the *same* as withdrawal of goods and services. In English the assumption is that withdrawal of love from someone is the *cause* for subsequently taking away goods and services. In English, if we have been summarily rejected, we assume that the person we thought loved us has had a "change of heart" (note the locus of state change is inside the body). Samoans have not been rejected until they notice that they are no longer on the receiving end of someone's attention, and it is irrelevant as to whether that person changed "on the inside" his or her opinion: one is simply cut off from one's "supply."

Mexican-American Immigrants

Eisenberg (1986) describes an ethnographic study of two little girls in California whose parents had emigrated from central Mexico just a few years before. The girls had access to extended families in both California and Mexico, and Spanish was the only language spoken in the home. Eisenberg followed the families for about a year, starting when the girls were about 2 years old, and her focus was on the function of teasing. Teasing is a curious sort of emotional exchange: Multiple levels of communication are involved, which may range from playfulness to sarcastic irritation, but teasing comments are meant to control the social and emotional behavior of the individual at whom they are directed by using mock challenges, insults, or threats. The two young girls, Marisa and Nancy, were often teased by adults, mothers, and uncles especially. Their mothers teased them about being crazy, about not loving them anymore, or about breaking up some other relationship their daughters had. The uncles were more likely to tease their nieces about being ugly or to make threats about injuring them. The teasing exchange was often to amuse others witnessing it and frequently was repetitious so that the child knew not to take it seriously and could begin to learn reciprocally to challenge the adult in the back-and-forth banter. Messages of social control were often evident, however, and I quote a passage below:

> [Nancy (N, 24 months) and her mother (M) are sitting on the stoop with their neighbor, Ceci (C), an older woman. Nancy pulls away when Ceci tries to hug her.]
>
> M: Oye, Nancy. Dale un besito a Ceci. (Listen, Nancy. Give Ceci a kiss.) [N whines and pulls away.]
>
> C: Un besito. [Sighs heavily, shaking head] Ah, pues, ya no te voy a querer. (A kiss. Ah, then, I'm not going to love you any more.)

M: [To C, shaking her head, clicking tongue] No le de manzana ni nada lo que quiere. (Don't give her an apple or anything she wants.)

C: [Shakes her head] Ya, no. Pues, porque ya no me quiere. (Not any more. Because she doesn't love me any more.)

[To N] Verdad que ya no me quieres? (Isn't it true that you don't love me anymore?) (p. 189)

Nancy's mother and neighbor collude to tease her about her refusal to hug Ceci and threaten not to give her things that she might want because, by implication, she does not deserve them if she does not demonstrate "love" for the gift giver. As the year went by, Eisenberg observed that Nancy did not develop as much skill at reciprocal teasing as did Marisa, in part because Nancy was often the target of the teasing and adults seemed more frequently to enjoy upsetting her. Marisa's exposure to teasing in her family was more playful, and she was given help by another adult or older child to facilitate her teasing rebuttal.

CONCLUSION

Social conversations are the primary vehicle in which children learn not only emotion-descriptive language but, importantly, how to use such language in their exchanges with others to achieve social–emotional goals. This skill of emotional competence is intimately linked to self-efficacy; with the acquisition of an emotion lexicon and strategies for using it with others, we can make our emotional experiences understood by others across time and space as well as use this skill to regulate the emotional qualities of our relationships with others.

As suggested by the research on scripts and narratives, children demonstrate skillfulness in learning their culture's routines for making sense of their affective experience by using fluid schemes and stories. These schemes and stories provide for an individualized conceptual elaboration of what exactly is emotionally salient for the child or adolescent. Unique and personal values, concerns, and expectancies are embedded in scripts and narratives. Near the beginning of the chapter I used the phrase "emotional thumbprint" as a way of metaphorically capturing the unique patterns in the narratives each of us tells about our emotional experience. Therapists, counselors, and probably effective teachers and parents try to comprehend those emotional thumbprints as a way to understand children's and youth's emotional experience with greater depth and accuracy. Being able to listen to and genuinely hear the emotion-laden stories of others is also functioning in an emotionally competent manner, and it is certainly part of the next skill of emotional competence to be discussed: empathy.

NOTE

1. Mei Yao Ch'en's (1965) poem in its entirety follows:

"Sorrow"

Heaven took my wife. Now it
Has also taken my son.
My eyes are not allowed a dry season.
When the rain falls and enters
The earth, when a pearl drops into
The depth of the sea, you can
Dive in the sea and find the
Pearl, you can dig in the earth
And find the water. But no one
Has ever come back from the
Underground Springs. Once gone, life
Is over for good. My chest
Tightens against me. I have
No one to turn to. Nothing,
Not even a shadow in a mirror.

Chapter 7

Skill 4: The Capacity for Empathic Involvement

Capacity for empathic and sympathetic involvement in others' emotional experiences.

In terms of emotional competence, empathic responsiveness may be one of the most significant components for promoting social bonds among people and fostering prosocial behavior. Without empathy as a component of emotional competence, one could conceivably demonstrate all the other "skills" of emotional competence in a Machiavellian or even sociopathic fashion. A good con artist knows how to use many of the skills of emotional competence described so far. He or she could readily infer the emotions of others and may be quite articulate in using emotion-descriptive language. Indeed, con artists may be very adept in creating empathic responsiveness in others toward themselves, but their own empathy is feigned.

Empathy, *feeling with* others, and sympathy, *feeling for* others, are emotional responses that connect us with others. On a larger scale, even society recognizes the importance of empathy and sympathy, for without them we would have no sense of mercy or clemency when dispensing justice. Empathy has also been referred to as one of the moral emotions, the others being guilt and shame (Zahn-Waxler & Robinson,

1995). The moral stance taken when we feel empathy (or guilt) upon witnessing another's distress is a felt sense of personal responsibility to ameliorate that person's distress. If we think of emotions as motivators of subsequent action, then feeling empathic toward someone's plight may nudge us toward becoming personally involved and doing something to help. But it is also evident that there are times when we feel empathy toward another's distress yet rather than doing something that might help the other, we turn our backs and focus on alleviating our own personal emotional upset. Consider the following vignette that contrasts these two responses upon witnessing others' distress.

Hannah and Maggie shared a big oversized multicolored umbrella as they walked home from middle-school in a rain storm that felt like solid sheets of water falling from the sky. They approached a mini-mart where they usually stopped to buy snacks. Next to the entrance, huddled under the overhang, was a woman with two young children. Their misery was made more acute by their obvious poverty. The girls paused, and while looking at them, Hannah sighed as she commented on how sad they looked. As they watched, the woman began begging for money from a man leaving the store.

Maggie grabbed her friend's arm and said tensely, "I don't want to go in there." Hannah responded firmly, "Oh yes we are!" and headed for the door. Hannah bought two half pints of chocolate milk and clutched her change. As they were leaving, Hannah turned to the woman and gave the umbrella to her. She handed the two cartons of chocolate milk to the kids, along with her change. The woman thanked her, and Hannah helped the younger one to open his carton as Maggie carefully kept Hannah positioned between herself and the family, her eyes downcast as she busily studied the wet cement.

As they continued on toward home, getting thoroughly drenched, Maggie said to Hannah, "I know you felt sorry for them, but she was so awful, making her kids go with her while she tried to get money. Why didn't she leave them at home . . . ?" Hannah responded, "I wasn't sure they had a home." Maggie pulled her coat over her head and muttered something about Hannah getting in trouble for giving away the umbrella. Hannah explained that she was certain her mom and dad would have done the very same thing.

Hannah's sympathetic concern for the homeless woman and her children was conjoined with a sense of personal responsibility to try to help. Her family held as a value that one should help others in need, and Hannah, while moved by the homeless family's obvious misery, was able to focus pragmatically on what she could do that would assist them. In contrast, Maggie appeared tense and reluctant to engage in any way with the family. Her preference would have been to walk past and avoid encountering them altogether, even if it meant forfeiting her customary snack after school. Afterward, Maggie may have tried to explain away her discomfort by suggesting the mother was "unfit" and that Hannah might be punished for giving away the umbrella. Such reactions, blaming the victim or censuring the helper, are also common responses in our media portrayals of crime or trauma victims. These responses are also part of the mind-set that short-circuits empathy such that it cannot be recruited to facilitate prosocial action. Hannah's emotional competence *and* moral character are such that she can use her empathic responsiveness to guide her as she aids others without becoming excessively distressed herself in the process.

Maggie's reaction would have been labeled *personal distress* by researchers studying differences among people upon witnessing others' negative emotional predicaments. Some scientists suggest that reactions of personal distress may indicate immaturity or an egocentric focus (e.g., Eisenberg et al., 1989). Others think that a personal distress reaction may occur when the observed individual's anguish, pain, distress, and so on are so intensely and vividly displayed that our boundaries between what is another's experience and our own become blurred (e.g., Zahn-Waxler & Robinson, 1995). People clearly differ in their thresholds as to what they respond to as intensely expressed emotion, and perhaps it is with low thresholds that the immaturity explanation makes more sense. On the other hand, perhaps personal distress is also evoked when we are confronted with an intense display of another's distress *but there is nothing we can do that is under our control* to intervene, to comfort, or to remedy the distress-causing circumstances.

A further significance about the differences among empathy, sympathy, and personal distress reactions is the subsequent behavioral response to the person experiencing anguish. When empathically responding, we might simply weep right along with the distressed person. When sympathetically responding, we might try to do something to comfort or ameliorate the difficult circumstances (e.g., helping and prosocial behavior). However, when feeling personally distressed by someone else's plight, we might avoid or rapidly depart from the situation as a strategy for ameliorating *our* aversive emotional experience (e.g., turning off the television when an especially gruesome newscast comes on about ethnic genocide, famine, or the ravages of disease in a refugee camp). I turn next to a description of the major developmental milestones in empathy and its accompanying prosocial behavior.

DEVELOPMENT OF EMPATHY AND SYMPATHY

For describing this aspect of emotional competence I have drawn heavily on Eisenberg and Strayer (1987), Zahn-Waxler and Robinson (1995) on the early origins of empathy and guilt, and Kurtines and Gewirtz (1991) on moral behavior and development. Readers are referred to these excellent sources for further elaboration. Beginning with early infancy, it is clear that very young babies respond to others' emotional–expressive behavior (see Chapter 5). Thus, this early attentiveness to emotional–expressive cues paves the way for later vicariously induced emotion, for we cannot be "induced" to experience another's emotional state unless we notice it and consider it salient.

Some researchers have also thought that the emotion "contagion" effect seen in early infancy is a precursor of empathy (e.g., one baby in the day-care center begins to cry and within a short time there is a whole chorus of wailing and weeping babies). Even as adults our emotional experience can be influenced by exposure to emotion-laden social interaction; we might recall feeling increasingly tense as others around us began to fret and show distress (try flying in a small commuter plane or maybe getting stuck in an elevator). Weeping along with our fellow audience in sentimental movies designed to be "tear-jerkers" may also be examples of emotion contagion (see also Hatfield, Cacioppo, & Rapson, 1994). Indeed, we may be prone to some degree of motor mimicry that is not even particularly emotional (e.g., yawning).

The consensus among researchers is that empathy and sympathy require the cognitive acquisition of a self distinguished from others and to some degree the ability to figure out the emotional state of the other (e.g., to recognize that some other person is *feeling something*). However, having the mental capacity for taking another's perspective and thus inferring his or her emotional state sounds emotionally detached, and empathic responding is in fact quite emotionally engaged. Sympathetic responding (or compassion or possibly pity if it does not contain elements of condescension) retains a greater degree of detachment from the other's emotional plight in a way that empathy does not appear to do so. Thus some other ingredient is also necessary to experience empathy.

Strayer (1987) is emphatic about the emotional involvement that is central to experiencing empathy: "An intelligent psychopath may have good role taking skills, but may use them only to manipulate others for personal gain. Again, the affective aspect of empathy is critical" (p. 225). She discusses the seeming paradox between empathy requiring a *merging* of self with another's emotional experience and simultaneously requiring a *differentiation* of the self from the other. Identifying with someone's emotional experience and projecting oneself into the emotion-eliciting situation are processes that facilitate our sharing in another's emotional response. But what keeps us from literally believing we are in the same situation and thus feeling exactly the same as the other person is knowing that we are, in fact, distinct from the other. We are not in the same emotion-eliciting situation. However, identification and projection can result in the person's becoming fixed on his or her own vicariously evoked emotion, akin to what may be happening in personal distress reactions when we are exposed to others' anguish or misery. For empathy to arouse sympathetic concern and pave the way for prosocial behavior, the focus needs to include the *other person* in conjunction with, yet distinct from, the self.

Four Phases of Empathy

Strayer (1987) described a view of empathy, derived from Theodore Reik's work (1949), consisting of four phases. She applied these four phases to describe what might occur developmentally as young children mature. The first is a less-than-conscious responsiveness to emotion cues, whether in a person's expressive behavior or in arousing contextual cues. Strayer suggested that this phase can occur in very young children (i.e., the emotion contagion effect mentioned previously), and it should broaden with age because of our increasing exposure to meaningful emotional cues.

The second phase requires an imaginal "introjection" of the other person into ourselves; in other words, we not only put ourselves in their shoes, so to speak, we can also "walk" in their shoes. The same sort of capacity may be evident in how young preschoolers can become completely absorbed in fantasizing themselves as superheros as they adopt karate stances or drape themselves in capes and the like. Readers of the *Calvin and Hobbes* comic strips may recall a strip in which Calvin imagines himself as a heroic adventurer and cannot comprehend why he is being compelled to eat some suspicious-looking food placed before him by someone apparently impersonating his mother. Calvin's imagined role expands into his everyday existence, including his perceptions and feelings. Strayer suggested that this second phase requires a permeable self-other boundary, for a rigid boundary would not allow for the imagined feeling of another's experience. She speculated that at this point some individuals experience personal distress and truncate the empathy process to attend to their own emotionally aversive state, whereas those with a more secure and differentiated sense of self may be able to sustain the vicarious emotional response such that they move toward the third phase.

The third phase is characterized by a "reverberation" or "resonance" between the imagined feelings of the other person and our own evoked similar experiences. This phase is truly the shared emotion phase, for the other's emotional state becomes "charged" with emotion meanings based in our own experience. This would also be the phase that is elaborated the most with development, as it is the richness of our own emotional experience that allows for the extent of resonance between another's feelings and our own. For example, many individuals experience empathy with others' sadness, for loss is something even young children come to appreciate. With more subtle feelings such as chagrin, guilt, or despair, I wonder whether as many of us would experience empathy with someone experiencing these emotions. When these feelings are vicariously invoked in us, not only do they require more complexity in their appraisal, but they are also likely to provoke self-reflection. That reflection could in turn elicit a self-focused aversive response, because as we contemplate our own prior experiences of chagrin, guilt, or despair, the reminiscence may confront us with shortcomings in ourselves. This topic warrants empirical investigation in an ethically sensitive manner.

The fourth phase is a resolution stage in which self–other boundaries are reasserted, thus permitting distance to reemerge between self and other, which is necessary for consideration about what sorts of action are best undertaken vis-à-vis the other person. It is in this last phase that helping or problem solving is initiated. With development, children acquire increasing sophistication in figuring out what sorts of action are best suited for a particular situation or a particular person (see Kopp, in press, for elaboration on children's planning strategies). Strayer (1987) proposed that it is in this final stage that empathy may shift into sympathy. She also noted that simply putting ourselves mentally in the role of the other could produce prosocial behavior similar to what emerges from the fourth phase, but empathy would not have been part of that process. An example of such emotionally detached prosocial behavior might be reading about flood or earthquake victims in the newspaper and subsequently sending a donation to the Red Cross for its relief efforts. One might feel concern for the stricken people, but one does not particularly feel a shared emotional impact upon reading about their plight. In sum, the emotional arousal of empathic processes *recruits* role or perspective taking to facilitate appropriate prosocial behavior rather than perspective-taking *spearheading* empathic experience with prosocial action following.

Cognition and Empathy

In a subsequent analysis of empathy in children, Strayer (1989) made an important developmental distinction between an empathic response that essentially is derived from the young child's focus on the emotion-eliciting *events* that are affecting another (e.g., watching child *A* hit child *B* and becoming distressed about witnessing the event of hitting) as opposed to an empathic response that stems from *participation* in the emotional reaction of the impacted individual (e.g., showing distress on seeing a crying child but without having seen the precipitating event). The former event-focused empathy relies on a rather concrete cognitive awareness of what sort of situations "cause" emotions; the latter participatory empathy requires cognitive awareness of the internal states of others. Thus, Strayer does include cognitive developmental complexity in her assessment of empathy, because representations, whether of emotion-eliciting events or emotion-experiencing people, determine the nature of the empathic response. Furthermore, what elicits an empathic response in children or adults depends heavily on the sorts of representations of which they are capable.

Using the Empathy Continuum rating scale, Strayer (1989) examined children's (ages 5, 8, and 13) attributions of emotions to themselves upon watching a variety of dramatic video episodes (a child exploring a house at night and frightened by a large shadow, a child unfairly punished when her brother lies to get her in trouble, a disabled child who cheerfully works at her physical therapy, etc.). She found age differences that indicated that the youngest children tended to attribute happiness to themselves more often than sadness or anger (although they were reasonably accurate in their attribution of these emotions to the video characters). Older children demonstrated the reverse pattern. For the fear video (scary shadow), both the 5- and 8-year-olds attributed fear to the character and to themselves, whereas for this emotion the oldest children reported that they felt less fear than the video character. The 13-year-olds appeared to respond in a more "empathically accurate" way to the angry and sad emotional experiences portrayed in the video scenarios, but they responded to the scary shadow video as possibly being somewhat immature. For the video with a cheerful disabled child character, the younger children said she was happy and they felt similarly, but the 13-year-olds were less sanguine, commenting about the difficulties she probably had experienced. Thus, the oldest children appeared to take into account *inferred* information about the video characters in how they cognitively and affectively responded to the video episodes.

Gender differences also occurred in the kinds of emotions that were attributed to the self while watching the video scenarios. Girls more often reported sadness and fear than did boys, who, in turn, more often reported angry responses than did girls. Strayer interpreted these sex differences as reflecting the nature of sex-role socialization and the effect of cultural display rules on what children were perhaps willing to report (see Chapter 8 for an extended discussion of display rules).

Strayer theorized that there is a change from overidentification with or "engulfment" by the circumstances surrounding another's emotional experience, namely, experiencing personal distress, to a more mature sharing in another's emotion. The former entails a blurring of self–other boundaries; the latter maintains an awareness that although we may feel similarly to the affected person, we are, in fact, not in the same situation. She posed the question of whether young children's self-reports of happiness after watching video characters feeling distressed are actually a way for the young child to control dysphoric emotions and thereby reduce the risk of engulfment in the sadness-producing stimuli themselves.

Strayer's work focused on how to elicit and measure empathy in children. Her Empathy Continuum is based on careful interviewing of the children to ascertain affective matching between the subject child and the video character as well as whether the subject child cognitively understands what the other character feels and why. She did not include in her assessment whether the children were willing to undertake any sort of prosocial behavior. Other approaches to measuring empathy in children have used children's likelihood to help others as part of the assessment for empathy. For example, one of the more frequently used scales is Bryant's empathy questionnaire (Bryant, 1982), which includes a mixture of items addressing general emotionality, expressiveness, and caring about others. The assumption in linking empathy with caring or helping behavior is that presumably one would not undertake altruistic action unless one was empathically moved. I turn next to this topic.

DEVELOPMENT OF PROSOCIAL BEHAVIOR

Considerable research has been done on children's prosocial behavior and its relation to empathy and/or perspective taking (e.g., Eisenberg, 1982; Eisenberg & Fabes, 1998; Eisenberg & Miller, 1987; Kurtines & Gewirtz, 1991; Underwood & Moore, 1982). Some research reflected inconsistent or little relationship between empathy and prosocial behavior (see Underwood & Moore, 1982). However, this inconsistency may be due to the nature of how empathy is measured. Using responses to pictures and hypothetical stories as indicative of empathy tends not to predict prosocial or altruistic behavior. Using physiological measures of arousal and self-report of feelings tends to have a greater relationship to subsequent prosocial behavior (Eisenberg & Miller, 1987). Social psychologists have also argued among themselves about whether empathy mediates altruistic behavior. For example, on one hand Cialdini, Brown, Lewis, Luce, and Neuberg (1997) carried out several studies with undergraduates and contended that their data supported a view of empathy as facilitating a projection of the self onto the distressed other ("self–other merging," in their terms), thus resulting in *self-interested* prosocial behavior. On the other hand, Batson et al. (1997) argued that higher levels of empathy do indeed elicit *genuinely altruistic* prosocial behavior. Their subjects did not report a projection of themselves onto the target, yet they felt empathy and subsequently were motivated to help the victim. In further support of their argument for empathy as mediating genuinely altruistic behavior, Batson et al. (1997) referred to research on humans' empathy with whales and subsequent altruistic helping of the animals (Shelton & Rogers, 1981). The point here is that presumably it is difficult for us to contemplate a self–other merging with a nonprimate species, yet we can feel empathy toward a threatened species and want to help them to survive.

From a developmental perspective, Zahn-Waxler (1991) located the origins of prosocial and altruistic behavior in the early attachment relationship between parent and infant. She noted that the social exchange and cooperative turn taking that has been observed between caregiver and infant "create a world of shared meaning, empathic understanding and appropriate linking of one's own emotions with those of others that then generalize beyond the parent–child dyad" (p. 156). For Zahn-Waxler, the love between parent and baby is essentially the crucible in which empathy and concern for others' well-being are forged. Thus, from a developmental viewpoint, it may well be that self–other merging is critical for an early sense of empathy and caring for the other. I suspect that with maturation, empathy and subsequent concern for others' well-being become more "autonomous" and do not always require the projection of the self's attributes, needs, and beliefs onto a target to feel empathy and want to help.

Hoffman (1978, 1982) was among the first theorists to link empathy with guilt and thus with early moral development. His argument is that empathy with another's visible distress develops first, but then as the young child realizes that he has caused the distress and that he had control or choice over his action, "his empathic distress may be transformed by the attribution of self-blame into a feeling of guilt" (Hoffman, 1978, p. 244). With guilt comes the motivation to repair the hurtful consequence, and a sense of personal responsibility begins to emerge. As I demonstrate later, this sense of being accountable for others' distress can be seen in children as young as preschoolers, and, at times, it may even be maladaptive.

Early research by Zahn-Waxler and Radke-Yarrow (1982) determined that not until approximately 18 months of age were children likely to show some solicitous behaviors, indicating a desire to comfort or help a distressed individual in their family (they would pat a crying sibling, try to get help from an adult, speak sympathetically, do something instrumental to help a distressed parent, etc.). Dunn's (1988) examination of emotions and social understanding in sibling and family relationships yielded further description of young children's "benevolence." In her detailed observations in the home, she found that a few children as young as 16 months initiated solicitous behavior toward a distressed sibling, but they were more likely at this young age to ignore or become distressed themselves. By 21 months of age Dunn found a number of children demonstrating comforting behaviors toward distressed siblings, but if they themselves had been responsible for their sib's distress, their most likely response was to exacerbate it. Indeed, the exacerbation of their sib's distress tended to increase during the 2 years the children were followed (to age 4). Interestingly, Dunn did not find age differences in the frequency of comforting/helping behavior; however, she did note that the older children tended to make more elaborate attempts at soothing, comforting, or helping.

Dunn also differentiated among types of prosocial behavior; she contends that not all prosocial behavior has its roots in empathy or even concern for others' well-being. Specifically, she found that helping was more likely associated with simply being sociable and wanting to engage other children in play. On the other hand, sharing with another child did seem to pivot on some degree of awareness of the other child's needs. She also found a sharp contrast between young children's helping and sharing behavior with fellow preschoolers—where it functioned as a strategy to engage others in play—and with one's sibling, where it occurred rarely (only 2–5% of all observed interactions in the home), perhaps indicating that there was less incentive to engage the sibling in play with these particular strategies. Indeed, "sharing" possessions was more likely to incite disputes between siblings than amicable play. Helping behavior, when it did occur, was more likely to be initiated by an older sibling toward a younger child.

Chapman, Zahn-Waxler, Cooperman, and Ianotti (1987) carried out a study that investigated a greater age span of children's prosocial behavior. They found that a further factor was also necessary for children to initiate helping behavior: The children needed to feel some sense of responsibility for alleviating the target person's distress. Chap-

man, et al. (1987) asked children (preschool through sixth grade) to respond to a number of stories in which two children were featured with
one of them experiencing a negative event. Those children who most
often attributed guilt or remorse to the story protagonists were more
likely to initiate helping behavior in unrelated contrived situations
(e.g., helping a mother to find a baby bottle after hearing an infant crying in the adjacent room). In other words, those children who had incorporated a cultural or familial value that sanctioned or even
mandated that "one should help others in need" were also the most
spontaneously helpful, but it could be that the hidden "threat" of guilt
was the primary motivator, as in "you are *obligated* to help others in
need, and if you don't, you are guilty of an immoral deed." (Perhaps
Hannah in the opening vignette had acquired this sort of mind-set
from her family.)

Strayer and Schroeder (1989) also investigated the relations between empathy, the type of emotion felt, and helping behavior in children ages 5 to 13. They found that older children were more likely to
use verbal methods of reassurance (e.g., "Don't be afraid now, it's all
right") than were younger children, but overall, the most common sort
of helping strategy was instrumental and goal oriented (e.g., "I'd help
her fix it"). They also found that happy or angry characters were least
likely to elicit helping responses, and fear and sadness most likely to
elicit helping.

What the preceding research suggests is that empathic arousal and
the more detached sympathetic response appear to function as motives
for initiating prosocial behavior, although they do not guarantee
prosocial behavior. Younger children may not be sure what would be
helpful for the affected person, and verbal interventions may not be
readily accessible to them. Among older children, youth, and adults,
factors that appear to counteract prosocial behavior, despite an empathic response to a target figure, are diffusion of responsibility, perception of the distressed person as "deserving" the miserable situation,
high cost–risk ratio of attempting to help, and conflicting demands,
such as in obeying authority figures versus alleviating another's distress
(Hoffman, 1977).

Thus far we have looked at empathy as witnessing someone's distress. We can also feel empathy with someone's joy, pride, or pleasure, but feeling empathically happy for someone does not usually
translate into subsequent helping behavior. This makes sense, because the happy "target" person presumably does not need help.
However, positive empathy may be associated with subsequent cooperation among young children. Empathic or sympathetic responses

that are characterized by sadness, distress, worry, and the like are typically the emotional elicitors that are involved in subsequent helping behavior.

In summary, by 18 months of age, many children show comforting behaviors toward family members and possibly other people with whom they enjoy a close relationship. Other prosocial behaviors, such as sharing and helping, emerge in the second and third years and may reflect a young preschooler's growing sociability. By age 4 to 5, children help and share more frequently than at younger ages, and their greater awareness of their peers' feelings, needs, and wants is reflected in these prosocial acts. However, as Dunn cautions, it is not evident that some act of self-sacrifice accompanies this prosocial behavior. Children take pleasure in playing with other kids, and knowing how to share and help appropriately facilitates this pleasurable exchange. Self-interest may then be the more prominent motive in prosocial behavior than "high-minded" moral and altruistic reasons. Yet concern for friendships and relations within the family speak to growing children's pragmatic understanding that their self-concern and others' well-being are intimately linked. Thus, the boundaries blur between self-interest and altruistic behavior toward others with whom they have close relationships.

Research on empathy among preadolescents and youth is scant. I suspect there are some significant transitions around preadolescence in how empathic responsiveness and relationship-promoting behavior interact. On the one hand, young adolescents can be insufferably egocentric and oblivious to others' emotional cues (especially their parents'). On the other hand, they can demonstrate the most exquisite sensitivity to their friends' emotional–expressive behavior. Thus, this age group might well show an increasing contextualization of empathic responsiveness, but empirically that is unknown. When looking for studies on adolescent empathy and prosocial behavior, I found that the relevant research on adolescents tends to focus on questions about moral reasoning rather than empathy and prosocial behavior (see Eisenberg & Fabes, 1998; Kurtines & Gewirtz, 1991). I have also noticed that in many high schools, the curriculum now mandates students to engage in some sort of community service project on an annual basis. It appears as though educators have arrived at this curricular decision to promote adolescent prosocial behavior, among other potential benefits. Whether involvement in community service programs does indeed foster a more generalized empathic and prosocial stance among the participating teens remains to be evaluated. This is clearly an area awaiting further research.

CHILDREN'S ATTEMPTS TO INFLUENCE
ANOTHER'S EMOTIONAL STATE

Intervening on someone's behalf is related to seeking to change how someone is feeling. This commonly takes the form of trying to cheer someone up, to calm someone down, or reassure someone who is scared. Strayer and Schroeder's (1989) research showed that verbal reassurance was more prevalent among older children. In this sense, trying to influence someone else's emotional state so that he or she feels better can also be viewed as prosocial behavior. Whether we are moved to do this because of empathy or sympathy with the other person's distress is unknown. However, being able to understand what the other person is feeling is critical, as is knowledge of any relevant personal information about the target person. There are also other occasions, clearly not prosocially intended, in which we attempt to influence another's feelings: for example, when we appease an irrational bully, tease someone to anger or to tears, or try to distract someone from their distress so that *we* do not have to feel badly anymore (the personal distress reaction described earlier). Few studies have been undertaken that have systematically examined children's attempts to influence others' feelings, and this area is wide open for research. In a couple of studies children have been interviewed about how they would go about altering others' feelings (e.g., Covell & Abramovitch, 1987; McCoy & Masters, 1985), but these investigators did not provide observational data on how children actually act during this emotion-influencing process. However, one of my studies did collect observations of children attempting to intervene and change another's feelings for the better (Saarni, 1992). Given my prerogative as author, I describe it in some detail here.

"Cheering Up the Sad Experimenter"

Eighty children across three age groups (7- to 8-, 9- to 10-, and 11- to 12-year-olds) met individually on two separate occasions with a woman introduced to them as a "market researcher." The first time she was visibly in a happy emotional state and engaged the children warmly; on the second occasion, a week later, she was in a sad, depressed state. Although she maintained facial regard and eye contact with the child, she adopted a slumped posture, did not smile, and spoke little and then in a flat monotone fashion. An "assistant" accompanied the children to and from their classrooms and prior to the second meeting asked the children to help cheer up her "colleague," who was feeling quite "down." All agreed to do so.

The children were videotaped throughout their interaction with the market researcher while doing a task for her. This allowed for the establishment of a base rate of emotional–expressive behaviors for when the children were with the market researcher in her happy state. This base rate could then be compared to what they attempted to do when trying to cheer her up in her sad state. As a check on the manipulation, a mirror was placed behind the children in a slightly offset position so that the video camera could also simultaneously capture the "market researcher's" expressive behavior toward the child.

Results indicated that the oldest children (11 to 12 years) were the most positive in their emotional–expressive behavior in both happy and sad sessions, and the middle age group revealed a curiously flat emotional profile in response to the two emotional state variations. In an exit interview these 9- to 10-year-olds indicated that they thought they had cheered up the sad market researcher by being very task oriented. Among the youngest children were those who did appear to become "engulfed" by the sad researcher's demeanor and looked as though they would very nearly cry, crawl under the table, or try to leave, but, overall, the 6- to 7-year-olds, as a group, did not differ that much from the 9- to 10-year-olds. Interestingly, it was the preadolescents, while showing the most positive behavior toward the sad researcher, who also revealed the most tension-filled expressive behavior (biting their lips, touching themselves, rubbing their fingers together, etc.). From an impressionistic standpoint, these oldest children seemed more self-contained and less influenced by the sad researcher's emotional–expressive behavior, despite the tension-laden nonverbal behaviors. The content of their conversation with her was also more often "upbeat," and they talked more than the children in the two younger groups, who tended to clam up when faced with the sad woman.

Few gender differences were found in this study, but older girls did smile more at the sad market researcher as a strategy to try to cheer her up. In contrast, some of the older boys appeared annoyed at the prospect of having to help cheer someone up, despite having agreed to do so (they drummed their fingers on the table, bumped around in their seats, etc.). Strangely enough, not one child ventured to ask the market researcher why she was sad, which may either be a commentary on how depression typically deflects social interaction or may reflect etiquette and authority conventions whereby children do not ask unfamiliar adults why they are feeling the way they do. In summary, this observational study raised many questions about the mutual interaction of emotional–expressive cues as well as the context's influence on the children (e.g., the effect on children when they are aware of being videotaped).

INDIVIDUAL DIFFERENCES IN VICARIOUSLY INDUCED EMOTION

Socialization's Influence on Individual Differences

Eisenberg, Fabes, Carlo, and Karbon (1992) and more recently Eisenberg and Fabes (1998) provide us with a review of studies that suggest some patterns about the kinds of children most likely spontaneously to behave in a prosocial manner. They note that preschoolers who are socially expressive (although not always in a positive fashion) and assertive, demonstrate sympathy, and are capable of reasoning about others' needs are most likely to help, share, and comfort others in distress. Compliant children, who shared or helped only when directly asked to, were more likely to react with personal distress when confronted with another's upset. They also tended to be rejected by their peers when they did comply (especially if they were boys). These children were generally less socially responsive, and their level of moral reasoning was unrelated to their degree of prosocial or altruistic behavior.

Socially Rejected Children

Upon thinking about these young children who did what others told them to do but were still viewed with contempt by their peers, I wondered whether they would become what older children call "wimps, geeks, and dorks." School-age children and young adolescents who bear these socially painful labels are often rejected and lonely. They have also been the object of study by Asher and his colleagues (e.g., Asher, Hymel, & Renshaw, 1985; Asher, Parkhurst, Hymel, & Williams, 1990; Asher & Wheeler, 1985). The children identified in these studies as lonely and rejected seem to fit the profile that Eisenberg et al. (1992) described for the preschool years. A subsequent study undertaken by Cassidy and Asher (1992) investigated relations between 5- to 6-year-olds' loneliness and their social status as rated by peers. Teachers also evaluated the children on behavioral adjustment. The loneliest children were, not surprisingly, rejected by their peers and were also rated by their teachers as showing *less prosocial behavior* and more shyness as well as being more disruptive and aggressive.

Thus, there seems to be some convergence upon a pattern of social skill deficit that may be linked with deficits in empathy and sympathy. These deficits in empathy/sympathy manifest themselves in inadequate prosocial behavior and personal distress reactions when faced with others' emotional upset or distress. Conceivably, for some children personal distress, experienced as negative emotional arousal, may consolidate into hostile attributions to the target child and result in aggression. This link needs empirical verification, but suggestions for the connection appear in work by Crockenberg (1985), Dodge (1986, 1989), Feshbach (1989), and Klimes-Dougan and Kistner (1990), and in Ascione's (1993) review on children's cruelty toward animals.

Family Influence

Eisenberg, Fabes, Carlos, and Karbon (1992) describe further a couple of socialization studies which suggest that family relations influence the development of sympathy: Sympathetic mothers produce sympathetic daughters and sympathetic fathers produce sympathetic sons (Eisenberg et al., 1991; Fabes, Eisenberg, & Miller, 1990). Modeling seems to be a key socializing agent here. Adult women who report empathy after watching distressing films also describe their families of origin in ways that indicate that positive emotions and sympathetic and vulnerable feelings were freely expressed.

Along similar lines, in the Eisenberg et al. (1991) investigation, parents' attitudes were assessed using the Parental Attitudes toward Children's Expressiveness Scale (PACES; Saarni, 1990b), which was modified for use with preschoolers. The parents of elementary school children who reported restrictive attitudes toward their children's emotional displays had children who seemed more inclined to experience personal distress rather than sympathetic concern when describing their reaction to another's distress. This effect was more noticeable when the parents espoused controlling beliefs about their children's emotional displays, even when the emotional displays simply expressed the child's own vulnerable feelings (e.g., sadness and anxiety). Parents who restricted their children's emotional displays only when their children expressed emotions that might hurt another's feelings—but not when their children expressed genuine vulnerable feelings—appeared to have more sympathy-oriented children. The most affected children appeared to be boys of mothers who endorsed controlling attitudes about their sons' display of emotions in situations in which only self-related vulnerable feelings were involved; these boys were the most likely to show personal distress reactions upon witnessing another's upset.

A number of studies have also reported links between children's empathic disposition and their parents' sympathy and disciplinary strategies. Strayer and Roberts (1989) found that empathy in young school-age children was positively associated with prosocial behavior in their families. Eisenberg, Fabes, Carlo, Troyer, et al. (1992) also found that mothers' encouragement of prosocial behavior and their own sympathy were related to their daughters' sympathetic behavior, whereas when expression of negative feelings was the "norm" in a family, the children were more likely to show anxious personal distress feelings when watching an evocative film. Eisenberg and her colleagues also found that parents who used an emotionally intense reaction when negatively disciplining their children tended to have children who were less likely to respond sympathetically (Miller, Eisenberg, Fabes, Shell, & Gular, 1989). A similar pattern was also found in adolescents: Warm parental communication was associated with adolescents who expressed more sympathetic responses (Eisenberg & McNally, 1993).

Krevans and Gibbs (1996) also found that parents who used inductive discipline methods with their children tended to have children who were both more empathic and prosocial. This effect of parental discipline was particularly strong when the parents expressed disappointment in their children's not living up to an ideal or standard of socially responsive conduct when the situation warranted it. The authors argued that when parents say to a misbehaving child that they are disappointed in the child's behavior because they *expected* the child to be able to live up to a standard, they are actually expressing confidence in the child to internalize this standard. This is to be contrasted with "ego attacks," which only humiliate or diminish the child's self-regard (e.g., "I can't believe how selfish you are!"). Finally, a longitudinal study found that empathic adults tended to have fathers who had been very involved in their care and mothers who permitted their children to express their dependency needs and vulnerability (Koestner, Franz, & Weinberger, 1990). This pattern suggests that sympathetic adults have grown up in families in which priority was given to the emotional needs and well-being of children.

Temperament Influence

Eisenberg and Fabes (1998) also contend that temperamental dispositions may be involved in personal distress versus sympathy reactions when faced with others' distress. The capacity to regulate emotional arousal so that it does not become too aversive when witnessing some other person's mishap or distress may be temperamentally influenced. When our own emotional arousal becomes aversive, we become self-focused rather than other-focused. The self-focus is not necessarily narcissistic or egocentric; it is simply that at that point people who are flooded with their own negative affect have to direct attention to coping with that onslaught of intense emotion within themselves. Turning one's focus toward the other is necessary for sympathetic concern and subsequent appropriate prosocial behavior to occur and is less likely to occur when a person is preoccupied with his or her own strong emotional state. The data that Eisenberg and Fabes reviewed suggest that those children whose temperament is characterized by negative emotionality and distractibility tend to be low in sympathy, whereas those children whose temperamental style showed more regulated emotion and longer attention spans were more likely to demonstrate sympathy.

Differences in Social-Emotional Adjustment and Empathy

Depression and Empathy

Zahn-Waxler, Cole, and Barrett (1991) concluded in their review on developmental patterns linking guilt, empathy, sex differences, and depression that girls may be more at risk for later development of depression (and females do indeed experience depression more than males in Western society) because of their greater concern for and involvement in others' problems and because of their tendency to feel at fault for negative events befalling those with whom they interact. Thus, when young girls show empathy and sympathy for others in distress, behave prosocially toward the distressed persons (e.g., provide helping, comforting, and sharing), and believe that they have some responsibility to intervene and assist others in need, they may be setting themselves up for depression in later life. But I think something else is needed besides the empathic prosocial orientation for depression to ensue. The following case, adapted from a student intern's experience, illustrates the links between an overdeveloped prosocial orientation, a vulnerable self-concept, and proneness to depression.

> Thirteen-year-old Angela worried a lot about what other people thought of her, although she was unsure just exactly what they did think. She always tried very hard to do what her friends might want from her, even if it ended up putting her at a disadvantage or hurt her feelings. For example, she had made a point of helping Chris, a guy she liked a lot, get a better grade on his English test by putting her paper at the edge of her desk so that he could copy some of her answers. Then she overheard him telling some other guys that he thought the new girl, Elyse, was really sexy and good-looking.
>
> After hearing him talk about Elyse, Angela felt deflated. She critically looked at her feet, her hands, her body; everything was too big. She used to think her face was all right, but it was really too round, and her lips were too fat. How could she have not noticed that before! Elyse was thin; no wonder Chris thought she was so fantastic.
>
> The next day Chris asked her if he could borrow her English

homework. Angela stammered and repeated her apology several times, "Oh, I'm sorry, I'd let you have it but I didn't get it done myself. . . . I feel bad that I don't have it for you; normally I'd have done it. . . . " Chris just said, "OK, OK, don't freak out about it," and he moved away to talk with some other kids. Angela stood there feeling like a jerk. She had just blown it. She dejectedly turned away and went outside to find a place where she could be alone.

Angela is faced with a pattern of compassionate altruism that is at her own expense. She has begun to define herself as someone who "always tries do what her friends want" and when she allegedly fails, she is a "jerk." By age 10 children are generally capable of comparing themselves with others (e.g., Higgins, 1991). In Angela's case, when she compares her looks to Elyse's and finds her body to be "deficient" relative to Elyse's appearance, she castigates herself severely. She does not consider how to remedy the ostensible deficiency in a pragmatic problem-solving fashion (e.g., changing her hair style, makeup, or whatever) or whether to dismiss the physical appearance comparison as unimportant relative to being smart and competent in school. Because Angela has focused on attending to others *at her own expense*, she has become very skilled at helping others but is skill-deficient at helping herself. Learned helplessness may be the outcome, which has been linked to onset of depression (e.g., Seligman, 1975). In contrast, a healthy dose of self-interest appears to inoculate young girls against depression, and as Zahn-Waxler et al. (1991) point out in their review, a masculine sex-role orientation (regardless of one's gender) appears to protect against depression as it is associated with greater emotional well-being and self-esteem. Not surprisingly, assertive self-interest is very characteristic of the masculine sex role in western culture.

Child Abuse and Empathy

Several studies have been conducted that examined physically abused children's reactions to distress in others (e.g., Klimes-Dougan & Kistner, 1990; Main & George, 1985; Hoffman-Plotkin & Twentyman, 1984; Trickett & Kuczynski, 1986). Physically abused children show a multitude of problems, but one that is obvious is their more intense and frequent aggressiveness compared to nonabused children. Their interactions with other children are frequently conflictual.

Main and George (1985) observed young preschoolers' responses to other children's distress in day-care settings. The target children were all from poor homes, with many of the households dependent on welfare and with only one parent in the home. Half of these children had been reported as having been maltreated; the other half did not have any incidence of maltreatment. The abused children (who were quite young: 1 to 3 years of age) showed no comforting gestures toward the child involved in the mishap; even worse, they sometimes moved in on the distressed child in a threatening and hostile fashion and attacked the crying child. Other times they began to fuss as well and even showed apprehension or anxiety toward the other distressed child. Diametrically opposed responses were shown by the nonabused children (who were also 1 to 3 years old): They looked at the distressed child and offered tentative touches or pats, about one third demonstrated active prosocial behavior toward the unhappy child. For this young age group, the proportion of prosocial behavior is about the same obtained with middle-class children; thus, the stress of poverty does not in itself affect young children's developing sense of empathy and concern for others. Rather, it is the emotional "nourishment" received by the infant from its caregivers that its feelings matter and are inherently important that contributes to the young child's emerging empathy and altruism. When a parent's "generosity of spirit" toward his or her child is impoverished, something sad and destructive grows between parent and child, and tragically this pattern is carried forward into future generations.

Delinquency and Empathy

Gibbs (1991), Bandura (1991), and Staub (1991) provide us with analyses of what appears to be going on in the minds of people who victimize others. Bandura and Staub examine the mind-sets of those whose victimization of others occurs in genocide, terrorism, and rape, and Gibbs focuses on delinquent youth. One could take Bandura's and Staub's positions and apply them to gang warfare, where one gang does seem to be bent on exterminating the other. Staub's review of rape and incest is also relevant to male delinquency: The need to feel powerful by coercing and degrading another person appears to underlie some delinquent acts. And it is evident that a deficit in feeling empathy is clearly one of the problems that contributes to the adolescent committing harmful acts.

First, such delinquents have impaired or distorted perspective-taking capacity; the intended victim is viewed as subhuman, worthless, dispensable, and inferior. Bandura states that the attribution, on some level, of the victim as *insensate*, as *un*feeling, is critical for short-circuiting the otherwise emotion-arousing response that would normally be evoked upon witnessing another's distress. Second, the attribution of *blame* to victims for what happened to them deflects self-evaluation and permits exoneration of the perpetrators' behavior toward the victim. Gibbs (1991) quotes delinquents as saying that the store owner "deserved" to get robbed because he had not secured the premises adequately. Robberies accompanied by subsequent ruthless shooting of the complying store clerk may well be similar to Eisenberg, Fabes, Carlo, Karbon, et al.'s (1992) finding that compliant boys were particularly rejected by their peers. Third, as Bandura argues, if harm doers can make a comparison with someone else's destructive behavior and view their own as less harmful, they can counter self-doubts and replace them with self-approving sanctions for the destructive exploits. Such a cognitive "switch" may be occurring with driveby shootings: The other drug "lord" did something bad to one's group, territory, or contacts, so now one not only seeks revenge but also condones it as a worthy act, despite the possible injury of innocent bystanders.

Not long ago a group of eight youths was arrested for abducting, gang raping, and beating two 14-year-old girls in San Francisco's Mission district. They were all members of a particular gang, and they believed that one of the girls was the girlfriend of a member of a rival gang. Although no evaluations of their construals or rationalizations for their behavior have appeared in local newspapers, I would guess that this horrible incident reflected much of what Bandura, Staub, and Gibbs described as underlying harmful, destructive, and exploitive acts. The girls were viewed as unworthy and as objects; their alleged association with the rival gang provided the comparison with the others' deeds as therefore justifying violent behavior. The girls were probably blamed, as in "they should have known better than to come into our territory unprotected," and responsibility was diffuse because there were many perpetrators.

Gibbs provides us with a brief review of treatment models for delinquents that focus on changing their cognitive distortions and providing them with social skills. He notes that the one program that also seemed to reduce subsequent antisocial behavior was one that integrated moral–cognitive developmental tasks with social skills training (Arbuthnot & Gordon, 1986). Such programs emphatically promote perspective taking on what others are thinking and feeling and thereby reduce projection, blaming, minimizing, dehumanizing, and mislabeling. In effect, they facilitate the normal process of empathy that would otherwise be short-circuited by distorted beliefs and attributions and self-exonerating biases.

The need to develop both delinquency prevention programs and emotional competency enhancement programs is well documented by

Weissberg and Greenberg (1998), who noted that the fastest growing group of criminal offenders consisted of juveniles. In their review of various prevention and enhancement programs, the topic of interpersonal negotiation skills (or related constructs such as interpersonal awareness, social problem solving, positive relationship-building skills) is repeatedly cited. I suspect that empathy and understanding others' emotional experience is central to the program components that address such social and relationship-promoting skills (see also Greenberg et al., 1995).

Gender Differences

In this chapter sex differences have already been touched on in several instances. For reviews of how gender and sex-role socialization may be linked with differences in empathy and prosocial behavior, interested readers are referred to Eisenberg and Fabes (1991, 1998), Eisenberg and Lennon (1983), Lennon and Eisenberg (1987), and Zahn-Waxler et al. (1991).

Eisenberg and Fabes (1991) concluded that when large gender differences are found, typically self-report measures of empathic responsiveness were used; that is, when given the chance to describe themselves, females are found to be more empathic than males' self-description. But when actual behavior is examined, gender differences tend to be inconsistent in prosocial behavior. The self-report bias shown by female respondents may reflect an internalized sex-role stereotyped belief rather than actual helping behavior. Eisenberg and Fabes (1998) further suggest that girls and women may be viewed as more sympathetic and hence prosocially oriented simply because they are less inclined to behave aggressively toward others. In other words, the relative absence of overt aggression may be equated with a prosocial, sympathetic stance, even though genuine sympathy and prosocial action are not experienced. Indeed, helping strangers has been found to be more frequent among males, but women do more long-term nurturing and helping of others in close relationships (e.g., Eagly & Crowley, 1986). Perhaps it is the *style* of how empathy and prosocial behavior are coordinated and expressed that differs among men and women rather than "how much" empathy one gender has relative to the other. By now, it should be clear that empathy and prosocial behavior are multidimensional, and it is not surprising that contextual factors, including one's scripts regarding sex role and one's self-definition, may influence considerably how one experiences empathy and concern for others' well-being in a particular situation.

Cultural Differences

Brislin's (1993) informative and readable book provides us with a variety of examples of how empathy is relevant to understanding people's emotions whose cultural socialization differs from our own . To be empathic to others' emotional experience in another cultural context is truly a test of being responsive to facial and nonverbal cues of emotion as well as taking into account common themes that have considerable cultural commonality (loss of family members, shunning by one's group or family for some shameful act, etc.).

Somatization is also common, and empathy to how one's body might feel when emotionally distressed can be an important cue for being responsive to another's distress. Brislin contends that people *learn* how to communicate their symptoms of distress in ways that are conventional or acceptable relative to their culture. For example, he describes Vietnamese–Chinese living in Hong Kong as referring to a "fullness in the head" to indicate mental distress, whereas Indians hope to elicit sympathy with their complaints about stomachaches, and many Mexicans are reported to experience memory problems when emotionally distressed. Thus, if talking about or expressing anxieties or depression is not culturally acceptable, it is hardly likely to elicit empathic responsiveness, and how will someone then obtain sympathetic support? Brislin suggests take the culturally acceptable route: somaticize, whether it is the liver, head, stomach, or heart that takes the brunt. North Americans somaticize their emotional anguish as well, and, indeed, one could argue that within the culture of gender, somatization is a more acceptable avenue for males to obtain sympathetic support than explicitly verbalizing or expressing their emotional distress. (Parenthetically, I rarely ever watch team sports on television, but occasionally I have caught some postgame interview with a member of the *defeated* team. Such individuals, who are males, are remarkable for their lack of complaining, whining, or feeling upset or dejected. The expression of vulnerability is not conventionally acceptable in this context—at least not if it is going to be televised—and instead one hears a litany of concern about thus-and-such's shoulder, back, knee, collarbone, or neck being a problem, namely, somatization.)

Another perspective on cultural differences in empathy and prosocial behavior is that of Snary and Keljo (1991). Their view is that nonindustrial cultures focus more on *caring* and tend to be more collectivist-oriented than do Western societies. They argue that individuals in these cultures appropriately use conventional moral reasoning rather than postconventional moral reasoning premised on universals and abstractions. These non-Western societies have cultural contexts that have built into them a collective responsiveness to the emotional well-being of their kin or tribe, and their moral system supports that orientation. Snary and Keljo contend that Western theories of moral development that stress abstract appeals to justice reflect our cultural values of individualism and are therefore biased or incomplete when applied to non-Western societies. In contrast, Turiel (1998) has argued that when we apply these broad descriptions of collectivist versus individualist characterization to non-Western and Western cultures, respectively, we miss the variation that exists within individuals and within societies. Moral reasoning is often contextualized or domain-specific, and individuals can "both participate in cultural practices and can stand apart from culture and take a critical approach to social practices" (Turiel, 1998, p. 914).

Finally, empathy is obviously differently conceptualized in different cultures. In Japan people are very conscious of how another responds to them; thus, empathy in this context might take the form of exquisite sensitivity to another's nonverbal behaviors as well as what behaviors are omitted from the interaction to infer the other's feelings. Quite different are the Ifaluk in Micronesia, who believe that people can directly cause others' feelings, and therefore an individual is supposed to respond to and, if need be, ameliorate another's feelings because he or she was responsible for these feelings being evoked (Lutz, 1987). If this is so, the cultural belief about how emotions come about would appear to facilitate prosocial behavior: The responsible party should intervene in another's feeling of distress.

CONCLUSION

In terms of emotional competence, when we empathically respond to someone else, we promote social bonds. These social bonds can take the form of *social responsibility*, as in the vignette about Hannah who gave her umbrella and change to a homeless family, or they can be manifested as one of the defining qualities of close relationships (e.g., we are more likely to feel empathic toward our friends). In short, experiencing empathy helps us to develop relationships with others that anchor us not just in self-serving reciprocal support systems but in greater endeavors of caring and collective well-being. However, I suspect that caring for others is best tempered with some degree of healthy self-interest. In the case of Angela, whose excessive preoccupation with helping others was at the expense of taking care of herself, we saw what may have been a fragile self-concept. In fact, it is not clear that she actually felt empathy with her friends' emotional experience; rather, she tried to "fix" things for them so that she would not be rejected.

With genuine empathy we can extend ourselves beyond our immediate time and space, truly a self-efficacious ability with implications for all sentient beings. We can observe the fear or loss in the eyes of strangers and reach out to comfort or help. For example, the tragic kidnapping of 12-year-old Polly Klaas from her own home in Petaluma in Northern California elicited from people around the country countless hours of donated labor and hundreds of thousands of dollars to help in the search for Polly. Upon the discovery of her body, the news media were filled with images of grief-stricken people clearly sharing in the anguish and horror experienced by Polly's family, although they had never met the family. The self-efficacy that is revealed in this empathic response to strangers or to those close to us is that we are *connected* to others in a common endeavor, whether that common endeavor takes the form of helping, comforting, sharing, or just listening to another's emotional experience. The paradox seems to be that empathy can be all too readily "turned off" or subverted with hurtful effects, as in the indifferent bullying and cruelty among schoolchildren, or with horrible and tragic consequences, as in village massacres in Algeria or when neighbors become one another's tormentors in the former Yugoslavia.

Ideally, our capacity for responding vicariously to another's emotional plight evokes our compassion and brings out the best in us. Given that some argue that our fellow primates are also capable of empathy (Brothers, 1989), perhaps empathy does say something about how our brains work too: We may well have evolved to be able to care for others, with our vicarious response to their expression of emotional distress as the mediating process for our acting altruistically toward others (e.g., MacLean, 1985). Empathy and caring for others are pivotal features of emotional competence; integrated with mature emotional competence is personal integrity and a moral disposition ("doing the right thing"; see discussion in Chapter 1). A well-developed moral disposition entails sympathy and a sense of obligation to promote others' well-being, as well as fairness and self-control, and I suspect that in this integration of empathy and ethics we can find the seeds of wisdom.

Chapter 8

Skill 5: The Ability to Differentiate Internal Subjective Emotional Experience from External Emotional Expression

Ability to realize that inner emotional state need not correspond to outer expression, both in oneself and in others and, at more mature levels, the ability to understand that one's emotional–expressive behavior may have an impact on another and to take this into account in one's self-presentation strategies.

For many people deception comes to mind when they think of "poker face," "emotional imposter," "emotional front or facade," or "saving face," and perhaps with a bit more contemplation, a somewhat self-conscious feeling comes up, for at one time or another we all realize we have concealed from someone else what we really felt. "But it was to spare the other's feelings," you may argue, and this is true, we often do not reveal our genuine feelings because they would have undesirable effects on others. However, we also frequently do not express our feelings straightforwardly because of our anticipation of undesirable effects on *ourselves* if we did so. Being able to separate our subjective emotional experience from our observable expressive behavior facilitates emotional competence when it is a strategy that permits us to strive for our interpersonal and emotional goals more efficaciously—assuming that the goals are in accord with our moral sense or disposition. Children begin to develop this separation of "inner" emotional state from "outer" emotional expression in the preschool years, and, indeed, by school entry some children can also talk about the process of doing so.

In this chapter I review what children learn about separating how they feel from what they show to others, and I argue that this is related to the sorts of interpersonal relations the child is involved in, the sorts of feelings being felt and how intensely, and the "social stakes" (or the risk felt) about showing how one really feels. Strategically maneuvering emotional–expressive behavior for social purposes (e.g., impression management) is briefly covered in a discussion of children's self-presentation skills. The chapter concludes with a discussion of cultural influence, which is considerable for this skill of emotional competence. In the sections that follow, I refer to this discrepancy between internal subjective feeling and external emotional expression as "emotional dissemblance." I also use the term "emotion management" to refer to children's regulating their experience of emotion by monitoring their expressive behavior. This last topic is a significant link to the next chapter on children's coping with aversive emotions and interpersonal conflict.

TYPES OF EMOTIONAL DISSEMBLANCE

Social psychologists interested in nonverbal communication have done much of the groundwork in investigating people's emotional–expressive behavior, its communicative impact, and its congruence with inner emotional state. I have divided my discussion of types of emotional dissemblance into two broad categories: The first is more rule driven, that is, there is more consensus and predictability in North American mainstream culture about the "when, where, and with whom" aspects of emotional communication, and the other is more situation dependent and tends to occur due to immediate need or expedience (such as avoiding getting into trouble).

Awareness of Cultural and Personal Display Rules

Display rules are essentially predictable social customs for how we express our feelings appropriately (Ekman & Friesen, 1975). All cultures have display rules, but they vary considerably in content and application. Display rules can take a couple of different forms (Ekman & Friesen, 1975). The first is *cultural* display rules: These take the form of social conventions or norms that prescribe how we should express our feelings, even if we do not feel the emotion that would correspond to the acceptable facial expression. Cultural display rules have the added advantage in that they are generally agreed to by most members of a culture or subculture and thus they permit smooth, predictable social exchange.

As an illustration, I conducted a study in which children were observed trying to monitor their expressive behavior to meet the cultural display rule of "look agreeable when someone gives you a gift, even if you don't like it" (Saarni, 1984). The children ranged from 6 to 11 years old and attended a parochial school that had explicit expectations for conduct; thus, they were more likely to be the sort of children who would be "motivated" to carry out this particular display rule. The children met individually with an ostensible market researcher, did a small task, and then received candy and money. This first session provided baseline data for their expressive behavior upon receiving a desirable gift. A couple of days later they returned to do another task and this time were presented with a "grabbag" of wrapped gifts. They received a dull and inappropriate baby toy for their effort. The videotapes of their unwrapping the baby toy and having to interact with the market researcher provided the following results: 6-year-old boys were uniformly negative in their expressive behavior; the youngest girls and both boys and girls of 8 to 9 years frequently demonstrated "transitional behavior"; I defined this as behavior that was not exactly negative, but the children did not appear to be adopting positive expressive behavior either. The transitional category also contained "socially anxious behaviors," such as glancing back and forth between the baby toy and the experimenter, touching one's face here and there, and biting one's lips. These children were aware that they could not just run out of the room (as some of the youngest boys attempted to do), but they also did not have a firm grasp on how to implement the cultural display rule of "look agreeable when you get a gift, even if you don't like it." Thus, they were tense and sought out social guidance, as when they glanced back and forth between the gift and the experimenter. By contrast, the oldest children (10 to 11 years), especially the girls, were most likely to express positive behavior toward the market researcher, despite receiving a dumb baby toy.

Cole (1986) replicated this study with several methodological changes and extended the sample to children age 4 years. She found that across this age span, children made an attempt to inhibit negative expressive displays when receiving an undesirable gift (which they had previously rated as indeed undesirable). She also found with a separate sample of 3- to 4-year-old girls that they smiled when in the presence of the examiner, regardless of the nature of the gift they received, but when the examiner was absent and they received an undesired gift, they did not inhibit their disappointment. Josephs (1993) also obtained this pattern of results with German preschool girls. This suggests that it is the *social* context that might be highly important here for understanding what sort of expressive display is revealed rather than an internal emotional state (for theoretical exploration of such effects, see Cappella, 1981; Fridlund, 1991; Zivin, 1985, 1986; for additional empirical confirmation see Jones, Collins, & Hong, 1991; Kraut & Johnson, 1979).

Cole, Jenkins, and Shott (1989) also examined facial expression control among elementary school age congenitally blind children. They found that these children also produced smiles when receiving a disappointing gift from an examiner, despite not being able to observe others' reciprocal expressive behavior. They were more likely than the comparison sighted sample to verbalize the need to deflect attention away from the disappointment by using conversational strategies (e.g., changing the subject).

Personal display rules are often more idiosyncratic, and their function differs from cultural display rules as well. Whereas the latter are for the sake of predictable and conventional social exchanges, personal display rules function to help us feel as though we are coping more adequately with an emotionally taxing situation. They are strategies that are often understood as coping efforts by others who know the individual well or who share similar cultural background (e.g., European-American females may cope with anger by becoming hurt or depressed, whereas European-American males may cope with hurt feelings by becoming angry; each gender often recognizes that about "one of their own" but may not as readily recognize cross-gender personal display rules as such). An example about a young adolescent is as follows:

> Fourteen-year-old Chris experienced a painful rejection by his first "girlfriend." When he ran into her at school and she was hanging out with another guy, Chris adopted emotional–expressive behavior that looked cool, impervious, and supremely self-confident. Inside he felt anger and sadness but did not reveal them. Chris felt that he needed to protect his vulnerability at having been rejected, and the adoption of the "calm, cool, and collected" expressive facade facilitated his sense of coping with the challenge to his emotional equilibrium upon seeing his former girlfriend again.

The personal display rule in this case was that if Chris felt hurt, vulnerable, and/or otherwise threatened, he would substitute the emotional–expressive behavior that was exactly opposite to what he felt in reality so that he would have at least the *illusion* of feeling relatively strong and invulnerable. Chris's substitution of a calm or stoic exterior, despite feeling otherwise, is commonly endorsed by preadolescents as an appropriate way to avoid being teased by others (von Salisch, 1991). Phrases such as "whistling in the dark" also capture our attempt to cope with aversive feelings by adopting a stronger-than-we-really-feel expressive facade.

What has not been researched is whether adoption of an emotional–expressive facade over time and with repeated good results contributes to an individual's beginning to feel less stressed, less vulnerable, and, indeed, genuinely what her initial dissembled expression communicated about her supposed internal emotional state. I think that what matters here is how others respond to emotional dissemblance and whether the expressive display is useful relative to situational demands. If others take it as a genuine emotional display and respond to an individual as though he or she were really "calm, cool, and collected," and if that sort of expressive display is effective for the situation (e.g., perhaps a situation requiring leadership and decision making while under pressure), then the individual receives *social feedback* that reinforces the adopted display as, in fact, reflective of his or her real self.

Direct Deception in Emotional–Expressive Behavior

In addition to cultural and personal display rules, people also exhibit ordinary deceptive emotional–expressive behavior. The key difference here is a relative lack of social consensus or predictability: An individual deliberately puts on a dissimulated facial expression, tone of voice, and so forth in a *particular and immediate situation* to mislead another about his or her emotional experience in order to gain some advantage or avoid some distinct disadvantage. For example, a girl who has set off the school fire alarm is not likely to express her glee at the commotion caused when she is around school authorities so that she will not be confronted as the possible culprit. This sort of directly deceptive emotional dissemblance would not be characterized by socially defined rules as to when to be employed. One is more likely to use directly deceptive emotional–expressive behavior when the stakes in a specific situation are clear. To illustrate, children may suppress their outrage at their teacher's unfairness, because if they did show their anger, they might experience even worse consequences from such a teacher; in contrast, they are likely to express vehemently their outrage at a peer's unfairness, and pity the poor parent who inadvertently appears to be unfair to his preadolescent.

A fairly large literature has begun to emerge on children's deception in recent years, and although the majority of it examines verbal lies, some studies have also observed children's behavior while they are lying (e.g., Chandler, Fritz, & Hala, 1989; Feldman, Jenkins, & Popoola, 1979; Josephs, 1993; Lewis, 1993a; Lewis, Stanger, & Sullivan, 1989). As an illustration, a series of studies by Josephs (1993) showed that young preschoolers were quite capable of deceiving others by adopting misleading expressive behavior, for example, pretending that sour juice tasted good. However, she found that they did not necessarily articulate this understanding. When the children were presented with stories in which the protagonist's facial expression and feelings could be discrepant, their interview responses did not indicate that they understood that such a dissociation between expression and feeling could occur. In other words, these young children demonstrated a tacit or pragmatic understanding of what to do behaviorally, but their verbalized knowledge did not reveal that they "knew what they knew" (or how they behaved).

In one of her studies, Josephs also determined that the children were capable of concealing a *positive* emotion, which had heretofore not been empirically or systematically examined. The children were seen individually by two research assistants. One assistant left the room, and Josephs arranged for the child to pretend along with the other research assistant that a glass of fruit juice was sweetened juice, when in fact it was quite sour, to trick the first assistant on her return. While this assistant was out of the room, the children were generally quite gleeful in their *Schadenfreude* (the German term for malicious joy or gloating) in anticipation of the reaction of the assistant on drinking sour juice. Thus, they had to conceal their positive emotional–expressive behavior for the ruse to succeed. Josephs found that the children showed many tension-related behaviors (e.g., hands over their mouth, a rather obvious attempt to conceal smiles and incipient giggles) and considerable glancing back and forth between assistants when the deceived assistant returned. However, some smiling did occur, and prolonged eye contact with the deceived assistant seemed to be a common strategy the children used to try to keep a "poker face."

DEVELOPMENT OF EMOTIONAL DISSEMBLANCE

Based on their collective social–emotional experiences over time, infants *gradually* learn to synchronize their emotional states and expressive behavior relative to an eliciting situation, but by no means do they necessarily begin life with an automatic "readout" of clearly discernible expressions that map onto reliably defined situational elicitors of emotion. Camras (1992) presents persuasive arguments and data for infants' acquisition of emotion *systems* of responses, including expressive behavior, which are heavily influenced by context. Her descriptions of her own daughter's early emotional–expressive development suggest that in seemingly neutral or even positive situations, a young infant may express a number of facial expressions denoting a variety of interpretive meanings (adult observers might judge them as indicative of anger, pain, sadness, disgust, or interest). For example, Camras's daughter, Justine, responded to her bath with facial expressions of distress, anger, sadness, and disgust (age 2 months). In short, the coordination of skeletal muscle patterning, situational "appraisal" (if we may call it that in the first weeks of life), and functional adaptation begins in a rather loose or haphazard fashion and progresses toward a socially defined *script* for what sorts of emotions are elicited by what sorts of situations and accompanied by what sorts of expressive behavior. (The reader might want to think about Lewis and Michalson's [1983] approach to components of emotions, described in Chapter 1, as being the potential constellation of emotion-related constructs that become coordinated with development.)

By the preschool years, if not earlier, young children also learn how to introduce disparities between their internal emotional experience and their external expressive behavior. Such discrepancies indicate that young children have begun to differentiate their inner emotional experience from what they express in their behavior—especially to others. Consider the following examples, which also capture the growth in sophistication of emotional dissemblance with increasing age:

> Katy (2.75 years): "I love Bubba" (said while she pinches her baby brother).

> Joey (3 years): "Mari did it!" (accompanied by an expression of indignation at being accused of throwing Marina's crayons into the toilet, which he had in fact done just minutes before).

> Marina (5 years): "When my mama gets mad, I show my sorry feeling, then she's not so mad."

> Paul (6 years): "You don't want to show them that it hurts, because then they'll think you're a crybaby."

> Cynthia (9 years): "When she just ignored me and invited the other girls instead to her party, I didn't show my hurt. I said to all

of them that she was stupid anyway, and I wouldn't want to go to her stupid old party."

Jared (11 years): "Well, it depends on whom you're with. Like I'd show how I feel to my friend Nick, but even with him I sometimes can't show or tell him my opinion because it might hurt his feelings."

Julia (14 years): "I used to think that I couldn't show my feelings to people unless they were my best friends or my parents, you know, only people I could trust. But now it matters to me how I feel; if the feeling is important or is about something important, then I'm going to show it, and that's just too bad if someone doesn't like it."

The preceding interview responses from children capture the richness of how children come to make sense of the fact that in our culture (and Western cultures more generally) we teach children a contradiction in values: "You should be honest," and at the same time, "your genuine ('honest') feelings may have to be expressed deceptively." There is a labyrinthine set of beliefs and expectations regarding what to express emotionally, where, when, and to whom. Impressively enough, by middle childhood children have learned and constructed for themselves a sometimes implicit, sometimes explicit, set of expectancies and contingencies for figuring out under what conditions which emotions get expressed and to whom. This growth in complexity of emotional expression is inseparable from the sorts of relationships children have. Thus, for example, children who grow up in homes with alcoholic parents or who are abused may well operate with a somewhat different set of expectations about how and with whom to express their feelings than do children who grow up in more functional families (e.g., Adams-Tucker, 1985; Copans, 1989; Putnam & Trickett, 1991). When we show our feelings indirectly or deceptively in our faces, our tone of voice, and our body movement, we are *dissembling* our emotional communication to others. Just as the children's comments show, dissemblance of feelings is related to whom we are with, to the social risks, and to what we are really feeling.

Forms of Expressive "Manipulation"

Perhaps the earliest form of this differentiation between internal state and external expression is the *exaggeration* of emotional–expressive behavior to gain someone's attention (a trivial injury becomes the occasion to howl loudly and solicit comfort and attention); readers who are parents are likely to think that this occurs in the second year, if not earlier. More systematic observational research supports this anecdotal view: Blurton-Jones (1967) reported that children, ages 3 to 4, in a free-play situation were more likely to cry after injuring themselves if they noticed a caregiver looking at them; they were less likely to cry if they thought they were unattended.

Minimization may be the next to appear; it consists of dampening the intensity of emotional–expressive behavior despite feeling otherwise. Socialization is likely to be highly influential here, as when we admonish children to calm down their rambunctiousness or control their upsetness. *Neutralization* describes the adoption of a poker face, but it is probably relatively difficult to carry off, and, indeed, Ekman and Friesen (1975) suggest that *substitution* of another expression that differs from what we genuinely feel is probably a more successful strategy (e.g., smiling despite feeling anxious).

Developing this skill of emotional competence permits fluidity in social interaction that clearly can be used to promote self-efficacy in interpersonal transactions. Whether we are trying to protect our vulnerability, enhance some advantage to ourselves, or promote the well-being of another for whom we care, being able to monitor our emotional–expressive behavior strategically is adaptive, and children learn to do so with increasing finesse as they mature (see also Saarni, 1989a).

Prerequisites of Emotional Dissemblance

As summarized by Shennum and Bugental (1982), in North America children gradually acquire *knowledge* about when, where, with whom, and how to express their feelings behaviorally . They also need to have the *ability to control* the skeletal muscles involved in emotional–expressive behavior. Significantly, they need to have the *motivation* to enact display rules in the appropriate situations. Finally, they also need to have reached a certain complexity of *cognitive representation*. An elaboration of a number of studies in which these issues were investigated follows.

Knowledge

In an early study (Saarni, 1979b), I interviewed elementary school children about when and why they would conceal their own feelings of hurt/pain and fear. The majority of their reasons referred to wanting to avoid embarrassment or derision from others for revealing vulnerable feelings. Getting attention, making someone feel sorry for himself, and getting help were also among the reasons mentioned for dissembling emotional–expressive behavior. Significant age difference appeared only when children were questioned about when would it be appropriate to express their genuine feelings, and older children were more likely to cite many *more* such occasions than younger children—suggesting that the older children (10 to 11 years) perceived the expression of emotion, whether genuine or dissembled, as a regulated act. The older children were more likely to make reference to the degree of affiliation with an interactant, status differences, and controllability of both emotion or circumstances as contextual qualities that affected the genuine or dissembled display of emotion. However, across all ages, the most common reason cited for when to express genuine feelings was if they were experienced as intense (and thus less controllable).

More recent research by Zeman her associates (Zeman & Garber, 1996; Zeman & Shipman, 1996) confirms and extends the previous findings. Using structured interviews and hypothetical vignettes, Zeman and Garber examined children's appraisal of how important the audience or interactant was for controlling the display of emotional-expressive behavior. Across all age groups (first, third, and fifth grades) children expected that they would control their expressive behavior more with peers than with parents (cf. Saarni, 1988). The reason that was most commonly cited for doing so was to avoid a negative social interaction. Older children also anticipated that they would be less likely to display negative feelings with their fathers and would be more likely to reveal sadness and pain to their mothers than to peers. Echoing Zeman and Garber, we clearly need more research that addresses how children experience disapproval for their genuine displays of negative emotion within these different relationships (mother, father, peer).

Ability to Implement Emotional Dissemblance

Control of skeletal muscles, especially in the face, is critical to being able to modify emotional–expressive behavior and thus dissemble the outward expression of our feelings. Children begin to be able to do this modification voluntarily at a young age (2 to 3 years), and it is readily apparent in their pretend play; for example, they mimic postures, expressions, vocal qualities, and the like of assorted fantasy characters. However, when it comes to deliberately adopting emotional expressions, posing of facial expressions proves to be difficult, especially negatively toned expressions (e.g., Lewis, Sullivan, & Vasen, 1987; Odom & Lemond, 1972). The difficulty in posing fear, disgust, sadness, and the like may be due to the fairly consistent socialization pressure in our culture to inhibit negative displays of emotion. A smiling expression is considerably easier for children to produce, but even then they may produce only partially "happy" facial expressions, perhaps partly due to self-consciousness. For example, trying to get a 5-year-old to "look cute while Grandma takes a picture" is likely to elicit crossed eyes, a tongue hanging out, and general clowning. By age 7, such a request might elicit a locked-jaw, square-looking smile with lots of teeth showing (if we are lucky). As Lewis et al. (1987) point out, when asked to produce a scared face, the young children in their sample produced *scary* faces instead.

Motivation

In a study with elementary school children, I investigated children's knowledge of how to manage emotional–expressive behavior and their expectations about what motivated story characters to undertake such management strategies (Saarni, 1979a). I used four stories that also had accompanying photos of children acting out the story line: (1) receiving a disappointing gift from one's aunt, (2) setting off the school fire alarm and then being intercepted by the principal, (3) showing off on one's skates and then falling down, and (4) being bullied by another child at school. In the final photograph, the protagonist's face was averted from the camera, and the children were asked how he or she felt and then to select from a set of four full-face portraits of different facial expressions how his or her face would look in this situation. No sex differences were found, although age differences did occur: Older children were more likely spontaneously to nominate the display of facial expressions that did not match the actual feeling of the story protagonist. With interview prompts, this age difference diminished somewhat.

When the children were asked to explain why the story character's feelings had not been genuinely expressed, four broad categories of motivation were apparent in their responses. Given that most human behavior has multiple determinants, similarly any given instance of emotional dissemblance may have more than one of these motivational categories underlying it. I elaborate on these four motivation categories next and also discuss them in the order in which they are hypothesized to appear in children's behavioral repertoires.

1. The first category of motivation is to avoid negative outcomes, as succinctly illustrated by a 6-year-old boy's response to an interview in another study: "He wouldn't show that he thought it [a trick played on another child] was funny, because he'd be scared that the kid would beat him up." This sort of rationale—to avoid some anticipated bad outcome—is generally found to be the most frequently offered as a justification for expressive dissemblance.

2. The second motivation category for dissemblance is to protect one's self-esteem or to cope more effectively with how one feels. An 8-year-old boy said the following: "He could show that he could stand up to stuff like that" in reference to being the target of criticism. When we adopt personal display rules, we may have as our motive the desire to protect our vulnerability, our self-image, or our self-esteem. This boy's comment alluded to being able to control stoically one's feelings, despite the threat to self-esteem implied by being criticized.

3. The third motivation category for expressive dissemblance concerns relationships. It has a more elementary version as well as a more sophisticated version. The simpler level is to dissemble one's feelings so as not to hurt someone else's feelings (see Chapter 4 for a discussion of my research; Saarni, 1987, 1989a), and even children of ages 5 to 6 years old are able to understand this sort of motive for dissembling their feelings (not that they reliably perform it, however). The more complex level of this motive category is to regulate relationship *dynamics*. This latter variant appeared most often in preadolescent children's justifications for expressive dissemblance in subsequent research (Saarni, 1991). Several of their responses follow: "He didn't want to let the other kids down, so he didn't show his disappointment [at losing the game that he had coached]"; "A friend would know that she felt sorry deep down inside but couldn't show it just then"; and "she knew her Mom had a lot a pride in her, so she tried to smile at everybody after she messed up" [during a solo gymnastics performance]. Concern for others' well-being is a prominent theme among such rationales, both simpler and more complex levels, and is generally associated with relatively close relationships or the desire to increase the closeness of a relationship.

An intriguing observational study carried out by von Salisch (1991) probed how children actually regulated a relationship by monitoring what they expressed. She developed a computer game that was rigged: The computer was cast as the "opponent" and a pair of children were to play as a team. If the airplane "crashed" on the screen, it meant the children had lost; however, its demise was in fact random but appeared to the children to have been caused by one of them. The participating children were 11 years old, and von Salisch was able to have the pairs consist of either best friends or casual acquaintances. In her analyses of the actual conflict episodes, the most frequent expressive behavior was smiling, followed by signs of tension, then contempt, and finally anger (only 3% of the expressions). In many cases the children also verbalized reproaches about the crash but then accompanied the reproach by smiling. With close friends the incidence of smiling was even greater than with acquaintances, and genuine smiles were especially notable in their reciprocity among girls in close friend pairs, even through these girls more frequently verbalized their negative feelings about their friend's game-playing skill (or ostensible lack thereof). The boys in close friendship pairs tended to verbalize less, but they showed more signs of tension than any other group. In essence, these preadolescent boys and girls used their smiles to reassure their friend that the *relationship* was still on firm ground, despite their reproaching the friend for his or her "incompetence" in making them lose the game against the computer. Clearly expressive behavior has among its functions more than simply the display of emotion; it is also a *social* message. Von Salisch's research shows us that children are adept at using this social function of emotional–expressive behavior to manage their relationships, and they do so in a discriminating fashion.

4. The fourth motivation category concerns norms and conventions; these are the cultural display rules that provide us with consensually agreed on scripts for how to manage our emotions. A couple of 9- to 10-year-old children's responses illustrate their notions of the norms for emotional dissemblance: "You shouldn't yell at a grownup" and "you should apologize, even though you don't feel like it." It is probably noteworthy that cultural display rules often have "shoulds" associated with them. Parenthetically, children may readily articulate culturally accepted scripts for emotional dissemblance, but that does not mean they will actually perform such scripts, such as apologizing when they would rather not. At least a couple of factors might account for why children do not consistently perform cultural display rule scripts, despite knowing them: First, the social stakes may not be sufficiently high for them to feel motivated to do so; and second their distressed, hurt, or angry feelings may be experienced as too intense to allow for emotional dissemblance. As mentioned earlier (Saarni, 1979a), intensity of feeling was cited by school-age children as the chief reason for genuinely expressing feelings.

These four categories for why we may be motivated to dissemble the expression of our feelings are not necessarily exhaustive, but they all have one significant feature in common: They are concerned with interpersonal consequences, and it is the varying nature of these social consequences that yields the differences among motives. Even the self-esteem motive for dissemblance does not occur in a social vacuum, for the self is embedded in a history of social relationships.

Cognitive Representation

As was already suggested by Josephs's (1993) research, a pragmatic or implicit knowledge of emotional dissemblance is likely to precede an articulated and verbalized understanding of expressive dissimulation.

Within the "theory of mind" literature, a large body of research has emerged concerned with children's understanding of real versus apparent phenomena, and this distinction has been applied to inner emotional state as "real" and external expressive behavior as "apparent." (One could quibble over the apparent distinction, because the social message of the dissembled expressive behavior may be what is "real.")

By school entry children generally understand that how they look on their face is not necessarily how they feel on the inside (e.g., Harris & Gross, 1988). Thus, relatively young children understand that the appearance of their facial expression can be misleading about the actual emotional state they are experiencing. By age 6 many children can provide justifications for how appearances can conceal reality, in this case, the genuine emotion felt by an individual. Harris and Gross (1988) examined young children's rationales for why story characters would conceal their emotions by adopting misleading facial expressions. A significant number of the 6-year-olds interviewed gave complex justifications that included describing the intent to conceal their feelings and to mislead another to believe something other than what he or she was really emotionally experiencing (e.g., "She didn't want her sister to know that she was sad about not going to the party"). Children younger than 6 can readily adopt pretend facial expressions, but they are not likely to be able to articulate the embedded relationships involved in deliberate emotional dissemblance.

These embedded relationships refer to how the self wants another to perceive an apparent self, not the real self. In other words, by age 6 children readily grasp that emotional dissemblance has as its basic function the creation of a false impression on others. However, the construct, "false impression," seems to have a rather negative connotation, and I think a more useful way to look at this development is to view children as acquiring effective *self-presentations*. These self-presentations are not false or phony aspects of the self but rather reveal the degree to which children embrace social interaction with flexibility and resourcefulness as they adapt the range of behaviors available to them in their expressive repertoire to the exigencies of the interpersonal transaction facing them. I consider this topic in greater detail next.

SELF-PRESENTATION STRATEGIES IN EMOTIONAL–EXPRESSIVE BEHAVIOR

Self-presentation in adulthood has a long research history (reviewed by Baumeister, 1982; Tedeschi, 1981; Tedeschi & Norman, 1985), and it has also been linked with coping with stress (Laux, 1986). Laux connects emotional well-being directly with self-presentation because if we manage our self-presentation (and thus our emotional–expressive behavior) to preserve our self-esteem in some threatening or otherwise stressful situation, then we will have coped more effectively with that situation and emerge from it *feeling better.* Thus, self-presentations that are simultaneously coping efforts can both be oriented toward changing the "person–environment transaction" and have an emotionally relieving effect (see also Lazarus & Launier, 1978).

DePaulo (1991) has provided us with a definitive review of what is known about the development of self-presentation, emphasizing nonverbal behavior. One important point she makes is that as children grow older, more of their peers and adult networks hold them accountable for being able to regulate and manage their emotional–expressive behavior. Thus, there is a continual reinforcement of motivation to manage how we present ourselves to others. At some point, it is likely that we acquire habitual nonverbal behaviors that reflect self-presentation attempts and may similarly reflect our chronic attempts to regulate our internal emotional experience (i.e., to make it more acceptable or more prestigious in the eyes of our audience). However, each of us needs to find a balance between adaptive self-presentation strategies and acknowledgment of what we are feeling. The following vignette captures this phenomenon:

> Fifteen-year-old Jason enjoyed a warm and affectionate relationship with his father until his dad was diagnosed with an inoperable brain tumor and died a short while later. In the first few weeks after his death, Jason was able to cry and emotionally express his grief around his mother and sister, but he revealed nothing of his sadness among his male peers at school. Some might not have even known that his father had recently died.
>
> Jason was big for his age, and he wanted very much to get on the varsity football team at his school; being overcome by tears or even just "misting up" was viewed as wimpy and unmanly among his social group and would get him teased. It might even get back to the coach who did the selection for the team and could cost him a place on the team if he didn't effectively shut down his grieving about his dad while at school. "Big boys don't cry" was definitely the controlling display rule of his peer group. Jason began to manage his expressive behavior with diligence.
>
> Jason maintained his stiff upper lip and his dry eyes throughout that school year. He did experience periodic bouts of nonspecific dermatitis. The following summer, when his boyhood pal, his dog, also abruptly died, Jason stoically excavated the hole in which to bury him. The next day Jason awakened to find himself covered

with scaly, itchy hives from head to toe, and it wasn't poison oak. Managing his self-presentation so well appeared to have penalized his autoimmune system, and, cruelly, it came out in a most visible manner, upsetting his careful attempts at self-presentation.

I return to this idea of "balance" in our emotion management in Chapter 11, in which I discuss capacity for emotional self-efficacy. However, what is apparent in this example is how important the social consequences of our emotional–expressive behavior are. An empirical demonstration of that significance may be found in a study in which I interviewed children from age 7 to 14 about how others would react to the presentation of an "emotional front." I also asked them about their preference for adults versus peers as recipients of their genuine emotional expressiveness as well as what the expected outcomes might be for children who almost never revealed their feelings versus those who almost always did (Saarni, 1988). I also asked them about how they thought they constructed an emotional "balance" for themselves between when to reveal their real feelings and when not to, but I reserve discussion of those results for Chapter 11.

The results of this descriptive study indicated that whether or not an emotional front was detected was highly related to the interpersonal context. Among the many significant effects and interactions, an interesting one was between girls and boys relative to an aggressive encounter: Should one cover up one's fear of a bully? Boys, by far, thought they should conceal their fear, even though the older boys thought it would be ineffective—bullies do what they want to do, regardless of someone's emotional dissemblance. The oldest girls more often thought the emotional front might well be perceived by the interactant but nothing would come of it, and the interactant would take the emotional front at face value. My inference here is that these oldest girls did not think that the story characters would risk "rocking the boat," so to speak, a finding which has its parallel in Rosenthal and DePaulo's (1979) research on women seeming to ignore or overlook increasingly deceptive cues in nonverbal behavior. (To confront another's emotional dissemblance carries some risk.) As far as preference for expressing real feelings to peer or adults, again the older girls tended to prefer their peers, whereas the youngest children preferred adults and the older boys were rather evenly divided. Examination of their justifications seemed to indicate that these preadolescent and adolescent girls found adults to be untrustworthy recipients (relative to peers) of their genuine feelings or that they would abuse their power with the girls if they did find out. It should be pointed out that this question specifically asked the children to exclude their parents from this comparison.

When asked about the consequences to children who almost always concealed their genuine feelings, a high proportion nominated outcomes that indicated that such children would be disliked, would be emotionally maladjusted, or would be hard to get to know. As one eighth-grader succinctly put it, "If she kept everything inside herself all the time, she'd consume all her anger, jealousy, whatever, and then one day she'd explode, commit suicide, and get emotionally disturbed." (Recall the "volcano theory" of emotion described as a type of Western folk theory of emotional experience in Chapter 1). For those children who were at the opposite end of this expressive spectrum (i.e., they "let it all hang out") about half of the subjects responded with the belief that such a youngster would be rejected by their peers. However, about one third of the expected consequences were positive in tone, that is, such genuine kids would be perceived as honest and more likable, and they could "get relief" (the volcano theory again). In summary, elementary school children and young adolescents view either extreme in emotion management as maladaptive, and they believe a flexible middle road makes the most sense when it comes to having satisfactory relationships with others.

Children's Influence on Others' Emotions

To orchestrate effective self-presentation strategies, children need to take into account their interactants' views and possible biases (e.g., unique personal information about their interactants; see Chapter 5). Having at their disposal the ability to manage their emotional–expressive behavior strategically makes it more feasible for children to try to influence others' emotional responses to them. Do children know that they can influence another's emotional reaction? Studies by Carlson, Felleman, and Masters (1983) and McCoy and Masters (1985) describe a developmental viewpoint. In the Carlson et al. (1983) study, 4- to 5-year-old children viewed slides of other young children displaying assorted emotional states; then investigators ascertained the children's accuracy of emotion judgment. The subject children were then asked "If *something* could change how [the child in the slide] felt, would you want it to, and if *you* could change how [the child in the slide] felt, would you want to?" As expected, targets feeling a negative emotion were selected by the subjects to have their feeling states changed whereas those feeling happy were not (or they suggested intensifying the happiness). Whether they themselves were to be involved in the change of emotion also led children to be more willing to endorse changing the target's emotion than if some external reason were to change the target's emotional state. Although this study tells us that preschoolers apparently can recognize that they can play a role in influencing someone's emotional state, we do not know their reasoning for *why* this might be desirable or strategic. The children were not asked to justify their responses or to nominate reasons for how or why they might be influential in changing another's emotional response. In any case, it is possible that preschoolers could not articulate such justifications.

McCoy and Masters (1985) remedied this ambiguity in a study in which 5- to 12-year-olds were interviewed in response to a series of slides depicting other children displaying assorted emotions. Accompanying stories were either social or nonsocial in nature and the emotional state of the child was explicitly stated. The subjects were then asked, "What could you do to make [character's name] not feel [affect given]?" Depending on the emotion in question, children nominated intervention strategies that would appear to require managing their emotional–expressive behavior; for example, nurturance was nominated to alter sadness and anger, and aggression was suggested to change happiness. Nurturing behavior would entail a variety of expressive behaviors in the brow (perhaps sad looking) and mouth region (perhaps smiling slightly) along with an appropriate comforting vocal tone, whereas aggressive behavior would include frowns, absence of positive expressions, threatening vocal tone, and gestures. The developmental difference in this study was that older children suggested more social and verbal nurturance strategies, which would presumably involve the expressive behaviors noted previously. The 5-year-olds were more likely to suggest material nurturance strategies to alleviate someone's sadness or anger (e.g., give the sad person some candy).

This study has a number of other complex findings, but for our purposes it is important that school-age children can readily articulate ways to alter someone's affective state. Older children were more likely to suggest *interpersonal* strategies, and if they had been interviewed further about how someone would *look* during these interpersonal interventions, this research might have shed light on their degree of awareness of how their emotional–expressive behavior would need to be managed.

Little research has probed children's spontaneous attempts to manage their own self-presentation behavior while seeking to influence another's emotional state. The research literature on empathy and helping behavior certainly suggests that children recognize how to comfort another in distress (see Chapter 7), but in that case the children are not necessarily trying to manage their own emotional–expressive behavior strategically. The study described in Chapter 7 about children's attempts to cheer up a sad research assistant (Saarni, 1992) may be relevant here in that it did capture children's spontaneous behavior in a naturalistic setting, but the study also highlighted the tremendous influence of contextual features on the interaction of two individuals. We turn now to this aspect of what goes on in the *system* of relationships, which children learn to recognize as the source of contextual cues that they need to attend to in order to develop flexible and effective self-presentations.

Recognition of Salient Contextual Cues

From an emotional competence standpoint, self-efficacy in difficult interpersonal situations can be promoted (1) if we are aware that our emotional–expressive behavior influences another's response, (2) if we then strategically try to manage our emotional–expressive behavior vis-à-vis the other for the other to respond in a way that is deemed more desirable, and (3) if we are aware of contextual cues that also influence the interaction (these contextual cues derive their meaningfulness from cultural scripts and thus can be quite variable).

Early work by social scientists studying nonverbal communication among mainstream North Americans determined two important contextual cues that influence adults' nonverbal expressive behavior in dyadic interaction. One cue was the status difference between the interactants and the other was how close the relationship was (e.g., Mehrabian, 1972). Typically, the nondominant person was more likely to control his or her expressiveness when interacting with a more dominant individual. In close relationships, nonverbal expressive behavior was likely to be less controlled and emotions more often genuinely revealed. As a downward extension of this research into childhood, I conducted a study with school-age children to examine how they took into account status (were the interactants equal in status or did they differ) and affiliation (was the relationship between the interactants a close one or not) as they predicted whether story characters' emotional–expressive behavior would be genuine or dissembled (Saarni, 1991). In addition, emotional intensity (strong vs. mild feelings) was included as a cue that influenced whether emotional displays were thought to be controllable or not.

The children's responses indicated that they did indeed take into account status similarity or difference and degree of closeness of relationship for predicting whether facial expressions would be genuine or dissembled. But if the feelings were intense, they were often predicted to be genuinely expressed, even though the story character had a lower status and there was little closeness in the relationship with the other story character. In terms of age differences, from ages 6 to 12, all children were aware that intensity of emotion and status difference between interactants would influence the protagonist's facial expression, but older children were more likely also to take into account degree of affiliation between the characters as a factor that influenced whether facial expressions would be genuine or dissembled.

The children were also asked to justify their predictions about facial expressions, and when these were analyzed, the most common rationale was to avoid negative interpersonal consequences. However, the variety of rationales increased with age, such that by ages 10 to 12 years, children gave a rich mixture of rationales, ranging from concerns about others' well-being to the desirability of observing norms and conventions, as the reasons for why facial expressions were thought to be either genuine or dissembled. Perhaps the point to make here is that children are keenly aware of the interpersonal effects that facial expressions have, and that certain social contexts "require" dissemblance while others are more appropriate for genuine expression of emotion.

INDIVIDUAL DIFFERENCES IN EMOTIONAL DISSEMBLANCE

Obviously we could examine a great range of individual differences in how children and youth go about managing their emotional–expressive behavior. Cultural display rules, by definition, show less variation, whereas personal display rules could be quite variable. Expedient deception has perhaps an even wider variety of options and patterns (for a recent review, see DePaulo, Kashy, Kirkendol, Wyer, & Epstein, 1996). As in the preceding chapters, I narrow the scope of this issue to patterns in emotional dissemblance related to gender and social maturity differences. In the case of cultural differences, I consider some representative studies that help to illustrate how to go about doing cross-cultural comparisons of the development of emotional dissemblance and emotion management.

Gender Differences

Some of the gender-related patterns in expressive displays have already been mentioned, and they would appear to reflect the influence of sex-role socialization on boys and girls in Western culture. The most frequently encountered difference mentioned in several studies already described in this chapter is that girls smile more than boys, especially in social contexts, and their smiles appear as part of early self-presentations that are geared to making social transactions more positive and agreeable. In most cases this probably is a functional emotion management strategy, but it can become overgeneralized by adolescence and adulthood to become a mask of polite smiling and "niceness" that can interfere with being taken seriously (e.g., Bugental, 1986; Bugental, Love, & Gianetto, 1971).

Interestingly, there may be no or few sex differences in children's *general understanding* of emotional dissemblance or of misleading displays (e.g., Saarni, 1979a; Gross & Harris, 1988). However, Terwogt and Olthof (1989) present data that suggest that knowledge of when to control emotional–expressive displays may be gender-related when the specific emotion is culturally sanctioned for one sex but not for the other. Specifically, girls in their Dutch sample said they would not express anger as readily as the boys would, and conversely, the boys were reluctant to express fear. The justifications for the girls included disapproval from adults for showing anger, and the boys worried they would be viewed as cowards by their peers if they expressed fear. Fuchs and Thelen (1988) also report that boys were loathe to reveal their sadness to their fathers but might consider revealing it to their mothers.

A recent study by Davis (1995) attempted to tease apart whether boys and girls differed in their emotion management strategies because of differences in motivation or differences in ability. The young elementary school children (grades 1 and 3) in her study went through the "disappointing gift" scenario described earlier, and their expressive behavior was videorecorded. The boys showed more negative expressive behaviors than the girls upon receiving the disappointing gift, an outcome that parallels earlier research (Saarni, 1984; Cole, 1986). However, in the next task Davis had the children play a game in which a desirable prize and an undesirable one were placed in two boxes, visible only to the child. The children were told to deceive the experimenter by pretending to like both prizes, and if they succeeded in "tricking" the experimenter to believe they really liked both, they would be able to keep both prizes. If they did not succeed, the experimenter took both prizes. Thus, for the children to get the attractive prize, they had to persuasively manage their expressive behavior to look positive for both attractive and unattractive prizes.

The results showed that the girls were more successful at suppressing negative expressive behaviors toward the unattractive prize than were the boys. Interestingly, the girls also revealed a greater number of social monitoring behaviors (e.g., rapid glancing at the experimenter) as well as tension behaviors (e.g., touching one's face) (see Saarni, 1992, and Davis, 1995, for the coding scheme). In comparing the children's expressive behavior in the two situations (gift and game), the children were given a clear incentive and were explicitly instructed to produce positive behaviors in the game situation. Indeed, compared to the disappointing gift situation, both boys and girls did reduce their number of negative expressive behaviors in the game situation. However, the girls' level of negative responses to both attractive and unattractive prizes was virtually indistinguishable. Instead, they appeared to monitor the social exchange more closely than the boys, which may have facilitated their expression management. Davis concludes that girls do have more ability in managing the expression of their negative feelings, and she suggests that individual differences (e.g., temperament) may interact with sex-role socialization to yield the gender pattern she observed.

An observational study by Casey (1993), which was also described in Chapter 4, is relevant here as well for its intriguing gender effects. She investigated the relations among children's ability to report their emotions and their ability to describe their own facial expression under two different social feedback conditions. The children, ages 7 to 12 years, were given a variety of tasks and then told that there was another child of their age and gender who might be brought in later to interact with them. The experimenter then left the room, and a video monitor in the subject child's room began to show this other child (a confederate) with the experimenter talking to him or her. The confederate child then gave either disparaging social feedback or positive social feedback about the subject child in the first room. The monitor then went dark, and the experimenter shortly returned to the subject child in the first room. The subject children were interviewed as to how they felt hearing the feedback, how they knew what they felt, and how they believed they looked in their faces when they heard the feedback. Their expressive behavior had also been videotaped throughout the whole episode, and thus their verbal reports could be compared to what they had indeed displayed. Although Casey was not investigating emotional dissemblance, she found that girls were facially more responsive to conditions of negative and positive social feedback than were boys. The latter tended to maintain a low level of constant negative expressive behavior under both conditions of positive and negative feedback. Casey argued that in comparison to boys, girls may embellish their facial displays to better regulate their social communications, and thus this skill may have contributed to their greater awareness and accuracy in also knowing how their faces looked upon hearing the feedback. Interestingly, there were few significant age differences in children's expressive behavior or their understanding of how they felt upon receiving the positive or negative feedback, but older children were more likely than younger children to report more sophisticated explanations for what they felt, which was an expected outcome.

Brody and Hall's (1993) excellent review of sex differences in emotion is oriented toward adult functioning, and they too emphasize that the type of emotion felt and expressed is itself influenced by sex-role socialization, via the family and peer group. Thus, they suggest that girls end up "cultivating" the expression of such feelings as happiness, shame, fear, and warmth whereas boys attend more to the expression of feelings of anger, aggression, contempt, and pride. Brody and Hall also contend that through a multitude of influences (which they describe in their review at length), by adolescence boys may end up expressing their emotions more through their physiology (e.g., Jason's dermatitis reaction described earlier) and their overt action (e.g., aggression, withdrawal, and avoidance). In contrast, adolescent girls may end up subjectively experiencing both negative and positive emotions more intensely, expressing them more intensely in facial and other nonverbal behaviors and using emotion-laden language more often.

I infer from their argument that girls' socialization provides them with proximal emotional–expressive behavior management strategies (i.e., language and facial expressions), which are useful for close interpersonal transactions in an immediate sense. On the other hand, boys acquire "invisible" emotion management strategies (i.e., resulting in physiological change but not especially anything noticeable in the face for communicative purposes) and distal behaviors with which to act on situations (to aggress, to avoid, to change, etc.). It sounds as though the old "instrumental males" and "expressive females" dichotomy is alive and well, at least in psychological research; however, I strongly suspect that boys and girls in the elementary school years, while showing some differences in emotion understanding, are in reality much more similar in how they understand the relations between what one feels on the inside and what one shows on the outside. Both boys and girls adroitly say, "It depends on whom you're with. . . . " With increasing age, socialization is likely to further "contextualize" emotion management so that our roles and scripts guide us as to how, when, and with whom we express our emotions.

Social Maturity Differences

Emotional Disturbance

Few studies have directly addressed the sorts of deficits or differences in emotional–expressive behavior management strategies that may exist for children who are functioning well in their social relationships as opposed to those who are not. Adlam-Hill and Harris (1988) undertook one study that empirically examined understanding of display rule usage among children identified as emotionally disturbed. They found that emotionally disturbed children of average intelligence showed a distinct deficit compared to their nondisturbed peers in understanding that internal emotional state and external expressive behavior can be incongruent. As a consequence, such children were also less likely to think that story characters would modify their facial expressions if showing how they really felt would hurt the feelings of another. Adlam-Hill and Harris speculate about why this deficit occurred and suggest that emotionally disturbed children may not understand how to protect others' feelings, or they may not be motivated to do so, or they do not even predict that the display of genuine emotion can affect another in the first place.

Insofar as emotion management, emotional dissemblance, and self-presentation may also be considered part of a larger "package" of coping skills, it would be expected that children with identified problems in coping with stress and conflict would not use adaptive emotion management strategies in an appropriate way or would do so only some of the time. Children with attention-deficit disorder would have difficulty scanning a situation for its relevant social cues and, characteristically, would demonstrate their impulsivity by seizing on one cue and reacting to it alone. For example, imagine an attention-deficit child receiving a disappointing gift from a well-meaning but misguided relative. To address the cultural display rule of "look agreeable when someone gives you something, even if you don't like it," such youngsters would have to inhibit their initial negative emotional reaction to the poorly chosen gift and instead direct their attention to their relationship with the relative and how they felt—both about their relative's feelings and how they wanted to be seen in the eyes of that relative (e.g., as a polite child), the latter representing the appraisal needed for an effective self-presentation.

Depression

If children nominate intense feelings as those least likely to be controlled and thus least amenable to management strategies, how would a depressed child make use of smiling displays to create smooth and engaging social transactions if he or she were feeling sad and hopeless? Not surprisingly, Harris and Lipian (1989) found that children who were hospitalized for acute medical conditions showed a regression or slippage in their understanding of emotion management. Harris and Lipian (1989) argue that the children's strongly negative and depressive emotional feelings "exert a pervasive filtering effect on consciousness. Other more positive concerns are either subverted to fit this one central preoccupation or are ignored" (p. 255).

At-Risk Children

Cole, Zahn-Waxler, and Smith (1994) investigated how 4- to 5-year-old children who had been categorized as at low, moderate, and high risk for developing behavioral problems (e.g., oppositional behavior or excessive aggression) would respond to the "disappointing gift" scenario. At-risk boys showed more angry, disruptive, and generally negative behavior during the examiner's presence than did low-risk boys. In contrast to boys, the at-risk girls showed a flattening of affect compared to the low-risk girls during the examiner's absence. Specifically, when the examiner was absent, the low-risk girls readily expressed their disappointment or aggravation with the lousy gift, but the at-risk girls expressed only minimal distress or negative behavior. These girls were primarily diagnosed as having attention-deficit disorder, and Cole et al. (1994) speculate that possibly their overinhibition of negative affect may be related to deficits in instrumental coping and appropriate emotion management.

Lonely Children

A fairly substantial research literature has emerged about lonely and rejected children (e.g., Asher & Coie, 1990; Cassidy & Asher, 1992; Parkhurst & Asher, 1992). Not surprisingly, lonely children are perceived as shy, but in addition there appear to be at least a couple of subgroups of lonely children: Some are aggressive and demonstrate minimal prosocial behavior and others are submissive and withdrawn (e.g., Parkhurst & Asher, 1992). Boys may be overrepresented in the former group (Cassidy & Asher, 1992), and children in the aggressive subgroup appear to be more often also rejected by their peers. From the standpoint of emotion management, we can infer that lonely, rejected children do not have the skills to be able to maneuver their self-presentations such that they can achieve more effective impressions on their peers. They may be using faulty social cognition in how they appraise what would be effective impression management, or they have an idea of what to do but have difficulty implementing it behaviorally. The latter may occur due to anticipatory anxiety about possible rejection, or if their shyness is characterized by general cautiousness, such a wary inhibited style may contribute to delays in emotional responsiveness toward others, and poor timing may impair their entry into social interaction. The fact that a low prosocial orientation has been found in a significant number of lonely children suggests possible deficits in empathic understanding of others or deficits in comprehending the emotional communicative behavior of others. Thus, lonely (and rejected) children may have deficits both at the *encoding* level of sending emotional–expressive signals as well as at the *decoding* level of receiving and comprehending others' emotional–expressive communicative behavior.

Autism

A more extreme group of emotionally disturbed (or different) children are those diagnosed as autistic. Harris (1989) argues that autistic individuals feel emotion but communicate it differently or maladaptively to others. In reviewing a number of studies, he suggests that autistic children do not take into account other people's *interior* state, namely, their beliefs, their feelings, their goals, and so forth. He contends that to do so, one must have the "ability to simulate or imagine the emotional state of another person by analogy with the state of the self " (p. 214). Autistic children do not appear to function this way, suggesting a fairly major cognitive deficit in their construal of their experience and environment.

Other researchers observationally tracked autistic preschoolers' spontaneous displays of emotion according to specific contextual categories and compared these patterns with those obtained from ordinary children; their results provided confirming evidence for Harris's contention (McGee, Feldman, & Chernin, 1991). These investigators found that the autistic children displayed about as many emotional expressions as the normal group, but the eliciting contexts were different indeed. Most of the autistic children's happy expressions occurred in solitary activity, whereas the typical children's smiles occurred in social activity with peers or adults. The normal children's angry expressions occurred most commonly when engaged in conflict with another child, whereas the autistic children's anger displays occurred in what otherwise looked like positive situations with adults. Not surprisingly, autistic children have considerable difficulty in social relationships, for their response to others' emotionally communicative behavior is not synchronized with their own emotional–expressive behavior. In essence, autistic children do not learn the cultural scripts or folk theories of emotion that other children do (see also Hobson, 1986). They do not know the steps to the "dance," and they march to the beat of a different drummer.

Cultural Differences

Mesquita and Frijda's (1992) review of cultural variation in emotions suggests that on the most general level, the majority of researchers agree that the phenomenon of "response inhibition, or the existence of some measure of emotion and expression control" (p. 198) is virtually universal. However, they also state that one of the most significant sources of variation in cultural experience of emotion lies in regulatory processes, whether these be the sort that prohibit certain emotions from being experienced and/or expressed or the sort that prescribe what one should feel and express emotionally under certain circumstances. Thus, on the more specific and descriptive level, cultures vary widely in terms of what one is expected to feel, and when, where, and with whom one may express assorted feelings. In short, folk theories of emotion are as variable as cultures are. To give some specificity to how these folk theories reveal themselves in children's responses to researchers investigating understanding of misleading expressions and display rules, I will describe several studies done with Japanese, African American, Italian, and Indian children.

Japanese Children

Gardner, Harris, Ohmoto, and Hamazaki (1988) evaluated Japanese children's (ages 4 to 6) understanding of whether facial expressions could be adopted to mislead another about their real feelings. The children were explicitly instructed that what a story protagonist would express would not be congruent with what she felt internally. Similar to an earlier study with British children, the 4-year-olds lagged behind the 6-year-olds in understanding that this distinction could be made. Gardner et al. (1988) interpreted their findings from the viewpoint common in the appearance-reality literature, which is that young children have a cognitive barrier, as it were, to comprehending simultaneous and mutual incompatibilities or contradictions that co-occur or are contained within the same object or event. It should be pointed out that this study required the children to *verbalize* their understanding; a tacit or pragmatic behavioral enactment of misleading expressions was not investigated (cf. Josephs, 1993). I think we need to be wary of the tendency to conclude from research such as this that young children are incapable of emotional dissemblance; it is most definitely not the case, but we do seem to be confronted with the fact that preschoolers have serious difficulties articulating that "they know what they know."

African American Children

Underwood et al. (1992) examined children's expectations of when to mask expressions of anger in response to videotaped hypothetical vignettes that featured a child interacting with either a teacher or another child. The children were all urban African American children in a low-income neighborhood; they ranged in age from 8 to 13. Children were asked to put themselves in the protagonist's shoes and respond with what they would do. They generally suggested genuine expressions of anger toward peers but were more likely to inhibit the expression of their anger toward teachers; this audience difference makes sense strategically, as teachers have authority over children, and the display of anger toward a peer is not the sort of expression of emotion that renders one vulnerable or "weak." If anything, in American culture, displaying anger may well facilitate impressing on one's peers that one is strong and invincible.

An interesting gender effect was also found, namely, that the preadolescent girls were *less* likely to expect themselves to mask anger toward teachers than were the boys of the same age. Underwood et al. (1992) speculate that in this American subculture, it may be resourceful for boys to present themselves as emotionally "contained" (e.g., stoic and unruffled) and for girls to present themselves as assertive. Underwood et al. also found that children who nominated masking anger also tended to do so if they felt sadness as well; in other words, negative emotions in general were proposed as being likely targets of masking strategies. Finally, the investigators thought they would see more usage of display-rule reasoning in this sample due to its being older than those used in other studies, but, in fact, many children preferred genuine displays of anger. What may be involved here is the nature of the emotion felt (anger) and the fact that displaying the anger was not sampled as occurring in close relationships (where it could hurt others' feelings whom one cares about), that the intensity of the emotion was not perceived as controllable (and therefore not "maskable"), and finally, that there may well be a bias for children to prefer genuine displays of emotion for themselves but to attribute dissembled displays to others (e.g., Karniol & Koren, 1987; Saarni, 1991).

Italian and British Children

Manstead (1995) investigated whether British and Italian children would differ from one another in understanding display rules; their supposition was that given greater socialization pressure in England to inhibit emotional expression, British children would both adopt and understand usage of display rules at a younger age than would Italian children. The participating children were ages 6 to 7 and 10 to 11 years old. Manstead presented the children with audiotaped vignettes about a disappointing gift and about disgusting food and then followed up with questions that asked the children what they would do if they were in the protagonist's position relative to expression management. The children were also asked about whether they could conceal genuine feelings from another (i.e., the appearance–reality distinction). The results indicated that the older age groups of both Italian and British children were more likely to suggest concealment of disappointment upon receiving an undesirable gift as compared to the younger children. In addition, the culture comparison indicated that British children were considerably more likely to ascribe concealment of disappointment to themselves than were the Italian children, with this effect being most pronounced among the younger children. By age 7, the proportion of British children suggesting inhibition of disappointment was nearly as high as at age 11, whereas a majority of the younger Italian children advocated genuine expression of disappointment upon receiving the undesirable gift. Relative to the appearance–reality distinction, Italian children were also less likely to contend that appearance of expression might not coincide with internal felt emotion than were British children. Thus, cultures that differ in their expectations about controlling certain emotions under certain circumstances also differ in the socialization pressure brought to bear on children to acquire such emotion management strategies.

Indian and British Children

Joshi and MacLean (1994) compared 4- and 6-year-old children in Bombay and England on their understanding that expressive behavior need not be congruent with subjectively felt emotion. They systematically varied child–child stories and child–adult stories, because children are more likely to endorse genuine displays of emotion with peers (e.g., see the study by Underwood et al., 1992, mentioned earlier). More than three times as many 4-year-old Indian girls than English girls endorsed the idea that children would inhibit or use misleading facial expressions to conceal a negative emotion when interacting with an adult. Indian and English boys did not differ. The authors emphasize a socialization interpretation of their findings, describing the sort of intense pressures applied to young Indian girls to adopt deferential and highly regulated decorum in the presence of adults. They also highlight the fact that this early acquisition of understanding that negative emotions are to be concealed from adults, especially by girls, is brought about not by greater concern for the feelings of others but by fear of punishment for acting improperly.

CONCLUSION

Self-efficacy and being able to manage one's emotional–expressive behavior go hand-in-hand. Without awareness and without ability to maneuver expressive behavior according to the interpersonal circumstances, we would be left with a rigid repertoire of communicative behavior. Even chimpanzees have more going for them than this (see Parker, 1990, for comprehensive reviews of self-awareness in other primates). We have social goals, whether to be liked and approved of or to impress others and appear confident and powerful; but these desires to influence others' responses to ourselves can be turned toward ethically admirable or malevolently manipulative purposes. Again I want to emphasize that emotional competence has among its criteria that self-efficacy be attained according to one's culturally relevant *moral sense* or disposition (see Chapter 1 for discussion). Given that the construct of emotional competence is proposed from a Western cultural perspective, these social goals would be guided by classical Western "virtues" of "doing the right thing," fairness, self-control, and a commitment to protecting the well-being of others. Mature emotional competence and moral character go hand in hand. Yet humans have foibles, and there are invariably situations in which we succumb to the immediate felt vulnerability of ourselves. We might then manipulate our emotional–expressive behavior to create an impression on others that we hope will get us "off the hook," so to speak. Emotional competence is not something that one acquires and then never loses; it is dynamic. Given that emotions are embedded in context, on occasion there are likely to be contingencies facing an individual that contribute to the individual's feeling compelled to protect him- or herself in the short run, despite the risk of long-term disadvantages.

From a developmental standpoint, the intermingling of emotional experience and social interaction is evident in children's acquisition of emotional dissemblance and emotion management strategies. There are highly adaptive and functional reasons for children to learn how to dissociate their emotional–expressive behavior from their internally felt, subjective emotional experience. One is being able to have reasonably satisfactory relationships with others; another is to be able to get others to provide support and validation; still another is to exert influence on others—as in impression management, persuasive communication, and the like. A reason that children are particularly likely to endorse is that it helps them to avoid getting into trouble, and finally, the omnipresent self-appraisal system has its antennae out to try to create experiences that strengthen or protect the self rather than undermine it (although sometimes attempts at self-protection are admittedly self-defeating). Coping effectively with interpersonal conflict and other situational stressors has much to do with how we regulate both our subjective experience of emotion and what we communicate expressively to others. And, of course, it has quite a lot to do with our sense of well-being as well. We turn next to how children acquire the emotional competency of coping with aversive emotions, taxing relationships, and stressful situations. And it is by no means clear that this next skill of emotional competence is ever truly "finished."

Chapter 9

Skill 6: The Capacity for Adaptive Coping with Aversive Emotions and Distressing Circumstances

Capacity for adaptive coping with aversive or distressing emotions by using self-regulatory strategies that ameliorate the intensity or temporal duration of such emotional states (e.g., "stress hardiness").

How do we know when we have coped effectively and adaptively with some upsetting situation that faces us? The answer to this simple question is more complicated than we might at first assume. For one, *we* may think we have coped adequately, but our interactant in the situation (e.g., a spouse, a friend or a coworker) may think we behaved childishly or, like the proverbial ostrich with his head stuck in the sand, avoided everything. Have we coped adaptively if the situation is resolved but we still feel upset? Have we coped adaptively if the conflictual situation is *un*resolved but we no longer feel so churned up about it anymore? We have to look at least at three perspectives in evaluating the degree of adaptive functioning in any given instance of coping: (1) from the standpoint of situational problem-solving and whether the resolution that is worked out is mature and functional; (2) from the standpoint of the emotional experience and whether we can acknowledge our feelings to ourselves, even if they remain unexpressed or otherwise "managed" (see Chapter 8); and (3) relative to the self-regulatory view, whether we come away with a sense of mastery and resilience, even if the situation itself is not especially under our direct control. In sum, coping involves the self, our emotional experience, and the physical and social environment. Although we can intellectually conceptualize these three constructs separately, in the ongoing stream of experience they are probably quite interwoven and inseparable. However, it is likely that if our efforts at coping include acting as though our self is not involved, or that our feelings are irrelevant, or that the situation is utterly futile, then our coping attempts will be ineffective. In short, to discount any of these three aspects of coping will probably cause further problems at a later time.

Emotional competence is evident in the capacity for adaptive coping insofar as all the preceding abilities or skills involved in emotional competence are also involved in effective coping. But what is intriguing about emotionally competent coping is that often it entails having to deal with our own feelings. The greater the degree of self-reflection available to the child, adolescent, or adult, the more likely that coping will include more levels, more variables taken into account, and more perspectives (e.g., other people's as well as different time perspectives). Such coping efforts may be more comprehensive and may lead to greater self-efficacy and emotional well-being in the long run, and accepting feeling badly in the short run may be part of the bargain. In other words, adaptive and emotionally competent coping does *not* necessarily mean that one feels better right away. I have always found very distasteful the phrase, "Don't worry, be happy." There is dignity in some forms of melancholy, and an individual's emotional disquiet may be entirely socially and morally appropriate. An example that comes to mind is when we have to make a choice that causes us to give up something dear to us (e.g., a friendship that is on the threshold of becoming romantic), but our decision is made with an eye toward issues of integrity (e.g., the friend is already partnered with another friend). We may also make a decision in support of our ethical standards that at the same time means that we must forgo some more immediate material or social rewards (e.g., foregoing a scholarship that has politically noxious strings attached to it).

REGULATORY PROCESSES

Before we move into the specifics of how children acquire coping skills, we need to define self-regulation and emotion regulation, for being able to modulate our degree of emotional arousal facilitates our coping with an environmental stressor or conflict. A person who is completely emotionally overwhelmed and immobilized may be closer to being in shock; however, some people have coped adequately with a terrible trauma *at the time it is occurring* and then afterward report going into emotional shock. For most of us, children included, some degree of being able to adjust the intensity of our feelings allows us to size up what is happening and how we are feeling. Then we are better positioned to be able to respond adaptively to the stressor or conflict. Indeed, many investigators now use the terms "coping" and "emotion regulation" interchangeably (e.g., Brenner & Salovey, 1997), and this makes common sense too: Effective coping is inseparable from effective emotion regulation and vice versa.

I have come up with the following definitions of self- and emotion regulation, which may seem surprisingly similar, and for good reasons: Emotions guide or activate the self's behavior vis-à-vis the situational context, and reciprocally, the self appraises one's situation for its meaning (e.g., relevance to one's goals) and therefore experiences emotion. This is essentially the *functionalist* view put forward by Campos (1994) and is similar to the relational model of emotion proposed by Lazarus (1991).

1. *Self-regulation*: The ability to manage one's actions, thoughts, and feelings in adaptive and flexible ways across a variety of contexts, whether social or physical. Optimal self-regulation contributes to a sense of well-being, a sense of self-efficacy (mastery), and a sense of connectedness to others. (See also Block & Block's [1980] ego resilience construct; Kopp, 1982.)
2. *Emotion regulation*: The ability to manage one's subjective experience of emotion, especially its intensity and duration, and to manage strategically one's expression of emotion in communicative contexts. Optimal emotion regulation also contributes to a sense of well-being, a sense of self-efficacy, and a sense of connectedness to others. (See also Block & Block's [1980] ego control construct; Thompson, 1994; Walden & Smith, 1997).

The term "regulation" itself implies a directed or governing control exerted by the individual. I am not certain that such directed control is necessarily conscious or verbalized or that even an awareness of a sense of intentionality exists. Newborns are capable of regulatory acts, even if we wish to label them reflexive, but many early "negotiations" undertaken by the newborn seem specific to particular environmental demands or "affordances," to use a term from Chapter 2.

Thompson (1990, 1991, 1994) has written comprehensively about emotion and self-regulation in the early years of life. He describes emotion in terms of its *dynamics,* among which are the intensity of emotion, the lability of emotional responsiveness (i.e., fluctuations in hedonic tone), latency (the time between a stimulus and an emotional reaction), persistence of the emotional response, and recovery (return to baseline). He sees the regulation of these emotion dynamics as crucial features of infant adaptation. These dynamic qualities of an emotional response obviously affect the infant's behavior (e.g., persistent crying vs. rapid recovery to a more calm state), but of interest to me is that these dynamics also influence the social interaction between infant and caregiver. These emotion dynamics may have their origin in the infant's temperamental style, but they rapidly come under social influence. One caregiver may be unfazed by her temperamental baby's low threshold for fussiness and distress; another caregiver may react to her similarly temperamental baby by becoming distressed herself. We can imagine that the first infant comes to expect a soothing response to its distress, whereas the latter infant may come to expect either avoidance or excessive intrusiveness by its caregiver. Thus, the infant invariably experiences social consequences to its emotional behavior from the first days of its life. As Thompson points out, the degree to which caregivers can help their infant to modulate its emotional arousal will facilitate its developing further regulatory capacities. Reciprocally, the degree to which the baby's caregivers escalate or ignore its emotional arousal, the more likely the baby will have a difficult time learning to cope with its distress and frustration.

Self- and emotion regulation would appear to be highly linked in Western culture, but are they in non-Western societies? In some cultures it is the contexts and content of what is regulated about the self and about one's emotional experience that differ. In other cultures rituals and observances offer possible solutions to distressing circumstances (e.g., sacrifices as appeasement of angry spirits). Support seeking and receiving solace from others might well be coping strategies that are almost universal in their adaptational value. I return to cultural differences in the latter part of this chapter.

Illustrations of Coping Strategies

Thus far, coping and emotion regulation have been presented in very abstract terms. Following are several vignettes about children's coping efforts from an investigation of children's expectations about the usefulness of various coping strategies (Saarni, 1997). The children were in two age groups, 6 to 8 years old and 10 to 12 years old, and they responded individually to a standardized interview involving these hypo-thetical vignettes. These stories also provide us with rather simplified descriptions of the usual coping strategies used in North American cul-ture and perhaps Western culture more generally. I present them in the order of my evaluation of the more adaptive coping strategies, which are discussed further. The coping strategy being illustrated is italicized. In the actual research project the children were not provided with this final sentence; they had to choose the "best" and then the "worst" strategy from a variety of alternatives.

1. Problem-solving strategy

One day Maria and Sandy were walking home from school. Be-cause they were late, Maria wanted to take a shortcut home, even though she knew there was this really horrible dog, a scary Dober-man pinscher, that lived along that shortcut. They decided to take the shortcut anyway. As they walked along, they heard the dog barking. Maria was afraid. *Maria said that she thought they had better turn back and go the other way; it would be better to be late than risk be-ing bitten.*

2. Support-seeking strategies

A. Solace seeking

Debbie and Allison were friends and were playing with Debbie's new ball. Allison really liked the ball and wanted to take it home overnight and bring it back tomorrow. But the next day Allison showed up empty-handed and told Debbie that her dog had chewed the ball up. Debbie looked worried and said, "I hope you'll get me another one," but Allison replied angrily, "Hey, it wasn't my fault! And my dog doesn't have a bank account to go buy you another one!" *Debbie then felt angry at Allison and ran to tell her Mom how angry she felt about what had happened.*

B. Help seeking (perhaps a blend of problem solving and solace seeking)

Luis was playing basketball during recess at school with his friends. When he bent over to pick up the ball, his pants ripped open. All his friends started to laugh, because his underwear was showing. Luis's face turned red, and he felt very embarrassed. *He pulled his sweatshirt down as low as possible and went to the school office where he phoned his grandmother to see if she could bring him some other pants to wear.*

3. Distancing or avoidance strategy

Jenny bought a special jacket that she had saved all her money for. She was pretty excited about finally being able to wear it to school, and she told her friend Alice about it over the telephone. When she got to school the next day wearing her new jacket, Alice started to make fun of the jacket, and all the other kids joined in. Stunned, Jenny felt incredibly hurt. *Jenny turned her back on the kids, and as soon as she was out of sight of the others, she rolled the jacket up and stuffed it into her backpack.*

4. Internalizing strategy

Ned had a crush on Julie, and as is often the case with 12-year-olds who have crushes, he communicated his interest in her by teasing her, in this case, about her "gigantic feet," after Julie accidentally stepped on his foot in the crowded cafeteria line. Now Julie was mad at him and didn't want to be around him. Ned felt badly; he felt sad about her not liking him anymore. *He went home and worried about what Julie was probably telling the other kids and how they would not want him to be their friend either. At school the next day he didn't talk much to anybody and blamed himself for alienating Julie forever.*

5. Externalizing strategy

Megan and Hannah were planning together what to do for Hannah's birthday party, which was going to be sometime the next week. When Megan said, "Just don't wear anything with your red hair that's going to make you look like a circus clown," Hannah got into a huff and went home. Several days went by, and Hannah passed out birthday invitations to everyone in class except Megan. Megan felt hurt, but she also thought Hannah couldn't take a joke. *During class Megan grabbed another kid's invitation, drew an ugly face on it and decorated it with red-colored scraggly hair, folded it into a paper airplane, and threw it at Hannah.*

Additional coping strategies, often referred to as *emotion-focused strategies,* may be variants of distancing or internalizing responses, or they may also be considered to be defense mechanisms (see Murphy, 1970; Schibuk, Bond, & Bouffard, 1989). The first three are more adaptive than the last three: (1) substitution or distraction from context or feeling, (2) reframing or redefining the negative context or negative feeling (projection or blaming someone else would also be included here, although they are not adaptive strategies), (3) cognitive "blunting" or information-seeking strategies (similar to repression and sensiti-zation), (4) avoidance of negative context or of negative feeling, (5) denial of negative context or feeling, and (6) dissociation of self from situation. These emotion-focused strategies may be more often used in situations in which we believe ourselves to have *little control* over the ex-ternal circumstances. A good example is having to undergo some aversive medical or dental procedure; all we can control is how we *view* the situation or whether we can distract ourselves from it.

Lazarus's (1991) comments about the appraisal of control are worth noting here. Accurate appraisal of *what* we have control over is important (at least in Western societies.) Believing that we do not have control when we do, probably leads to a poorer outcome than believing we do have control when we do not. Lazarus notes that fatalists (those who believe they have little personal control) are more likely to feel de-pressed. But as Lazarus notes, having or believing we have control is a two-edged sword, for control entails accountability: If one has control and a good outcome results, then one takes *credit* for it, and one's self-esteem and sense of well-being are enhanced. But the flip side of hav-ing control and the accompanying accountability is that if the result is unfavorable or harmful, then we are *blamed* for the event. Shame, guilt, sadness, and anger are all possible feelings that may be elicited when we feel blamed by others or by ourselves. The attribution of credit or blame in children's coping efforts has not been specifically investi-gated, but research on the self-conscious emotions of shame and pride by Lewis and his colleagues has some parallels, as does the work by Zahn-Waxler on the origins of guilt (see Chapter 2; Lewis, 1993a; Lewis et al., 1990; Stipek, 1995; Zahn-Waxler & Kochanska, 1990; Zahn-Waxler & Robinson, 1995; see also Lazarus & Folkman, 1984, for an adult-based model of how stress, appraisal of control, and coping are potentially integrated.)

A rather large literature has developed examining these assorted emotion-focused and problem-solving strategies in children, and I rec-ommend highly Aldwin's (1994) comprehensive book on stress and coping from a life-span perspective. Additional valuable resources in-clude Wolchik and Sandler's (1997) edited volume on coping interven-tions for children and youth as well as the earlier review by Compas, Phares, and Ledoux (1989); Compas, Worsham, and Ey's (1992) review of developmental changes in children's coping; Cramer's (1991) vol-ume on the development of defense processes; Miller and Green's (1985) chapter on children's coping with stress and frustration; and Sorensen's (1993) text on children's stress and coping using their dia-ries and artwork. Later in this chapter I return to the relative efficacy of problem-solving/support-seeking coping strategies versus emotion-focused strategies when I review several studies on depression in children and the effects of sexual abuse on children.

DEVELOPMENT OF SELF-REGULATION
AND EMOTION REGULATION

Very likely an infant first has to deal with emotion regulation: Its emotional arousal necessitates modulation. Ideally, the infant can access its self-soothing capacities, such as sucking on its pacifier or "shutting down" and going to sleep, and ideally its caregivers can also provide support and comfort to the infant (Kopp, 1989; Campos, Campos, & Barrett, 1989). As Eisenberg and Fabes (1992) have pointed out, an infant's arousability is an aspect of its temperament. When the infant has to modulate its arousal level, it is faced with having to regulate the intensity of its reaction. Thus, temperament and emotion regulation are intertwined, or at least they appear to be in infancy and well into childhood; I return to the influence of temperament on emotion regulation later.

From the perspective of how older children, youth, and adults regulate their emotions, Gross (1998) has described how we can look at regulatory efforts that are directed at the *antecedents* of our anticipated emotional reaction. Thus, we can reappraise or reframe the situation we are in to alter the meaning we attribute to it. By doing this, we alter our functional relationship to this context, thereby also changing our goal connection to it. This approach may be particularly useful when we need to curtail our emotional reaction, because it would otherwise cause more problems and conflict with other goals we have. For example, phobic reactions illustrate the failure of attempts to reappraise the stimulus situation; systematic desensitization is the intervention used to change the meaning of the feared situation by pairing it with relaxation. Gross also proposes that our regulatory efforts can be directed at *suppression of emotional responses*. This would entail our curtailing our emotional–expressive behavior, but it would still leave us with the original emotional experience—just its expression would be dissembled. Much of this sort of emotion regulation was addressed in the preceding chapter as part of self-presentation strategies.

Gross (1998) investigated the effects of these two strategies of emotion regulation on college students' physiological responses while they watched rather grisly medical films. Subjects who were instructed simply to suppress their emotional–expressive behavior had more elevated sympathetic nervous system activity in comparison to the subjects who were given instructions to watch the films with a detached, technical, or medical training perspective. In another study (Gross & John,

1997), college students were interviewed, and the results indicated that antecedent (reappraisal) and response-focused emotion regulation strategies occurred about equally, and the vast majority of the circumstances described by the students involved negative emotions as well as other people present.

Optimal self- and emotion-regulation development appears to entail the acquisition of a flexible repertoire of coping strategies. Specifically, optimal self-regulation stressing active problem solving and recruitment of social support (including gaining social approval) and optimal emotion regulation emphasize the capacity to tolerate intensity of aversive emotion to the degree that appraisal processes have an opportunity to make sense of what is going on (and thus allow for self-regulatory strategies). If appraisal indicates that control over the situational stressor or conflict is minimal or extremely risky, then adaptive emotional regulation may also involve distraction, cognitively reframing the meaning of the difficult situation, and moderate use of cognitive blunting or sensitizing, again depending on the degree of control over the stressor that an individual has. Avoidance, denial, and dissociation appear to be less adaptive coping strategies in that self- and emotion regulation are compromised for short-term gain but at long-term expense. The chronic use of avoidance, denial, and dissociation short-circuit opportunities for learning or problem solving; they *restrict* one's options rather than expanding them. I turn next to further discussion of the relations between temperament and regulatory behavior.

The Influence of Temperament on Coping and Emotion Regulation

The notion of temperament is multifaceted and fraught with many definitional and measurement problems (e.g., Campos et al., 1989; Derryberry & Rothbart, 1988; Goldsmith & Campos, 1982), but it is a useful construct for thinking about some of the influences on how children develop different styles of coping. I think of temperament as a collection of dispositions that characterize the individual's style in responding to environmental change (or the lack thereof). When this general definition of temperament is applied to how a person responds *emotionally* to change, we can examine differences in how emotional attention is directed, the intensity of emotional response, the threshold for arousal of emotional response, the duration (and other temporal aspects) of the emotional response, and even the proclivity for what sort of hedonic tone of emotional response is generated (i.e., negative vs. positive reactions to change). In short, these are the emotion dynamics described so lucidly by Thompson (1990).

Using temperament in this fairly global fashion as having to do with how we dispositionally tend to modulate our emotional reactions, we can examine how differences in temperament may influence coping efficacy. This approach was taken by Eisenberg and her colleagues in a couple of different research projects on preschoolers' coping efficacy relative to their social competence. In one investigation Eisenberg et al. (1993) looked at children whose emotional intensity level was rated by both their mothers and their teachers and then examined the children's social competence (adult ratings) and sociometric ratings (peer popularity). They also evaluated the children's coping strategies by having the teachers and mothers rate the children's likelihood of using assorted coping strategies (similar to those described earlier) in hypothetical situations. Among their very complex results were that greater social competence of boys (but not girls) could be predicted by their displaying adaptive coping strategies (e.g., problem solving) and not displaying excessive negative emotion. For girls, social competence could be predicted from their use of *avoidant* coping strategies rather than by their engaging in acting-out or conflict-escalating behaviors. For both boys and girls, high emotional intensity was associated with lower levels of constructive coping and with lower levels of attentional control (shifting and distractable attention vs. focused attention, as assessed by teachers). In short, those 4- to 5-year-olds who frequently showed high-intensity negative emotions were more likely to be distractable (with accompanying impulsive or disorganized behavior) and to demonstrate less constructive coping. They were also regarded by adults as less socially mature and by their peers as less attractive as playmates.

In a second study, Eisenberg, Fabes, Nyman, Bernzweig, and Pinuelas (1994) looked at 4- to 6-year-olds' emotionality (defined as intensity of reaction and negative tone of emotion), their ability to control their attention, coping skills, and their management of anger with their peers. The pattern of their findings was complex, with some results occurring only for teacher-rated behaviors but not for mother-rated behaviors. Gender of child was again a variable that affected some of the patterning of results. Overall, anger reactions that were adaptive, that is, the children used nonhostile verbal strategies to try to deal with the anger provocation, were associated with children who generally displayed low emotional intensity and higher social effectiveness as well as coping efficacy. This pattern was stronger for boys than for girls, and boys who used adaptive anger responses were also rated as higher in attentional control, namely, they were not distractable and impulsive. Girls who tended to escape the situation when angered were viewed by teachers as socially skilled; that is, the girls' avoidance of anger was apparently seen as not contributing to an escalation of conflict, a desirable outcome from teachers' standpoint. Although the authors were not studying sex-role socialization, it is noteworthy that teachers' approval of sex-typed behaviors (e.g., the girls' avoidance of conflict), even at this relatively young age, may be influencing children's subsequent style of coping with such gender role–laden emotions as anger.

Although the construct of temperament allows us to consider what children might "inherently" bring with them as they seek to cope with stressful circumstances, it is unlikely that temperament solely affects how adaptive their coping style is. Bear in mind that the social environment has also been modulating and *giving meaning* to the young child's emotional behavior all along, which includes such temperamental dimensions as intensity, hedonic tone, temporal factors, and the like. Cultures that value expressive restraint might ascribe rather different meanings to, for example, intensity of emotional response, than do cultures that do not have such an orientation. In the former, an especially intense response might be seen as indicating that something important must be going on for the individual; in the latter, an intense response might be seen as a minor exaggeration of the norm. In a moderately expressive culture as in North America, intense emotions seem to be variously characterized as romantic, excessive, out of control, zestful, energetic, genuine, and so on. The point is that in the long run adequacy of coping is best determined by whether people experience themselves as efficacious in the sociocultural context in which they find themselves. And that sense of efficacy must take into account the situation that demands a response, the individual self who makes sense of the situation, and the emotional experience elicited by that appraisal.

The Influence of Emotional Experience

Most research on children's coping has examined their choice of coping strategies from the standpoint of stressors, risk factors, or individual differences. Little research has been done on how the nature of the felt emotion itself might influence what sort of coping strategy is used, other than that the emotional experience is felt as aversive. One exception is Laux and Weber's (1991) work on adult coping as reflecting the kinds of intentions and goals that are embedded in different sorts of emotional experience; for example, if one feels angry, then coping strategies may reflect an intent to reclaim or defend an "entitlement."

The study I referred to near the beginning of this chapter also examined coping with specific emotions (Saarni, 1997). The participating children responded to a number of stories that featured five different negative emotions (anger, fear, sadness, shame, and hurt feelings, the latter viewed as a blend of anger and sadness). The stories were composed such that they all had moderate controllability of outcome, featured the protagonist as experiencing moderately intense emotions, concerned peer interaction, and were gender neutral. (The illustrations of coping strategies cited earlier were among the vignettes given to the children.) Assorted coping strategy options were also given to the children for how the story protagonist could deal with the negative emotion and stressful circumstances. The interview with the children focused on which coping strategy they chose as "the best," which strategy "the worst," their justifications for these choices, and how the story protagonist would feel after coping in either this best or worst fashion. The children were also asked how they themselves would have coped if they had been in the story situation.

The results indicated that although age differences appeared in the level of cognitive complexity for the justifications provided, little difference across age groups occurred in choices of best and worst coping strategies. Overall, children clearly preferred beneficial coping strategies such as problem solving and support seeking. Only for the vignette featuring hurt feelings did the majority of children pick distancing as the best coping strategy. Aggressive externalizing coping responses were most often selected as the worst option across all emotion categories. For the most part, children's justifications for their best coping choices emphasized the social and situational gains, and parallel losses were cited as justifications for the worst coping choice (e.g., externalizing).

Relative to how one would feel after coping in the best fashion, virtually all children reported that the protagonist would feel better, and only 11 out of 275 story protocols, less than 5%, contained reports of feeling badly, despite coping adaptively. After choosing the worst coping strategy, most children reported that the protagonist would feel even worse, but a small minority (10%) of the story protocols contained reports that the protagonist would feel better. These "improved" feeling states were generally about feeling relief at having lashed out at someone or enjoyment of vengeance.

When asked what they themselves would do, the majority of children again nominated problem-solving strategies, with some decline in the frequency of support-seeking and distancing strategies for the hurt-feelings scenario. Somewhat more children also indicated that they would personally be tempted to respond aggressively to retaliate against teasing children. Further research is needed on how children link desirable outcomes with emotional experience and, if they know what generally adaptive coping strategies are, what gets in the way when they do not employ them. One possibility is that self-appraisal, attribution of responsibility for the outcome, and controllability (one's own emotions as well as situational aspects) all interact to influence how children and youth cope in taxing circumstances. Further research is also needed to better understand what contributes to those children who expect that after coping by aggressing, they will feel better and, similarly, to those children who believe that after coping well, they will feel worse. The former may well turn out to be our playground bullies and the latter our depressed or abused children.

Hypothesized Relations between Attachment and Coping

Another possible influence on children's coping strategies is their early attachment experience with significant caregivers. There is relatively little longitudinal research in this area, although provocative retrospective accounts are available that suggest links between quality of attachment in early life with subsequent emotion regulatory "style" (e.g., Kobak & Sceery, 1988; Main, Kaplan, & Cassidy, 1985). I summarize here Cassidy's (1994) argument about the link between attachment history and emotion regulation.

Drawing on Bowlby's (e.g., 1979) and Main's work (e.g., 1990), Cassidy (1994) describes how the infant is biologically disposed to maintain proximity to the caregiver and thus learns to tailor its responses to the caregiver in light of his or her responses to it; that is, the infant can make use of reciprocal feedback in adjusting its strategies for facilitating closeness with the caregiver, an adaptive maneuver indeed. To illustrate, after a brief separation, securely attached infants respond to reunion with their caregiver with warmth, relief, and responsiveness on her return (mothers always seem to be the caregivers in this sort of research). They do not show the wariness, avoidance, or resistance that characterizes infants who do not enjoy secure attachments (i.e., infants who are insecurely or anxiously attached). Mothers of securely attached infants apparently reliably demonstrate sensitive responses to their infants' emotional signals, and thus their presence is a "safe haven" from which the infant can venture forth to explore the environment. That environment can, of course, produce taxing or difficult situations that require the infant or toddler to cope with it, and using mom as an ally and support base for when things get tough is an excellent coping strategy.

Cassidy (1994) goes on to say that for the securely attached infant, negative emotions such as anger and fear come to be associated with maternal sympathetic assistance, and that these negative feelings are associated neither with any sort of invalidation of the young child nor with denial of the negative feelings. In terms of emotional regulation, young children become able to tolerate aversive emotion temporarily and can begin to make sense of the frustrating or conflictful situations that face them and figure out a response.

A concrete example of a child learning to tolerate frustration might be useful here. Young preschoolers (2 to 3 years) have been known to bite a peer or sibling who has frustrated them. Most parents get nervous when they hear that their child has bitten another, for their adequacy as parents or as disciplinarians may be questioned. The family interaction described next is an adaptation of a story told to me by Manuel's sister (little Ricardo's mother).

> Rosa and Manuel wondered what to do with their daughter, 3-year-old Nita, who occasionally bit other kids when they took away something she was playing with or if she wanted what they were playing with. This morning Nita wanted the toy that her cousin Ricardo was holding; she tried to get it away from him, but he reliably yowled and protested. She grabbed him around the neck and bit down hard on his ear. His screaming was very loud, and Nita backed away looking afraid.
>
> Rosa thought maybe she should bite Nita sometime when she was acting up so that she'd know how much it hurt. (Believe it or not, some parents do advocate this strategy for stopping their children's biting.) But Manuel had a better idea. He took Nita aside and told her that he was going to tell her a story, and with that he placed her stuffed bear and Raggedy Ann in front of them. She was a rapt listener as he described how Bear and Raggedy Ann were friends but also got into fights. He pulled out a cookie and had Bear and Raggedy Ann "fight" over who would get the cookie. As they were struggling, he asked Nita what Bear and Raggedy Ann should do. Should Bear bite Raggedy Ann or vice versa? Nita readily volunteered that they should share the cookie. Manuel then had Nita pretend to be Raggedy Ann while he took the Bear's side, and he escalated the conflict as he said, "No, I won't share, I'm going to eat all the cookie, and you can't have any."
>
> He looked to see Nita's response, and she appeared to alternate between being close to crying and getting furious. He said, "I have more cookies in my pocket, Nita." Nita then said, as Raggedy Ann, to Bear, "Eat the cookie, my daddy has more and they are all mine!" And Raggedy Ann pounced on her daddy's pocket, and more cookies were produced. Manuel said to Nita, "If Raggedy Ann bites Bear, then it's hard to be friends, and she won't get more cookies from her daddy. When you bite Ricardo, like you did this morning, it hurt him a lot, and everybody got mad at you. Get something else to play with or share. Biting won't get you what you want."
>
> The next week Nita and Ricardo were once again in a conflict.

But this time Nita announced, "You're stupid, and I don't like you."

Maybe name calling wasn't the best way to deal with the squabble, but for Nita it was an improvement on biting and allowed her to withdraw and cool down. Ricardo, predictably, solicited her attention again within 5 minutes. Manuel's "scaffolding" approach to teaching Nita more socially appropriate ways to tolerate frustration did prove to be helpful to Nita, who bit another child only one other time after this incident.

If securely attached infants can use their caregivers as "safe havens" from which to venture forth to explore the physical and social environment, it is also likely that such caregivers provide a sense of stability for the child such that the child can also explore a range of emotions. For example, hanging onto mom or dad makes scary things tolerable and eventually "fun" (e.g., fireworks displays and amusement park rides). The caregiver's empathic sharing of emotions makes them acceptable and routine for the securely attached infant.

The anxiously attached infant, on the other hand, has often experienced its caregiver's rejection when it sought comfort for its distress. Such an infant learns that some emotions are not acceptable and maybe not even safe. The infant develops a wariness and avoidance of its caregiver and begins to regulate its emotions by minimizing their expression when in the presence of the caregiver. Cassidy cites a couple of studies that indicated that insecurely attached infants interacted responsively with their mothers when *not* distressed or needing care. But when experiencing emotional distress, they ended up suppressing their negative emotional display so as *to maintain* caregiver involvement. In other words, the infant's emotional regulation strategy seems to be, "Mom will stay with me if I don't raise any fuss." The cost, however, to the infant is constant emotional vigilance and suppression of normal distress, which, if it becomes a chronic pattern, is often maladaptive in other close relationships. This last point takes us to the next issue, does the quality of attachment with one's primary caregivers affect one's social and emotional functioning later in life?

Research undertaken by Kobak and Sceery (1988) on 18-year-olds suggests a link between their emotional functioning and their attachment style. When these young adults were interviewed about their family-of-origin relationships (George, Kaplan, & Main, 1985), the securely attached individuals emerged as less hostile, less anxious, and more ego-resilient; experienced less distress; and enjoyed more social support than the avoidant/attachment dismissing group or the excessively preoccupied group. Thus, relative to emotion regulation and associated coping efficacy, it would appear as though family-of-origin warmth, responsiveness, and empathy with the child's emotional experience contribute to the development over time of a competent coping style.

Do Families Make a Difference in Coping Competence?

Family Conflict and Dysfunction

Given the relatively few studies that have tracked quality of attachment to children's subsequent coping competence, the ways that families contribute to individual children's coping competence is far from being well understood. A larger body of research has examined the effects of marital conflict and anger on children's functioning—the latter having some links with how well children cope with the aversive feelings they themselves experience. Cummings and Davies (1994) have reviewed this area and, not surprisingly, the general conclusion they reach is that many children do not fare well when faced with frequent and intense marital conflict, an outcome echoed in other investigators' work (e.g., Emery, 1982; Grych & Fincham, 1990). If fighting (verbal and physical aggression) is common between spouses, the boys in particular appear to develop aggressive, externalizing behavioral problems. Daughters also demonstrate behavioral problems, but more of the girls also show distress, which may also account for why Vuchinich, Emery, and Cassidy (1988) found that girls were more likely to intervene in parental conflicts. Children find angry exchanges between parents very stressful, even when the children play no role in the dispute, and the immediate coping strategies children bring to bear on such a family crisis probably pivot on the child's perception of controllability of the dispute. If the child distracts the parents, will that stop the fighting, or does the arguing seem endless and futile and the only course of action to withdraw? Such a family environment is a painful one in which to grow up, and the impact on children's adjustment is generally negative, unless there are buffering factors such as extended family members who can offer the child respite and a safe haven.

Children growing up with depressed or psychiatrically disturbed parents have also been studied for how such a family environment influences children's emotional and social functioning. Obviously parental dysfunction co-occurs with the higher frequency of other stressful events for children (e.g., divorce, chronic unemployment, and spousal conflict). Goodman, Brogan, Lynch, and Fielding (1993) investigated the socioemotional functioning of children (ages 5 to 10) who had a depressed mother; the children were subdivided further into three groups: Some also had a disturbed father in the home, some were in mother-custody homes, and some had a well father in the home. They also had a comparison sample of children whose mothers and fathers were neither depressed nor psychiatrically disturbed.

Their results indicated that it was the combination of a depressed mother *and* a disturbed father that was associated with the greatest number of problems among *older* children. Apparently as the children matured, living in an emotionally strained household with two psychiatrically ill parents began to take its toll. Younger children did not yet demonstrate such negative effects. What their study also reconfirmed were the difficult effects divorce has on children when living with a depressed parent, particularly on self-regulation variables (e.g., Emery, 1988). Such children tended to be rated as undercontrolled: more often aggressive and impulsive. Given the vulnerability of single parents for experiencing stress, regardless of whether or not they are already depressed, it is not surprising that children of divorced parents often demonstrate behavioral problems. Children who had a well father and a depressed mother who were still married and living together did not differ from the children of well parents except for being rated by their teachers as somewhat less popular among their peers.

Although these researchers did not directly study coping competence, the implication I draw from their work is that when daily family life is fraught with tension, negative moods, unpredictable parenting, and spousal conflict, children's coping capacities may be excessively taxed with the result that they tend to use externalizing coping strategies more often. For all that we may know, perhaps their anger at their parents is expressed by projectively lashing out at "safe" targets such as siblings or peers, thus resulting in their being rated as undercontrolled rather than being able to express directly to their parents their outrage and sense of betrayal.

Parenting Style

Looking at more ordinary families, Hardy, Power, and Jaedicke (1993) examined several parenting variables (supportiveness, structure, and control) and children's coping with "daily hassles." Within their rather homogeneous middle-class sample, they found that only maternal supportiveness and structure were related to children's coping. Specifically, supportive mothers in moderately low-structured homes had children who generated *more* coping strategies across situations; mothers who provided more structure had children who used fewer aggressive coping strategies. Supportive mothers also had children who reported more avoidant coping strategies when the children perceived the stressor as uncontrollable. Hardy et al. (1993) concluded that children's coping is multifaceted and that for this age group (9 to 10 years old) distinctive coping styles or patterns were not discernible. However, it is noteworthy that parental supportiveness was found to be significantly related to the breadth of coping strategies. This relationship sounds consistent with the attachment link discussed earlier: Secure attachment facilitates exploration, some of which results in experiencing aversive feelings. If we feel that we have responsive support at home, it becomes much easier to try out different coping strategies in learning how to master assorted stressful encounters that we invariably will have in daily living.

Age Differences

Due to methodological variation, sample age differences, and rather profound contextual differences, we do not have a systematic empirical literature that tells us what coping strategies tend to emerge at what age for mainstream North American children. However, two general patterns have emerged with regard to age: As children get older, they generate *more* coping alternatives to stressful situations, and they become more able to make use of cognitively oriented coping strategies for situations in which they have no control (e.g., Altshuler & Ruble, 1989; Band & Weisz, 1988; Compas, Malcarne, & Fondacaro, 1988; Harris & Lipian, 1989; Miller & Green, 1985). Embedded in both of these age-related patterns is greater cognitive complexity that is associated with becoming older: (1) the ability to appraise *accurately* when a situation is simply not under one's control, (2) the ability to shift intentionally one's thoughts to something else less aversive, (3) the ability to use symbolic thought in ways that transform the meaningfulness of a stressful encounter or situation (reframing), and (4) importantly, the ability to consider a stressful situation from a number of different angles and thus consider different problem solutions relative to these different perspectives. As to when these two general developmental patterns in coping are clearly in place, I suggest that by 10 years old most children have a fairly well developed coping repertoire that includes the emotion-focused strategies of cognitive distraction and transformation. This assumes, of course, that the family lives of these children have been adequately supportive and that harsh traumas have not preoccupied the children's emotional resources such that inflexibility or dissociative processes have taken hold in the child's self- and emotion regulation.

INDIVIDUAL DIFFERENCES IN COPING EFFICACY

Gender Differences

Some researchers have found sex differences in children's coping strategies, usually in interaction with some other variable, and others have not found significant sex differences. For example, Altshuler and Ruble (1989) found no sex differences across the ages from 5 to 12 in children's nomination of coping strategies for situations involving uncontrollable stress (getting an injection and having a cavity filled). Compas et al. (1988) found that sixth-grade girls generated more coping strategies than same-aged boys for dealing with academic and interpersonal problem situations; by the eighth grade the boys had caught up and even slightly exceeded the girls in generating a greater number of coping strategies, but the difference was not significant.

Similar to other research on the *understanding* of emotional and cognitive phenomena, gender does not appear to be a major contributor to differences in cognitive construal of how coping or emotional processes work. However, gender may well show up in coping strategy investigations when children's and youth's actual coping behaviors are observed. The research earlier described wherein preschool girls' more frequent avoidance of anger provocation was rated as more competent by their teachers as compared to boys' use of nonhostile verbal involvement (Eisenberg et al., 1994) is an example. Girls' greater use of internalizing processes when emotionally disturbed (worrying, anxiety, self-blame, withdrawal, etc.) suggests coping strategies of a distancing or emotionally focused sort, whereas disturbed boys are more likely to be referred for externalizing behavior problems (aggression, hostility, stealing, etc.) (For a review on sex differences in aggression, see Eagly & Steffen, 1986; for sex differences in depression, see Zahn-Waxler et al., 1991.)

In their book, Golombok and Fivush (1994) conclude that differential sex-role socialization accounts for much of the gender-linked variation in emotional experience and behaviors, including vulnerability to emotional distress. Brody and Hall (1993), in their review of gender and emotion, similarly conclude that sex-role socialization contributes to gender differences in emotion-related processes, but they also contend that females' superior language skills in early childhood may be a factor that facilitates parents' talking about feelings more with their daughters, with the result that girls attend more and give greater significance to emotional experience. The result for coping competence may well favor girls when they are in uncontrollable circumstances; they may be more able to use emotion-focused strategies at a younger age than boys. Altshuler and Ruble's (1989) research did not confirm this, but their contexts for eliciting *verbal* reports of coping strategies were aversive medical procedures, a rather limited sampling of contexts. Ruble and Martin (1998) have also more recently reviewed sex differences in emotional functioning.

Interestingly, Compas et al.'s (1988) research did reveal that girls more often suggested emotion-focused coping strategies for academic failure as compared to boys, who suggested more frequently problem-solving coping strategies for academic failure; yet both boys and girls viewed academic failure as relatively more controllable than interpersonally stressful circumstances. If these young adolescent girls are reporting emotion-focused coping strategies for something they also view as comparatively under their control, then I would infer an element of denial, avoidance, or helplessness in such emotion-focused coping strategies. When something problematic is under one's control, but one acts as though it is not, further problems tend to ensue. By avoiding a conflict or stressor, by becoming helpless to do anything about it, by trying to pretend it is something that it is not ("Oh, who cares about homework anyway . . . "), in other words, by using emotion-focused coping strategies that at some level deny the reality of the problematic situation to be dealt with, we compromise our coping adaptiveness. This leads us to the next topic, whether social competence is associated with more constructive coping skills, and vice versa, are inadequate coping strategies associated with reduced social competence.

Social Maturity Differences

Social Competence and Constructive Coping

Most of us would conclude that it is not socially acceptable to beat someone up as a way to solve a dispute, nor is it socially effective to stay in bed all day and weep helplessly about not getting an invitation to so-and-so's party. Avoiding challenges and hard responsibilities (paying child support, asking one's sex partner to wear a condom, etc.) tends to be a lot more convenient and is certainly less hassle. Unfortunately, our media promote the social *effectiveness* of aggression for getting what one wants, despite its unacceptability, and learned helplessness is all too often promoted as well (particularly for female TV sit-com figures). Avoidance seems inherently reinforcing: One escapes from something onerous. What incentive is there for acquiring constructive coping strategies other than our desire to be a decent sort of person? One important incentive—in addition to such influences as family relationships and temperament—is that our peers will generally like us more if we use constructive coping strategies, and most children do want to be liked by their peers.

As mentioned earlier, Eisenberg et al. (1993, 1994) found that children in the age range of 4 to 6 were rated as more socially competent by teachers and also by their peers as more attractive playmates when they used constructive coping strategies (problem solving as opposed to aggression). An earlier study by Richard and Dodge (1982) with older children (second through fifth grades), who were also all boys, obtained parallel results. In their study of the boys' verbal reports to hypothetical stories, those boys who had been identified by peers and teachers as either aggressive or isolated children were found to generate fewer coping solutions to interpersonal conflicts as compared to boys nominated as cooperative and well liked. All the boys generated effective coping solutions on the first round, so to speak, but subsequent coping strategies nominated by the aggressive and isolated boys tended to be either aggressive in tone or ineffective. There was no statistical difference between the aggressive and the isolated boys, which seems surprising, since the latter were selected for their shyness and tendency to be alone. There were also no age differences. Thus, the authors' results extend Eisenberg et al.'s (1993, 1994) research in further confirming that children who are well liked tend to have broader coping repertoires that included a greater number of effective problem solution possibilities as opposed to falling back on aggressive or ineffective coping strategies after generating the first option.

Kliewer (1991) obtained rather different results in her study of elementary school age children. She found that children rated *by teachers* as socially competent were most likely to endorse using active avoidance of problem situations as a coping strategy. My hunch is that when teachers rate social competence, they are looking for children who do not give them a lot of trouble in the classroom. Thus, children who do not contribute to any escalation of conflict tend to be viewed as socially desirable and therefore as competent. Similar to the findings of Eisenberg et al., children who were highly emotionally expressive were also rated as using avoidant strategies less often. It appears as though children who are emotionally "in your face" come off as problematic to teachers, or they may be somewhat impulsive in temperament and tend not to weigh solutions to problems as readily as more reflective children might.

In a small but intensive study of 38 5- to 6-year-old children's coping styles and adjustment, Carson, Swanson, Cooney, Gillum, and Cunningham (1992) found that a passive–aggressive style of coping was most often associated with impaired social development. Similarly, impulsive acting out, dependency, externalizing, and internalizing behaviors and ratings were associated with adjustment difficulties. In evaluating the children's exposure to stressful events in their lives, the authors found some relationship between major stress exposure and social adjustment, but what seemed to be more directly linked to the children's social competence was the family's flexibility, support, and confidence in approaching major upheavals. These family variables may have influenced the children's emergent coping repertoire such that more adaptive coping strategies were developed and applied to other sorts of stressors experienced by the children and subsequently assessed in this investigation.

Finally, Allen, Leadbeater, and Aber (1987) interviewed adolescents ages 15 to 18 about serious dilemmas and problems (e.g., opportunity to make some money by delivering illegal drugs) and asked them to rate their likelihood of being able to respond competently (and morally) to such dilemmas. The youth were also asked about their own problematic behavior, such as illegal drug use, unprotected sex, and delinquent acts. Their results indicated that youth who admitted to more problematic behavior also had lower expectations about being able to respond competently to the hypothetical situations. Most interesting was the authors' interpretation of these results: They suggested that the youth's beliefs about what would be effective *for them* had parallels in the work on "internal working models of attachment" proposed by such researchers as Main, Kobak, and Cassidy, who were cited earlier. Namely, the quality of family relationships may be the significant link in what influences adolescents who get into trouble. However, this is not to say that economic deprivation, violent neighborhoods, racism and ethnocentrism, and cynical educational systems do not also play a significant role in why a young person may become involved in substance abuse, ill-considered sexual activity, or delinquent acts. Readers may also feel as though the once traditional mother bashing of psychological research has simply been replaced by family bashing. I am concerned that we not place "blame" on families that are hanging by their fingernails onto the proverbial cliff's edge as they glance below at looming poverty, threat of eviction or unemployment, and further violent victimization (see, e.g., Conger et al., 1993, for a study of economic hardship, families, and adolescent adjustment, 1993).

Depressed Children and Coping

Chronically sad children probably have good reason to be sad: An accumulation of losses, disappointments, humiliations, stressors, and unloving family relationships have taken their toll on their capacity to persist in enduring the onslaught of negative events in their lives. Hopelessness is a key feature of their depression, and while a minority of depressed children and youth are suicidal, those who do attempt suicide, do report considerable hopelessness (Asarnow, Carlson, & Guthrie, 1987). What is it about depression that locks a person into a cycle of persistent negativity, even when the external situation begins to improve? Research on depression, which has also been referred to as the "common cold" of mental illness, is considerable, much of it psychopharmacological in scope. Research on depressed children is also extensive, and much of that work indicates that depressed children also are likely to have other concurrent difficulties or disorders (e.g., anxiety disorder, adjustment disorder, conduct disorder, and attention-deficit/hyperactive disorder; Asarnow et al., 1987). Thus, it comes as no surprise that depressed children have a variety of difficulties in coping with stressors and with aversive emotions. After all, the diagnosis of depression entails a tautological argument: You are depressed because you cope ineffectively, and you cope ineffectively because you are depressed. This too may sound a bit like blaming the victim, and I wish to echo Compas et al. (1989), who exhort us to attend to the communities of our suffering children and to reduce the *sources* of stress rather than to focus so much on the deficits in coping demonstrated by a psychologically distraught individual. The "politics of stress management" are real and do indeed influence how our public revenues are spent.

Returning to what depressed children do when confronted by challenging circumstances, I describe the research program undertaken by Garber and her associates (Garber et al., 1991; Garber, Braafladt, & Weiss, 1995). In the first study Garber et al. (1991) asked 30 children between the ages of 8 and 17 to nominate what they would do to change an aversive feeling. (Age and gender patterns were not reported, if there were any.) The psychiatric clinic-referred depressed children were more likely to suggest avoidance or negative strategies to alter the bad feeling (e.g., "I'd go to my room" or "I'd kick the wall"). The nondepressed children, who had been referred to a medical clinic, more often reported using problem-focused and active distraction strategies (e.g., "I need to get a hook to put on my door that would be too high for my little brother to reach so he couldn't come in and mess my stuff up, and then I wouldn't be getting mad at him all the time" or "I really hate going to the orthodontist, so I take my Walkman and listen to my favorite tapes while he messes around in my mouth"; examples are mine; they are not quoted from Garber et al.).

The depressed children did not differ from the nondepressed youngsters in suggesting ways to maintain or prolong positive emotional states; rather it was when feeling negative emotions that the depressed children appeared to get "locked into" a negative expectancy mode that biased them toward using coping strategies that were more likely to be self-fulfilling choices. That is, these sorts of ineffective coping behaviors were more likely to have the consequence that the depressed children would find themselves isolated or in trouble with others.

Garber et al. also note that few children nominated seeking social support for when they were feeling badly, nor did they often report using cognitive reframing strategies (transforming the meaning of the difficult situation mentally, using counterarguments to refute irrational beliefs, etc.). The latter does not surprise me, because adults find it similarly difficult to cope with negative feelings by reminding themselves that "it could be the silver lining of the dark cloud" or whatever that trite statement consists of. However, not seeking social support is surprising, since seeking comfort or assistance is what younger children would be expected to do. I wonder if this individualistic orientation is not culturally based, for I suspect that in non-Western cultures, where kinship systems play a greater role, going to one's elders or to religious leaders would be undertaken when feeling badly. It is also quite possible that negative feelings would be experienced somatically in a number of non-Western cultures, and thus comfort and help would be sought for the physical complaint. Of course, somatization occurs in our society as well, but all too often our culture's beliefs about the desirability of emotional stoicism makes it even more burdensome for many children and youth who feel vulnerable and distressed and yet feel compelled to be miserable in silence and alone.

In the later study, Garber et al. (1995) expanded their sample size and used the Children's Depression Inventory (Kovacs, 1980) to evaluate whether or not children were depressed. Without going into detail here, their results indicated that depressed girls significantly underutilized problem-solving strategies as compared to nondepressed girls, and the depressed boys used more negative externalizing responses. The former choice of the depressed girls suggests that they avoided the stressful or conflictful situation, and the boys exacerbated it. Both strategies would tend to leave the depressed child in ongoing stressful transactions. In addition, Garber et al. found that although depressed and nondepressed children rated assorted emotions that they would feel in stressful situations equally intensely, the depressed children did not anticipate that emotion-regulation strategies would be helpful or constructive. It may be that for depressed children a sense of futility "corrupts" any remnant of self-efficacy they might have otherwise experienced upon trying to regulate their aversive feelings.

Coping in Sexually Abused Children

Not seeking social support and *not* undertaking adequate problem solving in situations over which one has some control are among the serious risk factors affecting victims of sexual abuse. A chilling report by Long and Jackson (1993) on college-age women's retrospective accounts of how they coped with sexual abuse as children indicated that they experienced more symptoms (depression, anxiety, hypersensitivity, etc.) in adulthood the more they reported using emotion-focused coping strategies (e.g., "I went on as if nothing happened"). About 52% of their sample had been molested by nonfamily members; the rest were victims of incest. The authors also asked the women to report age at onset of abuse and their sense of control over the abusive situation. These two factors together were significant predictors of the number of problem-solving coping strategies used, although when entered in the multiple regression analysis singly, only age of onset was significant: The older the woman was as a child or youth when the molestation first occurred, the more likely she used problem-solving strategies.

The authors found that 21% of their sample reported never having used any problem-solving strategy at all, whereas only 2% of the women reported *not* using an emotion-focused strategy; 79% never sought help from someone else. My inference here is that the younger children are when victimized sexually, the greater the likelihood of their feeling powerless and believing they have no control over events happening to themselves. When we add to this the risk and scariness of significant others shaming the child for having been molested (instead of believing and supporting the child), then avoidance, denial, and dissociation seem to make more sense *in the short run*. This apparently is the outcome for many incest victims and perhaps also for boys molested by males, for these acts of abuse seem to be particularly insidious in shaming a child and have as an outcome children bearing in silence their anguishing "secret" (e.g., Briere, Evans, Runtz, & Wall, 1988; Friedrich & Reams, 1987; Gelinas, 1983; Peters, 1988). For the former, incested girls, repeated victimization often occurs or their children may also be molested (e.g., Goodwin, McCarthy, & DiVasto, 1981); for the latter, molested boys, identification with the aggressor develops for some and some may become the next generation's perpetrators (e.g. Ryan, 1989).

The significance of seeking support and of being believed and affirmed as worthy comes through in a number of investigations (e.g., Adams-Tucker, 1985; Conte & Schuerman, 1987). Consensus appears to be that the maladaptive sequelae of sexual abuse are mediated by what happens *before and after* the abusive incident (e.g., Alexander, 1992; Cole & Putnam, 1992). If disclosed, is the child supported and cared for, or is she castigated and humiliated or even threatened as the cause for why the family is broken up, evicted, unemployed, and so forth? Alexander (1992), in particular, provides a thought-provoking review of how attachment relationships with primary caregivers mediate the conditions in which abuse is more likely to occur: The parents have problematic attachment histories that impair their parenting, and those attachment histories may be maladaptive because the parents themselves were also abused (see also Cole, Woolger, Power, & Smith, 1992). When sexual abuse occurs within the immediate family, virtually by definition we are looking at severely impaired attachment relations, for even if neither parent (or stepparent) is the perpetrator, it suggests that the quality of relationship between child and parent is so strained that the child does not feel that he or she can safely report distress and upset to either parent when an older sibling, stepsibling, or relative is the offender. Such a youngster is then left feeling unable to control the abusive situation and must rely on emotion-focused coping strategies to manage his or her affective upheaval.

As noted above by Long and Jackson (1993), the heavy reliance on emotion-focused coping strategies was associated with a greater number of self-reported psychiatric and psychosomatic symptoms in adulthood. In summary, sexual abuse—as do all forms of child maltreatment—takes its toll on children's ability to cope flexibly and resourcefully. Because intrafamilial sexual abuse is particularly double binding, young child victims may be at even greater risk for becoming rigidly dissociated from what is happening to them; the self is fragmented along polarized "good–bad" dimensions, and emotion regulation and self-regulation become distorted (see also Calverley, Fischer, & Ayoub, in press). For some, multiple personality disorder may result; others become offenders or escape into substance abuse. Alexander (1992) would argue that what needs to happen to interrupt the generational transmission risk pattern is a corrective therapeutic experience that directly addresses the maladaptive attachment relationship style that has developed between child and parents or, in adulthood, between intimate partners.

What are the coping strategies of incested and abused children in non-Western countries? How do coping strategies vary with structural and demographic variables (access to kinship systems, degree of poverty, physical threat due to warfare, etc.)? Culture is a profound contextual variable that mediates the meaning of child maltreatment; thus, in some cultures a raped child might be forced to become an outcast, to be a prostitute, or even to be killed. In other cultures, beating of children is "routine," and clitoridectomies are performed on young girls as an approved ritual. In the next section I briefly discuss some ideas about the cultural context in which to appreciate the efficacy of coping strategies and how they relate to emotional competence.

Cultural Differences in Coping Strategies

Consider how culture influences the meaning of emotion, the self that experiences emotion, and the social script that surrounds the emotion-eliciting event in the following examples:

> Ten-year-old Chuck had lost his older brother, age 13, in a car accident about a year ago. He and his brother had shared a bedroom, and in spite of some competitive sibling rivalry, Chuck had adored Willy. When Willy died on the operating table, Chuck had been at home with his grandmother; his mother called to tell him. Chuck had cried a lot then, but a few weeks later, with his dad's approval, he had moved most of Willy's things out of the bedroom to the garage. He kept a couple of photos of the two of them together on his bulletin board. As the weeks went by, Chuck sometimes felt sad, sometimes regret, and sometimes guilt, the latter when he relished having the whole room to himself. He turned more and more to his friends and in the spring got really involved in baseball. Now, a year later, he had to look at the photos to remember what Willy looked like. Willy had not liked baseball.

> Ten-year-old Aki had lost his older brother, age 13, in a car accident about a year ago. He and his brother had shared a bedroom, and in spite of some differences in opinion, Aki had adored Kazuo. When Kazuo died on the operating table, Aki had been in the waiting room with his parents and little sister. They had all wept together and held one another close. An altar was put together commemorating Kazuo, and photos of him were in evidence throughout the apartment. Aki often stopped in front of the altar and felt the loss of his big brother and tried in many ways to recreate his brother's presence for himself through prayer and adopting some of Kazuo's behavior. He hoped fervently to become like his big brother as a way of honoring him and keeping the relationship within him.

These two examples are intended to illustrate how a similar event, death of a sibling, takes on different emotional meanings relative to cultural context. The result is differences in coping with both the feelings one experiences and the social relationships surrounding the emotion-eliciting event. Mainstream North American culture tends to discourage negative emotions such as sadness and fear, perhaps especially for males, although anger is seen as empowering of the self and is therefore acceptable. Thus, Chuck's mourning of his brother is fairly short-lived, and his autonomy and being different from his brother are encouraged. Another culture, in this case, Japanese, may view sadness as justified and even ennobling; sadness conveys honor for the deceased and acknowledges one's connection to them. The idea of "getting over" one's grief is an anathema.

Kitayama and Markus (1994) argue that the Western cultural goal of self-actualization is a "manifesto" for the self to separate itself from others and "to seek, find, and express one's own internal attributes" (p. 12). This cultural definition of self as *agent* has a number of implications for emotional experience and coping with aversive feelings. A self construed as an agent in determining the individual's "destiny" means that a major focus is on *control* of the external world and on *self-esteem* maintenance. For coping efficacy, the inference is that if one exerts control effectively in Western culture, one is also probably more often using problem-solving strategies when dealing with stressors. It may mean that what will prove to be "competent coping" *in Western culture* is being able to appraise a stressful situation in terms of what one can control about it and then to resolve the problematic situation functionally and maturely (see the beginning of this chapter). In short, what is competent about coping is inextricably tied to cultural values.

As Markus and Kitayama (1994b) also point out, North Americans are notorious for outscoring all other nationalities in what they refer to as *false uniqueness*; in other words, North Americans (and this includes quite young children as well) think they are better than most others. It is as though this inflated view of the self is a buffer against having to experience aversive emotions and cope with stressful situations that carry some risk of diminishment of self-esteem. However, if one is a member of an interdependent or collectivist culture (see discussion in Chapter 2), as many Asian cultures are sometimes described, then to present oneself modestly and with humility will facilitate one's harmony with others. Self-esteem or, perhaps better, a sense of well-being is to be found in promoting smooth relationships in which everyone feels in attunement with one another. Western culture might view this as self-sacrificing, but it is seen as relationship enhancing for an interdependent culture, for it is the connection with others that is of greater significance. Competent coping in a collectivist or interdependent culture might more often take the form of support seeking; possibly there is less need to see oneself as having to gain control over the external situation, and therefore there is greater use of coping strategies that provide distance from or avoidance of the stressor. This area of psychological research has only recently been addressed from a cultural comparison viewpoint, but research by Xinyin Chen and his colleagues

(Chen, Rubin, Li, & Li, in press) confirms that children and adolescents in mainland China who were rated by their *peers* as shy/inhibited proved to be socially competent and well adjusted. This outcome is just the opposite of research on European–North American children and youth, where it has more often been found that the shy/inhibited personality is associated with adjustment difficulties and greater prevalence of internalizing problems (e.g., Rubin, Chen, McDougall, Bowker, & McKinnon, 1995). However, consistent with research on Western children, Chen et al. (in press) did find that there were maladaptive outcomes for aggressive boys.

Weisz, Sigman, Weiss, and Mosk (1993) undertook another research project that is relevant to culture and coping among children. They studied parental reports of behavioral and emotional problems among young adolescents (11 to 15 years) in Kenya (Embu tribe), Thailand, and the United States, the latter being subdivided into African Americans and Caucasian Americans. Their sampling procedures were carefully undertaken (all families were rural and had rather modest economic and educational backgrounds). Their question was, to what extent do cultural values, mediated by socialization practices, translate into differential rates of children's problems? They hypothesized that the Thai and Embu children would show a greater incidence of internalizing or overcontrolled problems such as fears, somatic complaints, shyness, and so on, whereas the more autonomy-promoting culture of the United States would produce children who were more frequently cited by parents for their externalizing or undercontrolled behavior. Indeed, that is what they found, with some interesting subpatterns. Embu children are especially exhorted to be obedient and compliant, and when they evidenced problems, they were frequently somatic. Embu parents more often reported vomiting, sleep problems, and aches and pains. The children were also reported more often by parents as being perfectionistic, compulsive, feeling guilty, or acting young for their age. Caucasian American children topped the sample in incidence of total number of problem behaviors, but they particularly "excelled" at showing undercontrolled behaviors, such as being disobedient, impulsive, having poor peer relations, bragging, and bullying others. Thai children had the lowest mean number of problems compared to the other three cultural groups. When somatic complaints were excluded from the analyses involving undercontrolled and overcontrolled composite scores, the only cultural group that continued to have significantly more under *and* overcontrolled problems were the Caucasian American children, relative to the Embu and Thai children. There was no significant difference between the Caucasian and African American children in this analysis.

I infer from this study that our culture's emphasis on "being your-self," as opposed to learning to become part of the group and thereby respecting one's elders, being obedient, and showing deference and re-straint, may contribute to American children's *not knowing what to do* when faced with a stressful situation. They have to figure out how to cope rather than having available to them well-established cultural prac-tices that everyone agrees to as being the acceptable way to deal with difficult situations. Thus, North American children appear to have a greater likelihood of acting either in an emotionally overwhelmed, in-timidated, or defeated fashion, or they externalize their distress and be-have aggressively and defiantly toward others. Finding the balance among effective coping, feeling connected with others, and developing the valued Western autonomous self is a developmental task or hurdle we are just beginning to appreciate from a cross-cultural perspective. Perhaps one way to look at this task is that North American children may have to work harder because of the ambiguities they face in deter-mining all the nuances of our cultural scripts surrounding emotions, relationships, and stressful events. There are not very many clear-cut answers for youngsters figuring out how to cope with feelings they may not even know how to label, much less how to deal with the multiple complexities of a stressful situation and the people involved in it. (See also Frijda & Mesquita, 1994, for a parallel analysis of Dutch and Turk-ish young adults; the Dutch sample demonstrated a much lower con-sensus than did the Turkish as to whether other people would have similar feelings if they were in a similar situation.)

CONCLUSION

As children mature, their growing cognitive sophistication, exposure to varied social models, and breadth of emotional–social experience con-tribute to their being able to generate more coping solutions to prob-lematic situations. The older they are when faced with severe trauma, the more able they are to see the situation from various perspectives (including those held by other people who may be part of the problem-atic situation) and figure out a way to resolve it. With maturity, they be-come more accurate in their appraisals of how much control they really have over the situation and of what risks might accompany taking con-trol of a difficult situation (e.g., intervening in a fight). Effective coping in Western cultures involves acknowledgment of one's feelings, aware-ness of one's self as having some degree of agency, and a functional ap-praisal of the problematic situation and one's role in it. By late childhood or early adolescence, Western children who have enjoyed secure attachment within their supportive families, are self-confident, and have escaped severe trauma should generally be capable of this sort of emotionally competent coping. (Note that these are rather significant contingencies that may be all too *in*frequent when one considers the incidence of divorce, poverty, community violence, and abuse in American families.) Indeed, there are occasions when the adolescent with this optimal background "regresses" to less mature forms of coping (e.g., when vulnerability-inducing emotion is experienced as extremely intense and the situational parameters are unfamiliar), but, overall, the capacity for emotionally competent coping should be accessible.

Of course, a further caveat is in order: When the challenge that we have to cope with is social (and most challenges are), the degree to which the other interactants are emotionally competent also contributes to whether the problematic situation is *mutually* efficaciously coped with. We may act maturely, take responsibility for our role in a problematic situation, and try to negotiate with the other, but if the other is not in any condition to be able to respond reciprocally and appropriately, our personal control may be limited and our optimal coping may take the form of problem solving that deliberately makes use of distancing. When we must deal with a child in the middle of a tantrum, then distancing may take the form of a time out; an enraged adolescent might be distracted and a verbally abusive individual is best avoided. Emotionally competent coping is not easy and does not necessarily leave us with feelings of well-being, but when integrated with our moral sense of fairness and "doing the right thing," we will come away from even very taxing situations with having tried our best.

Chapter 10

Skill 7: Awareness of Emotional Communication within Relationships

Awareness that the structure or nature of relationships is in large part defined by how emotions are communicated within the relationship, such as by the degree of emotional immediacy or genuineness of expressive display and by the degree of emotional reciprocity or symmetry within the relationship; for example, mature intimacy is in part defined by mutual or reciprocal sharing of genuine emotions, whereas a parent–child relationship may have asymmetric sharing of genuine emotions.

This next skill of emotional competence integrates all the prior skills and capabilities described in earlier chapters with the older child's growing awareness of how emotions are communicated differently, depending on the nature of his or her relationship with the other. At first glance, this may seem to be a parallel skill to recognizing that we maneuver our expressive behavior to manage our self-presentation effectively (see Chapter 8). However, this skill highlights that children (or more likely by now preadolescents or adolescents) recognize and use emotional experience *to differentiate the organization of their relations with others*. This skill requires individuals to take into account several aspects

249

of the relationship's dynamics: (1) the *interpersonal consequences* of their emotional communication within the relationship for themselves and for the other,[1] (2) how they maintain the relationship quality (e.g., equilibrium) or alter it (e.g., by deepening or attenuating it), and (3) how they apply power or control within the relationship.[2] Several examples illustrate what I mean:

> Joan, age 12, looked angrily at her friend, Tasha, and said, "You took my library book and lost it! I can't believe you'd do that!" Tasha, quite chagrined, responded, "Joanie, I am really sorry, and don't worry, I *will* replace it." Joan replied, more gently now, "OK, I know you didn't do it on purpose."

> Susan, age 12, looked angrily at her sister, Christa, and said, "You took my library book and lost it! I can't believe you'd do that!" Christa, irritably, responded, "For crying out loud, Susan, it's only a book! Back off and I'll take care of it." Susan replied, "Well, don't think you can borrow anything from me again!"

> Rachel, age 12, looked angrily at the other girl, Connie, and said, "You took my library book and lost it! I can't believe you'd do that!" Connie, with considerable hostile sarcasm, responded, "Oh, look at her have a temper tantrum! I'm so scared I might just pee in my pants. Oh, she's so fierce, maybe she'll bite like a mad dog. Tough shit about your book." Rachel replied, "You're gonna' get it for this! I am fed up with you, so here's something for you to cry about," as she swung her backpack hard into Connie.

Here, the same event was placed in different relationships, with the protagonist feeling anger in all three cases. The outcomes were, however, quite different because of the differences in the nature of the relationship. In other words, experiencing anger (or any emotion, for that matter) is hardly a uniform transaction interpersonally. With a good friend, communicated anger is more likely to elicit remorse and attempts at resolution of conflict and restoration of relationship equilibrium. With rivalrous siblings, anger might elicit instrumental "repair" but less remorse, and the relationship is likely to continue its pendulum swing of on-again, off-again sibling squabbling alternating with harmony. With an overtly hostile relationship, anger is likely to elicit further escalation of conflict and hostile deprecations, and the transaction is likely to intensify in negative and retaliatory ways. As a result, power may be abused within such relationships, resulting in aggression. Emotion communication lies at the heart of the relationships we have with others and may well even define the parameters of the relationship.

This area is virtually devoid of systematic developmental research. However, among the few exceptions is a study by Whitesell and Harter (1996) on anger between close friends versus anger experienced with a more casual acquaintance. In their study, preadolescents (11 to 12) and adolescents (13 to 15) responded to an interview in which they were to imagine that they and either their best friend or a casual acquaintance were engaged in a variety of hypothetical situations. Attribution of blame, violation of expectations, and emotional reactions were elicited. Invariably, the children and youth more often blamed the casual acquaintance for what had been anger provoking than they did their friend. In fact, many of the children said they themselves must have somehow contributed to the upsetting situation. As for violation of expectations for how a friend should act, only the adolescents reported that they would feel more distress if a friend treated them in this fashion versus a mere acquaintance. Emotional reactions to the friend's aggression were more complex than when an acquaintance was the aggressor. Multiple feelings were typically reported when the friend was insulting and hurtful but less often for the casual acquaintance. Whitesell and Harter (1996) interpreted their findings as follows: "Thus, in dealing with a friend's aggression, children may feel sad that the self has been insulted, sad that the relationship is threatened, angry that the friend has done this, afraid that the relationship will suffer, and so on. When a classmate or casual acquaintance is involved, on the other had, self-centered concerns would be more likely to prevail *because no important relationship is involved*" (p. 1356; emphasis added). This study is among the few I touch on in this chapter, but I also draw upon relevant material in social psychological or clinical research with adults.

From an emotional competence perspective, self-efficacy would be served if we were aware of how we communicated our feelings with others and recognized that we communicated differently depending on the nature of the relationship. With awareness, we would be better able to gauge our goals vis-à-vis a particular person (or set of people) and to alter our emotional communication in order to fine-tune the quality of the relationship and its boundaries. Not surprisingly, this is exactly what many couple therapists do when working with distressed spouses: They seek to enhance the respective partners' awareness of how their emotional communication affects the other and whether they achieve what they want within the relationship with that sort of emotional communication (e.g., Fruzzetti & Jacobson, 1990; Gottman & Porterfield, 1981; Greenberg & Johnson, 1990; Lindahl & Markman, 1990). It is also what management trainers seek to do in their workshops for sensitizing managers to how they communicate with their subordinates or what organizations do in training their employees for "customer service" (e.g., see Hochschild's [1983] analysis of flight attendants' emotion management training). Finally, awareness of emotional communication is one of the core features of training programs for counselors and therapists, and countless volumes have been written on how to cultivate, refine, and dovetail one's emotionally expressive communication with clients (e.g., Teyber, 1985).

From a developmental standpoint, children demonstrate qualitatively different styles of emotional communication according to different relationship structures before they begin to acquire explicit awareness of emotional communication as part of how relationships are defined. For example, Underwood et al. (1992) found that school-age children said that they would not show their anger to teachers but would to their peers. Likely justifications might have included such comments as "you'd get in trouble," or "the teacher would think you were talking back," which would indicate that children recognize that with an authority figure (e.g., a teacher) expressing anger directly has undesirable repercussions. Whether such children could say that it is the difference in power and status that affects how anger is communicated in North American culture is unlikely, but many adolescents probably do have this degree of insight and could verbally construct some of the relationship parameters that define how certain emotions get communicated. (For a review of status, power, and dominance in *nonverbal* interaction among adults, see Edinger & Patterson, 1983. For a theoretical discussion of power and dominance in *verbal* discourse wherein dominance is evident in asymmetric initiative–response contributions to conversations, see Hermans & Kempen, 1993.)

In addition to the status–power–dominance cluster that influences much of North American emotional communication, whether verbal or nonverbal, the other major variable is degree of closeness or affiliation between interactants. Mehrabian (1972) also referred to this as responsiveness, and this cluster, closeness–affiliation–responsiveness, captures the degree of warmth and liking between people. Combined with the dominance cluster, we get asymmetric relationships such as between parent and child, where a high degree of closeness exists alongside clear power or dominance differences. Indeed, when we speak of a "parentified child," we often think of a parent who has abdicated the dominance of the parental role (and often its attendant responsibilities as well). In such a role reversal, the parent's style of emotional communication with his or her child typically reveals the parent's immaturity and may predict later adjustment difficulties for the child because of the relationship's reversed asymmetry. As their parents move into their elderly years, many adults have found to their surprise that they must now adopt an asymmetrically greater degree of power in their communication with their aging parents; they had become accustomed to symmetrical communication during earlier adulthood.

In intimate adult relationships we would expect not only a high degree of closeness but also that the dominance variable would be symmetric or balanced, with partners equally sharing status or power within their emotional communicative style. In this latter pattern we may see the characteristics of intimate emotional communication: trusting self-disclosure of vulnerability which elicits empathic responsiveness and reciprocal vulnerable self-disclosure (Fruzzetti & Jacobson, 1990). School-age children use parallel reasons for evaluating when they would express their genuine and vulnerability-inducing emotions: "If the other person is my friend, then sure" (Saarni, 1988). Equal or balanced status and power combined with a high degree of closeness make for an emotional communicative style that consists of a *mutual* exchange of more frequent genuine displays of emotion and a preponderance of positive emotional expressiveness.

This notion—that awareness of emotional communication within relationships is central to how we define relationships—is closely related to interaction rituals (e.g., Goffman, 1967), processes of interpersonal negotiation (e.g., Selman & Demorest, 1984), and the report and command features of metacommunication (e.g., Saarni, 1982; Watzlawick, Beavin, & Jackson, 1967). I comment briefly on each of these topics as related to emotional communication.

INTERACTION RITUAL

There is often a predictability in our styles of emotional communication within certain relationships, and the consistencies appear to be related to our goals in the relationship transaction. Many of these goals appear to be what Goffman referred to as "face-work": how to save face, how to project oneself favorably, how to restore interpersonal equilibrium when someone else loses face, and so forth. Such interactional goals contribute to what a given cultural group professes as etiquette, "proper" demeanor, and obligatory social behavior. For example, consider the old adage, "children should be seen but not heard." Clearly this was for the convenience of adults, but it was also viewed as proper demeanor for children when in the company of adults, who, by definition, were authority figures. Thus, by their adopting this obligatory social behavior, children expressed their deference to authority and illustrated their "good moral upbringing," thereby also putting their parents in a favorable light for others to see. Although we currently do not think children should only be seen and not heard, remnants of this obligatory social behavior can be seen in negative judgments of a parent whose child is throwing a temper tantrum in a public place, that is, the parents have ostensibly done an inadequate job of upbringing if their child is screaming so loudly.

A more complex view of interaction rituals may be found in Sarbin's (1989, 1990) theoretical work. He used the idea of *narrative emplotment* to describe the predictable course of unfolding events when we experience an emotion. A coherent, meaningful script that includes setting, time, characters, intentions, events, roles, and so forth can be constructed for emotions if they are viewed through a dramaturgical metaphor: Who was present or conspicuously absent, who did what to whom, what occurred next, how did various characters respond and counterrespond, how did contextual constraints influence the course of events, and what was the outcome or "ending." Hermans and Kempen (1993) argue that these narratives of emotion are learned as patterned wholes, but I suspect there is more fluidity in these emotion narratives than these theorists suggest. I find more appealing Lutz's notion of open-ended folk or ethnotheories of emotion, which when embraced by a particular individual can change as a function of unique experiences that an individual might have (Lutz, 1987). An example that comes to mind is the likelihood of change in immigrants' expectations for *what* to feel, *how* to express a feeling, and toward *whom* as they acculturate to their new society. In my opinion, the various constructs of narratives, scripts, interaction rituals, and folk theories of emotion all tend to converge toward a general theoretical position that regards emotional experience as an intersubjective phenomenon (i.e., socially shared) that is deeply entwined with the circumstances of one's *existence* (including one's past, one's future expectancies, as well as the immediate present).

INTERPERSONAL NEGOTIATION

The idea that emotional experience is manifest in socially shared transactions is explicitly addressed in Selman's interpersonal negotiation model (Selman & Demorest, 1984, 1987). Processes of emotional communication within relationships are relevant in that he and his colleagues premise their model on how the interactants define a problem between them, and problems between people are invariably emotion laden! The way the problem is perceived can range from elementary (the problem is defined in terms of the wants of the person viewed as having the most power) to complex and mature (the problem is defined as a shared or mutual concern, taking into account both persons' needs or wants). A problem also implies a goal, whether it is to restore relationship equilibrium or to achieve some instrumental or task outcome. Whether the problem is defined in either an elementary or a complex fashion, its definition influences the nature of the goal as well, which in turn sets the stage for emotional communication within the dyadic relationship. However, it is also possible that the stream of influence can operate in the reverse direction as well: The nature of the dyadic relationship determines the quality of emotional communication, which in turn defines the goal and how the problem between the two persons is delineated (as illustrated by the research of Whitesell & Harter, 1996, described previously). I suspect by the time one reaches adolescence, both interpersonal negotiation and relationship-dependent emotional communication can function as starting points for how people try to manage their relations with others. As an illustration, consider the following vignette (adapted from a real case):

Fifteen-year-old Georgia was a star volleyball player for her school, a private and elite school. Georgia was on an academic merit scholarship and was also a member of an ethnic minority group in a school that leaned toward European American homogeneity. The coach for the team often adopted a very dictatorial style and criticized the team's efforts zealously. After the team lost a game to another school, the coach lashed out at the girls, and Georgia, outraged at his disrespect toward the girls, spoke out. Her team members started to applaud, and the coach exploded and shouted she was off the team for the rest of the semester.

The next day Georgia asked to meet with the headmaster to discuss what had happened. She was very nervous as she waited outside his office, but she also felt what she had said was justified, and the coach was in the wrong. She also wanted to get back on the team. The principal beckoned her to come into his office, and sternly asked her why she had such an "attitude" and brusquely stated that such attitudes were not acceptable at the school. How she could have been so insolent when she was a scholarship recipient was beyond his comprehension; imagine, jeopardizing her scholarship. . . . Georgia realized that this man and the coach were a unified front against her, that they could not or would not see her perspective. Their tactics with her were to bully her. She realized she would need others who were more powerful to back her.

After conferring with her family, Georgia and her parents filed a grievance against the school with the Office of Civil Rights of the United States Department of Education. Shortly thereafter, she received a letter from the school reinstating her on the team; the whole team, including the coach, would be going on a week-

end retreat to develop better communication and team cooperation. And the principal apologized for not hearing her side of the
story. Georgia astutely recognized that threat and counterthreat by
"bigger guns" was the name of this game.

Georgia decided to go to another school the following year.
She realized that at her former school, social interaction was nar-
rowly defined by ascribed power and status. As she told a newspaper reporter, "If you didn't have much power or status, you had to
act deferential and put up with others' arrogance and conceit. It
was such a putdown." She said she wanted to be able to relate to
others more flexibly and more openly and thus had chosen to
transfer to a public school.

Georgia wanted and expected complex interpersonal negotiation,
characterized by mutuality and the interactants' taking into account
one another's needs and wants. The coach and headmaster operated
from a power standpoint and thus used lower-level negotiation tactics
characterized by one-sided assertion of their wants and viewpoints.
Georgia realized that she would have to reciprocate their negotiation
strategy by finding a representative for her side that was more powerful, and she successfully met that challenge. From an emotional communication standpoint, Georgia viewed the deprecatory harangue
from the coach as disrespectful: It was a communication style that invalidated a relationship she believed should be premised on teamwork
and cooperation. The coach and headmaster viewed Georgia's communication style as not befitting a lower-status individual addressing a
higher-status person. Regrettably, higher-status individuals are all too
frequently thoughtlessly insulting to less powerful people and may even
view such an emotional communicative style as "justified."

As a further illustration, the reader has probably overheard parents in public places address their children in an insulting or humiliating fashion. Such parents may even feel their way of speaking to their
child is justified: "I don't want her getting a big head" (i.e., "I don't
want her assuming that she has any power in this relationship") or "She
needs to know her place" (i.e., "She belongs on a lower level than the
parent"). Recipients usually experience power-assertion emotional messages that are devoid of responsiveness or warmth as negative, and the
recipient of such emotional communication can rebel and challenge
such communication as Georgia did. But more often, less powerful
people grudgingly comply, fume with resentment, or become passive–
aggressive in return. It is not surprising that the greatest source of
stress reported by American workers is their workplace supervisor
(e.g., Karasek & Theorell, 1990), who probably uses power-assertion
emotional communication without any warmth or responsiveness

(which by definition implies taking into account the other's needs and wants) toward his or her subordinate employees.

METACOMMUNICATION

This term may be most generally defined as referring to "a message about a message." If we now think of emotional metacommunication, we would be referring to an emotional message about an emotional message. Family systems theorists have long used the notion of meta-communication to make sense of the complex interactions in families. Satir (1967), for example, believed that metacommunication conveyed three features about an interaction: (1) the sender's feelings and atti-tudes about the communication itself (e.g., "the message I sent to you was a loving one"); (2) the sender's feelings and attitudes about him- or herself (e.g., "I am a good mother"); and (3) the sender's feelings, atti-tudes, and intentions toward the receiver of the communication (e.g., "I want to take care of you in the best way possible"). How do all these complicated metacommunications get across? Very simply: Our emo-tional–expressive behavior that accompanies our verbal behavior in-forms our interactants as to what is going on. Inconsistencies and incongruities between verbal and nonverbal behavior occur frequently, and these "mixed messages" probably reflect different appraisals and meanings within the relationship transaction. For example, a genuine smile accompanied by anxious and hesitant vocal expressiveness may indicate the individual's liking of the interactant, but the person is also concerned that her affection may not be reciprocated by the inter-actant. The smile expresses the individual's positive appraisal of the interactant whereas the anxious voice derives from the individual's anxiety-eliciting cognitions about the anticipated evaluation of herself in the eyes of the other.

Systems theorists also use the concepts of report and command in their analyses of complex communication (Saarni, 1982; Watzlawick et al., 1967). Report refers to the content of the message—its literal mean-ing, so to speak. Command, however, refers to the relationship context between the interactants and is intended to take into account the pro-cess of *influence* within the interpersonal transaction. Following is an expansion of the example about smiling accompanied by an anxious tone of voice to illustrate report and command:

Sara, age 11, had moved with her family during the school year, and, as a result, she found herself starting a new school at the be-ginning of February. She was a good student and didn't worry much about the teachers, but she was concerned about how she'd make friends all over again at this new school. She worried that she wasn't especially good at sports, and her braces seemed to have taken over her entire mouth, and she felt self-conscious talking with her mouth visibly full of metal. As a result, she came across to the other kids as shy and quiet.

Valentine's Day was looming, and Sara busied herself during art class making a gorgeous Valentine for her best friend at her former school. Some other kids noticed it and started giggling about what sort of boy it was for. Sara replied simply, "I miss my friends at my old school, so this is for one of them." Virginia came over to her desk, and said, "Well, that's a lucky friend; your valentine is really beautiful. I wish I could make one like that for my mom." Sara offered to share some of the sequins she had brought from home with her, and soon Virginia was busily creating a fancy Valentine herself—with Sara's further offers of sequins and lace scraps.

Valentine's Day was on a school day, and when she arrived at her desk, Sara found a lovely plump chocolate truffle. She looked around her, delighted and pleased, and Virginia caught her eye. She came over and said, "My mom just loved the Valentine I made for her. I gave it to her this morning before she went to work, and she was going to put it on her desk for everyone to see. My dad divorced us, so she's pretty lonely now." Virginia's disclosure was not lost on Sara, and she felt her self-consciousness melting away. She smiled broadly, braces and all, at Virginia, and asked in a hesitant voice, "Is that chocolate from you? Would you like to have a bite?"

Virginia and Sara became good friends, and Virginia good-naturedly joked with Sara about her braces and pointed out that at least 10 other kids in the class had "teeth armor" as she called them. By the end of the semester, Sara felt she had her niche again with her peers.

In this dialogue the report features of Sara's and Virginia's communication have to do with missing friends, making Valentines, mom's reaction to the Valentine, Virginia's family's divorce, and questions about the source of the chocolate and whether Virginia would like some to eat too. These report features are the "surface" content of the communication, but what is significantly communicated here are the mutual relationship-building gestures expressed by the two girls. Sara's initial disclosure about missing her friends elicited interest from Virginia, and Sara responded by sharing her craft supplies. Subsequently Virginia demonstrated reciprocal "object" generosity by giving Sara a chocolate truffle and reciprocated an even more personal disclosure, that her parents were divorced. The dovetailing of disclosures and reciprocal sharing illustrate a process of mutual influence: As each girl extended herself a little bit toward the other, her gesture was reciprocated in kind and thus validated. The spiral of mutual liking was strengthened, and their friendship was initiated.

This example was essentially positive in tone and outcome, but it is not difficult to imagine families in which children's expressions of feelings are met with disapproval, contemptuous and humiliating reproaches, and even punitive responses. Sarcasm is an especially obvious example of how the command feature of deprecation of the other is conveyed by the emotional–expressive behavior of the communicator, although the report feature may seemingly be innocuous (e.g., "Oh, those jeans seem a little loose on you," directed by a parent to her overweight son whose jeans are straining at the seams).

Finally, command features convey our feelings about our feelings as when we verbally communicate our emotional experience to another but qualify its meaning by our accompanying emotional–expressive behavior. An example that comes to mind is when we describe to a friend some embarrassing incident and while we tell the story we smile and laugh ("I was struck by foot-in-mouth disease again"). Our positive expressive behavior reveals (or is intended to reveal) that we do not really feel that the embarrassment was important in the overall scheme of things, and we are not shamed by our embarrassing behavior.

Report and command features are essentially conceptual tools that give us a way to characterize our emotion-laden communication within our interpersonal exchanges. Self-efficacy and emotional competence are furthered when we can be aware of others' implied messages that are not necessarily directly verbalized. In short, we have more information with which to guide our responses to others if we can recognize in their communications both the direct report features and the implicit command features. If we are also aware of our own report and command features in our interpersonal communication, we can reflect on our feelings about our relations with others with greater insight and with greater awareness of how we affect others. For example, we may have intended our loud voice to express how emphatically we feel about some issue, but when we notice the target child cringing and turning away from us, we realize that our communication was "received" or comprehended as sounding angry. We can then correct that unintended effect and clarify what we had meant to say to the child. We might also learn that a loud voice for emphasis may not be the best command feature to use and that other expressive gestures with our hands or face might be more precise in conveying what we intended. We turn next to several studies about children's acquisition of emotional communication within relationships.

DEVELOPMENT OF CHILDREN'S EMOTIONAL COMMUNICATION STRATEGIES

When we interact with a young infant, we can create, with the infant, cycles of mutual influence in our own and the infant's nonverbal emotional–expressive behavior (e.g., Cappella, 1981; Stern, 1985). These cycles of mutual influence have been referred to as reciprocal social dialogues and affective attunement, and they function to help infant and caregiver to develop together shared perspectives and understanding. "Intersubjectivity" is another term used to designate how we experience with someone a mutually felt emotional response, and not surprisingly, empathy plays a role in this notion of being able to share an emotional experience. These concepts (i.e., reciprocal dialogues, affective attunement, and intersubjectivity) are important developmental precursors for children *to experience* in their family relationships in order to recognize that our emotions have interpersonal effects and influence. Without such experience, children would not be able to undertake different sorts of interaction with others outside their family and vary their emotional communication according to the nature of the relationship they have with that person (e.g., taking into account dominance and affiliation differences). They would not recognize that their emotional communication influences the other, and that this process is mutual. If their emotional communication style goes against social consensus as to what is appropriate, they will indeed experience social consequences such as rejection and teasing, or attempts by the other to "teach" them to send their signals differently. The latter situation is not unfamiliar to adults who have traveled to another country whose culture is quite different from their own; they may feel that they are committing countless social blunders and may become aware of others' attempts to guide them toward appropriate social behavior.

Social Dimensions in Dyadic Relationships

An early study by Mendelson and Peters (1983) examined whether children took into account what they knew about the nature of a relationship between two people when predicting the emotions that would be communicated in a dyadic interaction. Only 13- to 14-year-olds consistently used relationship structure (e.g., friend/not-friend, parent/not-parent) to make sense of how both hostile and affectionate behaviors were communicated. Children at ages 9 to 10 took into account only hostile behavior in their predictions about the sorts of emotions that would be communicated, and affectionate exchanges were not often used as indicators of how close the relationship was.

A study I undertook attempted to examine more systematically children's views of social dimensions within interpersonal relations and how they affected children's expectations for genuine or dissembled emotional–expressive behavior in hypothetical vignettes. The vignettes varied according to whether (1) the status between the interactants was the same or the interactant was in the dominant status position relative to the child protagonist, (b) the relationship between the story characters was relatively close versus distant or unfamiliar, (3) the emotion felt was or was not intense, and (4) the facial expression of the protagonist was genuine or dissembled (Saarni, 1991; see also Chapter 8). The 113 participating children ranged in age from 6 to 12 years (first, third, and sixth grades). Eight vignettes were carefully constructed to vary status, affiliation, intensity, emotion type and dissembled versus genuine expression; they were also accompanied by schematic illustrations. An extended interview of each child included comprehension checks and systematic questions that probed how changing (1) the status difference between the two focal interactants, (2) the degree of affiliation between them, or (3) the intensity of emotion felt by the child protagonist would influence whether the facial expression displayed by the protagonist would be dissembled or genuine (i.e., congruent with internal subjective feeling state). Following are two of the vignettes with sample interviews for the richness shown by the children in their constructions of "social reality."

The following story (featuring "Fara" for girls, or "Fred" for boys) entailed high-intensity emotion (anger) experienced by the protagonist, who displayed a genuine facial expression and had low affiliation with the interactant, albeit of the same status as the interactant.

"THE PIANO"

Fara had to perform a song for her music class. She was told to do it with a girl named Marcia, whom she did not know very well. Marcia said to Fara that she could play the piano while Fara did the singing. After Fara agreed to Marcia's plan, they both promised to learn their parts at home. However, on the day of the performance, Marcia had not learned her part on the piano, and Fara was left to sing by herself all alone in front of the whole class. Fara felt so furious with Marcia for not sticking to her promise to learn her part, that she felt she could burst with anger. Fara looked hard at Marcia and frowned angrily.

The child respondent is a sixth-grade 11-year-old girl.

Comprehension Questions

    1. Tell me, did Fara know the other girl, Marcia, very well or not?
       "No."

2. How did Fara feel?
   "She felt mad."
3. How did Fara look on her face?
   "Mad."

Interview Questions

Some kids think that Fara would have controlled her anger and just shown a straight serious face if this story were a little bit different.

1. Do you think that if Marcia were an adult, like a teacher's aide, Fara would have then shown a straight face, or would she have still frowned angrily? [*This probe alters the status dimension between the protagonist and interactant.*]
   "Her face would've looked just sort of blank."
   Why?
   "Because, like, an adult could have benched her if she looked mad."
2. Do you think that if Marcia were a close friend, Fara would have then shown a straight face, or would she have still frowned angrily? [*This probe alters the degree of affiliation between the protagonist and interactant.*]
   "She would've frowned."
   Why?
   "Because the girl knows Fara could go tell her mom on her and she'll be in big trouble for not keeping her bargain."
3. If Fara was really only concerned that she do her best and was not interested in what Marcia did or did not do, would she have then shown a straight face when Marcia didn't do her part, or would she have still frowned angrily? [*This probe alters the intensity of emotion felt by the protagonist, in this case diminishing anger.*]
   "She'd have a straight face."
   Why?
   "She was confident in herself and she could do it anyway without the other girl."
4. Going back to how the story was in the beginning, what would you have done if you were in Fara's situation yourself?
   "I'd just look blank."
   Why?
   "Because the teacher could walk in just right at that moment, and then there'd be a problem."

In the following story (featuring "Holly" for girls, or "Henry" for boys), the protagonist experienced low-intensity emotion (amusement) and had low affiliation with and same status as the interactant.

"THE DOG"

Henry had a dog named Joker, who really liked to get into mischief. One day he took him to the park where some kids were eating their lunch. Henry did not know these kids. One guy was talking fast and waving his arm around, and in his hand was a roast beef sandwich. In a blink of an eye that dog Joker ran up to the guy and snatched the sandwich right out of his hand. Joker then ran back to Henry to show off his prize and gulped the sandwich down in one bite. When the guy saw that Henry was the dog's owner, he went up to Henry and asked for an apology. Henry thought Joker had actually been more funny than bad and felt like smiling, because he felt the whole thing had looked pretty funny. However, pretending he felt badly about his dog's behavior, Henry put on a straight face and apologized to the guy.

The child respondent is a first-grade 6-year-old boy.

Comprehension Questions

1. Tell me, did Henry know the boy whose sandwich Joker took?
   "No."
2. How did Henry feel?
   "He thought it was funny."
3. How did Henry look on his face?
   "He looked like he was a little bit sad about it but he wasn't really."

Interview Questions

Some kids think that Henry would have shown that he felt it was a pretty funny situation and therefore smiled if this story were a little bit different.

1. Do you think if the boy were older than Henry, Henry might have smiled, or would he have kept his face straight? [*This probe alters the status dimension between the protagonist and interactant.*]
   "He would keep his face straight."
   Why?
   "Because he'd be scared that the kid would beat him up."
2. Do you think that Henry would have smiled if he had known the boy, or would he have kept his face straight? [*This probe alters the degree of affiliation between the protagonist and interactant.*]
   "He'd keep a straight face."
   Why?
   "He'd want to keep his friend happy. Laughing at him wouldn't be very nice."
3. If Henry felt his dog's snatching the sandwich was the funniest trick he had ever seen him do, would he have then smiled even

as he tried to still apologize to the boy, or would he have kept his face straight? [*This probe alters the intensity of the emotion felt by the protagonist, in this case, intensifying it.*]
"*He should have a straight face and apologize.*"
Why?
"*Because he wants to keep the other boy from getting mad at him.*"
4. Going back to how the story was at the beginning, what would you have done if you were in Henry's situation yourself?
"*I'd feel sorry and apologize.*"
[Probe: And how would you look?]
"*I'd look sad.*"
Why?
"*Because the dog took the sandwich, and that's not very nice.*"

The complex patterns of how the child subjects believed the facial expression would change in light of these manipulations of social–relational contexts and their justifications for the expected expressive display produced endless analyses. Overall, what emerged was that as each of these three contextual features (i.e., status, affiliation, and intensity) was made to change, it interacted with the remaining two, and the older children in particular attempted to take these multifaceted changes into account as they predicted the facial expression. About 67% of the older children's responses were consistent with what experts on adult nonverbal communication would have predicted: If two out of three context features were typically associated with dissemblance (i.e., low-intensity emotion, higher status of interactant, and low affiliation between interactants), then dissembled expressive behavior was expected by a clear majority of the older children. If two out of three (or all three) context features were linked with genuine expressions (i.e., high-intensity emotion, similar status between interactants, and high affiliation between interactants), then a genuine expression was usually anticipated by the older children.

The dimension of closeness or degree of positive affiliation has also been addressed in a research on empathic responsiveness. Strayer and Roberts (1997) examined literal physical distance from others and the degree of empathy school-age children felt toward these other individuals. They used hypothetical videotaped vignettes and had the children move photos of the actors or actresses on a grid closer or further away from themselves depending on their subjective comfort with the character. They also evaluated the children's empathic responsiveness toward the assorted vignettes' characters. The relationship between degree of empathic responsiveness felt toward a character and how close his or her photo was placed to the self increased with age. The authors argued that "as empathic responses grow in complexity and strength, their effects in other areas (such as personal distance) should become clearer and stronger" (p. 399). Interestingly, punitive adults and children who lied to gain an advantage over another vulnerable child elicited the least empathic responsiveness. More likely to elicit empathy were characters who endured undeserved hardship. I turn next to a discussion of several studies that examined children's use of relationship knowledge in emotional communication.

Relationship Knowledge

In their review of research on children's concepts about the family, Pederson and Gilby (1986) described children's and adults' views of what the functions of a *family* were. Not surprisingly, children and the adults were most in agreement about families providing the necessities of living, but a close second in proportion of agreement (65% of the children and 100% of the adults) was that families were supposed to provide positive emotional experience, including love, caring, support, and happiness, for their constituents. The point here is that broad consensus exists across both children and adults about the quality of emotional communication that characterizes and virtually defines at least one relationship structure, namely, family relatedness. Interestingly, the children and adults did not nominate "to produce biological offspring" as a function of families. I infer from this research that how social and *emotional* ties are communicated is critical for defining the concept of *family* in Western culture.

Complementing the preceding research but focusing on psychopathology within families, Cook, Kenny, and Goldstein (1991) evaluated 70 families seeking outpatient counseling. These families included a troubled adolescent as the "identified patient," and all the families consisted of two parents, thus limiting the degree to which their results can be generalized to single-parent families. Their goal was to examine reciprocal communication patterns in these families to shed light on how dysfunctional interaction comes about. In their complex analyses, they determined that adolescents and to some extent fathers bore much of the responsibility for both initiating and reciprocating the interpersonal expression of emotional negativity. Mothers were more apt to reciprocate their adolescents' negativity. But the major outcome was the statistically robust feedback loop or vicious cycle in which these families were caught: Adolescents communicated negatively with their parents, who in turn reciprocated with negativity, thus eliciting still more affective negativity from their sons and daughters, and so on.

Whereas Pedersen and Gilby's subjects emphasized *warm* emotional communication as a function of families, these families also emphasized emotional communication, but it was decidedly negative in tone and had deleterious effects on family members. Thus, emotional communication does indeed characterize a major function of families, but such communication can range from destructive to enhancing for both the individuals involved as well as the family as a *systemic* whole.

A recent study on school-age children's understanding of secrets examined the effect of relationship understanding on children's willingness to pass on a secret to their mother or to a good friend (Watson & Valtin, 1997). Secrets are by definition emotion-laden communications (in my opinion), and secret keeping and secret sharing are underresearched from the standpoint of the emotional functions they play for children. Although Watson and Valtin were more interested in children's understanding of interpersonal intentions vis-à-vis the nature of secrets, their results are important here for how they revealed children's use of relationship knowledge in choosing whether or not to share a secret. First, the children were generally able to distinguish among different kinds of secrets (i.e., innocent, dangerous, guilty, and embarrassing secrets), and the distinction among these categories of secrets interacted with children's willingness to share the secret with either mother or their friend. The age of the child also affected the pattern of results such that the youngest children (5 to 6 years) were more likely to tell mother more secrets than the older children. Indeed, the older children were more likely to share secrets with their friends—as an expression of, maybe even testimony to, their friendship—than with their mother. The exception was sharing of embarrassing secrets (i.e., wetting one's pants) by the older boys: Few would confess this to their friend, whereas the older girls were more willing to share "bodily loss of control" with their same-sex friends. Humiliation and fear of loss of reputation were among the reasons cited by the older boys for not telling a friend, but they might tell their mother because she could be counted on *not* to embarrass them. As for guilty or dangerous secrets, older children felt a clear sense of tension about whether to maintain their friend's secret as an act of trustworthiness, even as they also worried that perhaps an adult "should" know about the guilt-laden activity (i.e., theft) or dangerous event (i.e., lighting a fire in an empty garage). As one girl put it, "Mother is like half a friend—so sometimes you can share some secrets with her" (Watson & Valtin, 1997, pp. 448–449). From the standpoint of understanding how relationship structure affects our emotional communication, the older children were more consistently concerned with how trust defined a relationship, and, by implication, with trust comes a degree of reciprocity and mutuality.

Good friends should be able to trust one another, and similarly in well-functioning families mutual trust exists as well. Emotional communication is profoundly affected by the degree of trust one feels toward another with the result that the greater the trust, the more likely one will disclose information about one's experience that is emotionally vulnerable. Emotionally vulnerable information about oneself or another is invariably anxiety-provoking, and it takes a mutually respectful relationship for anxiety-laden exchanges to be reassuringly heard.

Another of my studies, described in brief in Chapter 8 (Saarni, 1988), is also relevant to how children use relationship knowledge in their acquisition of this emotional competence skill. I investigated children's beliefs about how others are likely to react when they present an "emotional front," (i.e., when they dissemble their emotional–expressive behavior so that their genuine emotional state is not directly revealed). The children were in three age groups: 6 to 7, 10 to 11, and 13 to 14 years. They first answered a series of questions about four photo-accompanied vignettes, and the pattern of responses varied considerably according to context. Relevant to our concern here is that when their responses were coded for whether the interpersonal consequences of the emotional front were evaluated as positive or negative, several significant age effects occurred relative to how the children took into account their knowledge about the relationship between the interactants. The two older groups of children believed that it would produce desirable consequences if they dissembled their disappointment over an unwanted gift to an aunt (e.g., "Her feelings won't be hurt"), whereas dissemblance toward a hostile bully would simply be ineffective—bullies are presumably not deterred by adopting a tough emotional front. The youngest children had a more negative view of dissembling to an aunt; their responses focused on the story character not getting what he or she wanted for his or her birthday. They also believed that dissembling to bullies would produce positive outcomes (e.g., "Then he won't keep on bothering you," if they covered up their fear). Greater experience with hostile relationships (such as with bullies) may have produced more cynicism among the older children. Across age groups, a majority of children thought it would be a good thing to dissemble their hurt when falling down after showing off on a skateboard because saving face in front of their peers was considered important. Children at all ages also thought the outcome would be negative for the protagonist child for having set off the school fire alarm, despite presenting a false front of mock innocence to the principal.

When the children were asked what the interpersonal outcomes would be if the story characters showed their real feelings (and appropriate photos of genuine facial expressions were then shown), they made significantly different responses for the fire alarm and the bully stories depending on age. Older children thought the outcome would be more positive if they showed their apprehension to the principal (i.e., they could cut their punishment losses with an authority figure, so to speak, if they admitted to the misdeed); younger children expected mostly negative consequences. For the bully story, more of the older children believed the outcome would be *highly* negative if one expressed one's genuine fear (note that earlier a dissembled expression also elicited negative consequences, but in this case genuine display of fear was thought to exacerbate severely the outcome of the interaction with the hostile bully); more of the younger children thought that there could be positive consequences (e.g., "Someone might help you if they see you are afraid"). Across age groups, children thought the interpersonal consequences would be negative if they revealed their genuine disappointment to a misguided aunt (e.g., "She'd think you were rude" or "next time she wouldn't get you anything for your birthday") or if they expressed their hurt after showing off, because then they risked being teased by their peers (as one 11-year-old put it, "If you're going to show off, you'd better not mess up, because if you do, you'd really look stupid" and by implication, if "you do mess up, you'd better make a joke out of it").

These data indicate that children evaluate how emotions are communicated in relation to the nature of the relationship between interactants and in relation to social goals or motives. Expectations for strategic social–emotional behavior are also discernible in some of the children's beliefs, such as the need to save face in some situations (e.g., after hurting themselves while showing off) or to allow another to save face (e.g., smiling at a misguided aunt for choosing such a poor birthday gift). Although this study did not investigate children's views of reciprocity or symmetry in relationships, the ready acknowledgment of interpersonal consequences that are *contingent* upon emotional–expressive behavior suggests that children implicitly use notions of reciprocity in some of their expectations (e.g., "I'll not show how I feel so that you won't have to experience a negative feeling").

Finally, von Salisch's (1991) study, which was reviewed in Chapter 8, is also relevant to this emotional competence skill. Recall that her friendship pairs played a computer game that had been rigged so that it would appear as though one of them had caused the pair to lose the game. With their close friends, the children smiled very frequently, even as they uttered verbal reproaches or expressed contempt for their friend's "failure" in the game. Their smiling was often reciprocated, and the dance of smiles seemed to function as a mutual reassurance that the relationship between the children was maintained and not threatened—despite the occasional reproaches and expressions of contempt. Not only did the children's smiling behavior express positive feelings, it also contained important social messages about relationship durability (or equilibrium) and about how the interactants defined their relationship by their style of emotional communication. Imagine the outcome if one of the participants had suddenly stopped reciprocating the smiles.

Related results from younger children also suggest that friendship tends to elicit compromise or attempts to resolve conflicts (e.g., Hartup, Laursen, Stewart, & Eastenson, 1988) and that reactions to well-liked "provocateurs" are more controlled (Fabes et al., 1996). Not surprisingly, child friends also have more disagreements and conflicts and may even criticize one another more (e.g., Gottman, 1983): If friendship is also characterized by children as a relationship in which genuine feelings are more likely to be expressed (e.g., Saarni, 1979b), then that also includes negative reactions as well as positive ones.

How children's emotional communication within relationships changes with transition into adolescence is an area needing more systematic investigation. Among the few studies available is one by Zeman and Shipman (1997), who examined 5th-, 8th-, and 11th-grade children and youth. These authors found that it was the 8th-graders (13 to 14 years old) who demonstrated an emotional distancing from their mothers and tended to expect more negative consequences to their sad or angry emotional behavior. By 11th grade (16 to 17 years), these older adolescents seemed to be more accepting of their emotional experiences and anticipated more support and acceptance from others, although they were very clear that expressing anger toward their mothers was not likely to be acceptable. In sum, these teens managed their emotional experience (sadness and anger) relative to social context (peers and family), but it was done in light of their own developmental needs and goals. Thus, the young adolescents were "busy" pushing their families away while the older adolescents seemed more comfortable with how they managed their emotions as they may have already established some degree of emotional independence from their parents.

We also know that the notion of reciprocal influence is cognitively better understood by adolescents, but to what extent they demonstrate their understanding of mutuality in interpersonal negotiation when experiencing conflict or negative emotion appears to depend on their social maturity (e.g., Selman & Demorest, 1987). The media's reports of driveby shootings in revenge for some slight or turf encroachment may indicate some sort of primitive reciprocity as in "You hurt me, I'll hurt you back and worse," but this is not what is intended by Selman and his colleagues (e.g., Selman, Beardslee, Schultz, Krupa, & Podorefsky,

1986) when they emphasize the *collaborative* nature of mature adolescent negotiation. How alienation, futility, and dashed dreams affect adolescents' strategic use of emotion communication in close relationships is not known, although there is a good possibility that underdeveloped emotional communication within the family is part of what contributes to adolescents' experiencing alienation, futility, and marginalized outcomes (e.g., Straus, 1994). On the other hand, several studies have indicated that when children and young teens are asked about what would happen if they expressed aggressive retaliation toward friends, they responded with anticipations of guilt, negative self-evaluations, and questions about the legitimacy of their own action (e.g., Perry, Perry, & Weiss, 1989; von Salisch, 1996b).

Given the paucity of empirical research in examination of children's awareness of how emotional communication varies within relationships, this chapter does not have the usual gender, social maturity, and cultural influence subsections. Instead, I would like to consider more generally in the next section how emotion is contextualized within social transactions and by adults' perception of children's social–emotional behavior. I conclude with a comment on culture's influence on such social–emotional transactions.

EMOTIONS WITHIN SOCIAL TRANSACTIONS

Conflict and Anger

I was particularly intrigued by a study undertaken by Shantz (1993) that emphasized children's own narrative constructions of the events that contributed to peer conflict and their role in the conflict. This study used a clinical interview strategy with 7-year-old boys and girls. Upon request, the children were readily able to recall a recent conflict or fight that they had had; the interviewer followed up with a variety of probes about its onset, what issues were disputed, what strategies were used, what emotions were experienced, how the fight or argument ended, and what "lesson" they learned from the dispute. The children fingered the other child as the instigator in 51% of the stories and themselves only 8% of the time; 41% of the time they were unsure as to how the fight got started. Two major issues contributed to almost all the disputes for this age group: The need to control another person's behavior (66%) and/or the possession of objects (33%). Of greater interest here is the first issue, and, indeed, being put down by another (20%), being hit (20%), and, to a lesser extent, violations of friendship expectations (16%) were all significant causes of dispute. Not surprisingly, the most frequent emotion reported was feeling mad or angry, followed by bothered, upset, or sad. Data were not provided as to whether mad/angry feelings were more often felt for the personal put-down dispute and sadness for the friendship violation, and although such an attribution would make sense, it needs to be empirically examined in this age group. Shantz does suggest that when children reported feeling bothered or upset, they may have been referring to feeling sad; it is possible that this emotion may be difficult to access or to report due to the vulnerability of the self that is implied (see also Fuchs & Thelen, 1988).

Conflicts were ended either by external agents (peers, yard-duty teacher) or by the children involved in the conflict themselves. The majority of these conflicts were perceived by the children as having win–lose outcomes, a smaller set was seen as having no resolution, and only a modest number (14%) were seen as being collaboratively resolved or resulting in compromise. The vast majority of children (80%) did not talk with their friend or acquaintance about the fight, some offering as a rationale that they wanted to avoid the topic so as not to provoke the conflict again.

In terms of what lessons were learned from the conflict, 76% of the children dutifully reported having learned something (Shantz notes that this probe pulls for a certain amount of social approval seeking from the adult interviewer). More children reported learning to *inhibit* behavior rather than to change it. Most of the "lessons learned" were of a very concrete behavioral sort (e.g., "I won't play with him again"), and a much smaller number of reports concerned the nature of the conflict itself or the friendship with their disputant. Those children who reported not learning anything from the conflict were a minority (24%), but the reports of their conflicts were distinctive for several reasons: (1) Their conflicts were much more likely to involve aggression; (2) the conflicts were clearly defined as ending with one person winning and the other losing, and (3) 75% of these sorts of conflicts were reported by boys. It is interesting to speculate whether these little boys were constructing in their own conflicts (or rather the narrative description of their conflicts) a rendition of what they watch on television or play out on electronic games. However, this sort of dispute structure may also simply be a pervasive characteristic of the socialization of boys in Western culture, and media merely replicate the cultural expectations for male behavior (see also Golombok & Fivush, 1994). Recent research by Herrera and Dunn (1997) suggests a different view. They found that when mothers emphasized their own needs when in conflict with their young child, their child was less likely to use constructive conflict management strategies with his or her peers. Thus, how parents and children manage their conflicts between them may well prove to be once again the foundation for how children generalize their social interaction strategies outside the family (see also Parker & Herrera, 1996, for an investigation of abused vs. non-abused children's friendships; not surprisingly, the abused children's friendships were more conflict laden).

What I find significant about Shantz's (1993) study is how children construct their stories about their conflicts. Their stories begin with clear causal events that initiate conflicts and subsequent outcomes, and emotions appear to be both part of the cause of the social dispute and part of the outcome. It is the self that experiences strong emotions which activate the self to engage in some goal-directed fashion to bring resolution to the emotion-eliciting *and* conflict-causing events. The outcome of the conflict, whether one loses, wins, or compromises, is also marked by emotion: on the one hand, sadness, upsetness, anger, and wariness, and on the other hand, pleasure, pride, relief, or excitement. Awaiting further systematic research is how the experience of these emotions is embedded in different relationship structures (e.g., friend, not-friend; family versus peer) that are further contextualized by gender role. As an illustration of what such research might entail, readers are referred to Roecker, Dubow, and Donaldson (1996), who undertook a comparison of school-age children's and young teens' coping with observed conflict between adults versus conflict between peers; the former elicited more internalizing reactions.

Cross-gender conflicts among school-age children and youth have been infrequently studied, but one exception was a study carried out in Germany by Oswald, Krappmann, Chowdhuri, and von Salisch (1987). They found that a shift occurred between ages 10 and 12, with the younger group relatively sex segregated on the playground. However, the older group increasingly reported more friendships with the opposite sex and were observed to "parade" in front of opposite-sex groups, apparently trying to impress the others. In addition, whereas the 10-year-olds were remarkably unhelpful with opposite-sex children, by age 12 there was a noteworthy increase in cross-gender helping. Finally, Golombok and Fivush (1994) in their review suggest that aggressive girls are more apt to play in mixed-gender groups but at the same time are also more likely to be rejected by their peers. Along with such studies as von Salisch's (1996b) described earlier, this area of research represents a fertile field for investigation.

Adults' Perception of Children's Emotional–Social Behavior

Few studies have explicitly examined the influence of particular patterns of children's emotional–expressive behavior on adults. More frequently, research has looked at how child behavior more generally elicits caregiving, attention, or, in some cases, abuse (e.g., Bell, 1974; de Lissovoy, 1979). However, implicitly, a great deal of research on children's emotional–expressive behavior has also involved such behavior's influence on adults: It is the adult interviewer, coder, or experimenter who is influenced by the child subject. But, of course, that is not the focus of most studies, and it may not even have been considered relevant to how research outcomes were interpreted. But an early study undertaken by Bates (1976) suggests that as investigators, we ought to be more aware of how children's emotional–expressive behavior may influence our judgments and ratings of them.

Bates (1976) examined the effects of children's emotional–expressive behavior on adults' perception of them. He used four 11-year-old "confederate" boys to act out scripts with young adults; these scripts varied in nonverbal expression of "positivity." For the high-positive script the boys looked at the adults' faces 75% of the time and smiled as frequently as seemed appropriate. For the low-positive condition they were to maintain facial regard no more than 25% of the time and not smile at all. (There were a number of other interaction conditions included in this study which I do not address.) Of interest here is that high-positive expressive behavior on the child's part elicited from the adult subjects significantly more positive facial expressions, more positive tone of voice, and more verbal interaction. If the adult was a woman, these positive response variables were even higher.

In addition to coding the adults' expressive behavior in response to the child, the adult subjects were also asked to evaluate the child's intellectual abilities and social skills. Significant effects were once again found for positive expressive behavior: The confederate children trained to display the positive behavior were judged to be more intellectually able and much more socially skilled than the low-positive children. The many studies that have been done since Bates's work have unfortunately not looked at how the children's positive expressive behavior is a significant contributor *in itself* to ratings of social competence (when made by adults). In short, "being nice and agreeable" (translate: smile a lot and make eye contact) is likely to make grownups like a child and evaluate the child more favorably—even if the child's peers disagree (think of how negatively children view "the teacher's pet").

Parenthetically, in the context of trying to untangle child and parent influence in incidence of physical child abuse, Bugental and her colleagues (Bugental & Shennum, 1984; Bugental, Blue, & Lewis, 1990) investigated how "difficult" children elicit dysphoric emotional responses and negative attributions from adults. The emotional–expressive behavior of these "difficult" children was characterized as unresponsive, which, in turn, was based on their relative lack of eye contact with adults, slow verbal response, and atypical gestures, facial movements, or noises emitted. These children did not smile much either. Such children were viewed by many adults as hard to be around, and their responses to such children included coercive action or helplessness.

Relative to emotional competence is Bates's discussion of reciprocal feedback loops that get started in social interaction: A positive initiation is reciprocated by a positive response, which in turn elicits further positive overtures, and so forth. The same sort of feedback loop apparently works for negative emotional–expressive behavior as well: Negative behavior from person A elicits a reciprocal negative response from B, to which A responds with more negativity, and B reciprocates again with negativity, and so forth (e.g., see Gottman & Levenson, 1992; Harris, Gergen, & Lannamann, 1986; Katz & Gottman, 1993). Bates's study is strongly suggestive of how powerfully a positive self-presentation can influence others' reciprocal response to oneself. Insofar as a child or adolescent has social goals that she wishes to reach, knowing how to adopt a positive "emotional front" may well be very efficacious and allow for sufficient success at reaching one's goals. The result may be that the emotional front is no longer a posture adopted to mask apprehension or social anxiety; instead, the confident positive expressive self-presentation becomes a genuine portrayal of the self's view of the self.

Culture and Emotion within Relationships

A quote from Kenneth Gergen (1990) seemed most fitting for this topic: "emotions are not the possessions of individuals, rather, emotional performances are embedded within relational scenarios. What we term emotional understanding emerges as the result of judging the individual's adequacy within a recognized scenario" (p. 602). Upon reading Gergen's essay, I recognized that his arguments for how to understand emotion meaning systems cross-culturally could be applied to *emotional development* in our own culture. The quote captures the main thrust of his argument, for he is adamant that emotional expression can only be understood in the context of unfolding events and the nature of the relationship between interactants. He refers to this as an emotional performance within a script or scenario, although he does not mean that the performance is play-acted or pretended; rather, each culture or subculture defines for its members *intelligible* paths for the sequence of emotion communication. It is the traversal of these paths, which both the actor and the audience understand as meaningful (i.e., intelligible), that he considers to be the emotional performance. Applying his argument to emotional development, I infer that we get more competent or adequate (to use his term) as we understand and apply these culturally defined emotional scripts to our social interaction in functional ways. But it is really the *relational space* between people that is best characterized as "competent" or "adequate." Depending on the relationship dynamic between ourselves and another, our emotional "dance" together may be adaptively harmonious, only moderately connected, or nonsensical. The first demonstrates affective attunement, and the last resembles some of the performances exhibited by characters in Sam Shepherd plays (although these dramatic enactments eventually unfold as intelligible to the attending audience).

An example drawn from Whiting and Edwards's (1988) comparative study of children growing up in six cultures illustrates the sorts of problems produced by the lack of shared meaning systems about emotional communication. The scene that follows is of a 10-year-old Mixtecan child who lives in the Indian barrio of Juxtlahuacan and speaks her native tongue but attends a Spanish-speaking school in town; the teacher has been correcting the pupils' notebooks.

> Rosa . . . walks down the aisle toward the teacher. When she gets to her, the teacher is talking to another boy. In silence Rosa raises the notebook in her hand and puts it in front of the teacher's face in order to have her attention. The teacher takes the notebook. Rosa, standing next to her, leans her head against the teacher's body with her look fastened upon the teacher. The teacher distractedly returns the notebook. The little girl takes it, and remains looking for a moment and then turns around and returns, walking slowly to her bench . . . [and] puts her notebook away. (p. 249)

In the Mixtecan culture, children use considerably more visual and motoric modes to communicate their intentions than Western cultures do. The result described previously is an *in*adequate interaction between a child and her teacher: Neither the child nor the teacher grasps the goals of the other's style of communication. The child wants the teacher to evaluate her notebook and tries to communicate her desire by looking at the teacher and leaning her body against her; the teacher may perceive the child as intrusive or immature in her attention-getting behavior and thus does not examine her schoolwork. We can guess how such ineffective interactions eventually turn out: Rosa will likely drop out of school, experiencing it as an alien place. The teacher's prejudice toward the local native people will be reinforced, and Rosa may not acquire the skills of the dominant Spanish culture that will allow her to become bicultural and thus economically more successful in her country. Indeed, Whiting and Edwards (1988) describe the conditions in Rosa's school as verging on chaos, presumably due in part to the paucity of *mutually intelligible* social–emotional scripts for interaction.

CONCLUSION

Although I have not directly addressed "social competence" in this chapter, it is important to comment on how this skill of emotional competence might fit into the literature on social competence. I have found Rose-Krasnor's analysis of that large literature most helpful and will apply it here (Rose-Krasnor, 1997). In her review she notes that social skills, peer popularity as measured by sociocentric ratings, friendships (or lack thereof), and interpersonal problem-solving approaches have only low to moderate association with one another. Some of this is due to different kinds of data collected and from different sources, but I think her argument is a good one: These different facets of social interaction should *not* correlate highly with one another precisely because they are at entirely different levels of analysis. She has thoughtfully partitioned this large body of social competence research and theory into what she calls a prism (or a pyramid). At the apex is *social effectiveness,* which she considers to be transactional, context-dependent, and a performance-oriented organizing construct. At the middle level of this prism is what she refers to as the *indices* of social competence, and it is at this point that promoting the goals of oneself and of others are balanced. She contends that social interaction consists of a continuous dialectic between self-oriented goals and other-oriented goals (and I concur). The former appear in the self's taking initiative in relationships and the latter in seeking connectedness with peers and groups and in meeting societal expectations for desirable interpersonal behavior. At the bottom and broadest level of this theoretical prism are discrete social skills such as perspective taking, social problem solving, empathy with others, emotional regulation, appropriate communication, and so forth. Twenty-nine such skills were once proposed as reflecting social competence (Anderson & Messick, 1974). Individual differences and cultural variability are most noticeable at this broad and multidimensional level.

I think that the emotional competence skill proposed here, namely, awareness of emotional communication within relationships, would *by analogy* be at the base of a corresponding pyramid for emotional competence. But the analogy is only a partial one, for I see awareness of emotional communication within relationships as having embedded within it an awareness of goals for oneself as well as for others. Thus, Rose-Krasnor's perspective on social competence would seem already integrated with the fairly mature emotional competence skill I have proposed here. However, her approach to the social competency field is a productive one and certainly provides considerable organization to an otherwise unwieldy and diverse body of empirical data and theoretical perspectives (e.g., she cites 13 differing accounts of what exactly is social competence). It may well prove to be an approach that would ultimately also benefit the rapidly accumulating research on emotional development and emotional competence (e.g., Garner, 1996). Indeed, I would look forward to an integration of both social and emotional competency approaches.

Our thinking about how emotional experience develops has in recent years increasingly embraced a social contextual view of emotion processes. Yet at the same time among the more intriguing contemporary research are studies on how relationship histories (both long- and short-term) influence emotional development. This suggests that richly descriptive longitudinal research may be our best source for understanding both the continuities and the discontinuities in emotional development and emotional competence. Unfortunately, this also tends to be the most expensive research to undertake.

Parke (1994) succinctly summarized a number of trends and unanswered questions in emotional development. He too emphasized that the important questions lie in examining how emotion processes unfold within relationships as opposed to artificial laboratory "interactions." Relationships with parents, siblings, other kin, peers, teachers, and extrafamilial caregivers are probably the most common relational patterns experienced by Western children. Within each relational pattern children learn how status, intimacy, gender, and age roles influence the communication of emotion. The socialization of emotion, by definition, occurs within relationships, and in a sense, the medium *is* the message for understanding emotion processes. The subtlety and richness of our awareness of how our emotional communication differentiates our relations with others reflect our socialization experiences. However, the immediate contextual demands to which we respond in our interpersonal worlds color that awareness as well.

NOTES

1. In self-presentation, the focus tends to be more on consequences for oneself *or* for the other; the emphasis here is on the relational "space" between the interactants.
2. Alternative concepts here include ascendancy, superordinate versus subordinate status, initiative, assertiveness, and so forth.

✿ Chapter 11

Skill 8: The Capacity for Emotional Self-Efficacy

Capacity for emotional self-efficacy: The individual views him- or her-self as feeling, overall, the way he or she wants to feel. That is, emotional self-efficacy means that we accept our emotional experience, whether unique and ec-centric or culturally conventional, and this acceptance is in alignment with the individual's beliefs about what constitutes desirable emotional "balance." In es-sence, we are living in accord with our personal theory of emotion when we demonstrate emotional self-efficacy as well as in accord with our moral sense.

ACCEPTANCE OF ONE'S EMOTIONAL EXPERIENCE
AND SUBJECTIVE WELL-BEING

This last skill of emotional competence brings us full circle back to the self: The capacity for emotional self-efficacy refers to our viewing our-selves as feeling the way we want to feel. This does not mean that we al-ways feel happy; at times, we feel badly, even downright miserable. However, we judge our feelings to be appropriate to the circumstances, and we believe our emotions are justified, for they serve our interests in an adaptive manner. In short, it may be highly adaptive to feel quite distraught about some event, as it mobilizes the self to take action to remedy the painful situation. On some occasions we learn from our distress not to put ourselves in a particular risky situation again; on other occasions we take care to provide a "safety net" for ourselves so that we do not repeat our distress or despair to the same degree. Individuals with a capacity for emotional self-efficacy know how to cope with aversive emotions by regulating their intensity, duration, and frequency through appropriate and adaptive action. They do so with the belief that they will generally be effective in such regulation and can tolerate and not be overwhelmed by negative emotion. This belief may be given additional support by their having the moral conviction that they are navigating a morally acceptable course, albeit an emotionally difficult one.

Depressed people may feel justified in their emotional response of sadness and hopelessness, but their efficacy in coping with negative emotional states is poor. Similarly, battering spouses may view their anger as "justified," but their sense of efficacy in coping with anger and aggression is also poor (Saunders et al., 1987). Indeed, most depressed people would rather not feel depressed, and most battering spouses would rather not feel that their anger is *out of control* (Dutton, 1998; Sonkin, 1988). Perhaps this is the key issue for emotional self-efficacy: feeling relatively in control of our emotional experience from the standpoint of mastery, positive self-regard, and acknowledgment of our moral commitments. Such individuals do not feel overwhelmed by the enormity, intensity, or complexity of emotional experience, nor do they react to emotional experience by inhibiting, distrusting, or "damping down and numbing it out." Issues of emotional regulation are relevant here, as is the question whether some kinds of emotional regulation are dysfunctional and ultimately maladaptive (see also Lazarus, 1991; Thompson, 1990; and Chapter 12).

The capacity for self-efficacy probably entails some understanding of how one's personality interfaces with one's emotional experience. Insight into one's foibles, talents, vulnerabilities, and strengths can be melded with emotional self-efficacy to generate a sense of self-acceptance. I suspect a healthy dose of self-irony and tolerance for ambiguity goes along with emotional self-efficacy as well, but I have no empirical evidence for this.

Harter's (1986b) work on self-worth and how it mediates emotional and motivational systems within people is relevant to emotional self-efficacy. Using path-analytical techniques with data from older children, she found that global self-worth strongly influenced affect (defined here as happy vs. sad), and affect in turn influenced motivation (defined as energy and interest vs. their absence). Her model suggests that the overall evaluation of the self is laden with feeling, and it is this feeling about who we are as a person that energizes us or renders us lethargic. It should also be noted that the determinants she used for global self-worth consisted of social support, positive regard from others, and competence in domains viewed as important to the self.

The notion of emotional self-efficacy maps onto Harter's model very well. If we experience ourselves as generally well regarded by others who are significant to us, and we believe we function competently in the activities important to us, then the feedback we get from our behavior and relationships reinforces our belief in our self-efficacy. Assuming that people want to be efficacious, that is, they generally desire to succeed in their endeavors and attain their goals, then upon goal achievement, they will likely feel happy (or contented, or relieved, or perhaps even elated and joyful) (Lazarus, 1991).

Lazarus (1991) refers to the transitory *state* of happiness as related to but different from *subjective well-being,* which is more *trait*-like and thus has some degree of continuity over time. He emphasizes the subjectivity of this assessment of well-being, for it is based on people's expectations relative to their typical level of affective adaptation. For example, if our life is hard and something delightful happens one day, we might experience a lot more happiness at that moment than someone whose lifestyle is customarily easy and the same "delightful" event occurs. On the other hand, our life may be so unrelentingly bitter that we cannot appreciate positive events. We can look at subjective well-being from a figure/ground perspective: Subjective well-being constitutes the "ground" relative to daily events that elicit our emotional response; the latter constitute the foreground or "figure" relative to our sense of well-being. This background subjective well-being may function as a mood-like buffer when we have to endure a truly and unbelievably bad day (e.g., the car breaks down in the middle of rush-hour traffic, we step in dog feces, a panhandler screams epithets at us after we give him a dollar, and when we finally get home, not only has the washing machine leaked all over the floor but the answering machine has 23 messages on it). At that point, we need all the subjective well-being and emotional self-efficacy we can dredge up in our 30 seconds of introspection before tackling the washing machine and the phone messages. In Lazarus's (1991) words, we need a *positive appraisal style* if we are to cope with a truly bad day and still come out with our sense of emotional self-efficacy intact, albeit somewhat tattered.

Lazarus's critique of empirical research on subjective well-being is interesting, for much of the self-report questionnaire work on which it rests is data driven and weak on theory. In particular, as Lazarus (1991) notes, there is often a "bottom-up, response-centered" (p. 409) approach that looks at ratios of aggregated positive to negative experiences as indices of relative well-being, but this research often neglects to take a top-down approach, for example, by examining more global outlooks on life as suggested by the phrase "positive appraisal style." Feist, Bodner, Jacobs, Miles, and Tan (1995) examined whether subjective well-being consisted more of the daily details of living as opposed to a more dispositional or general attitudinal outlook on life. They evaluated monthly a sample of young adults (median age was 24; most were female, and the majority were Caucasian, Christian, and single) for a period of 4 months on a variety of self-report measures that included both general beliefs that would index a positive appraisal style as well as more specific "daily hassles" and health complaints. Using structural modeling techniques, the authors concluded that neither a dispositional nor a "daily details" model explained how we experience subjective well-being. Instead, our sense of well-being reflects both a general outlook on life as well as the extent of our daily hassles and complaints. In short, both contribute to (or diminish, as the case may be) our perceived sense of well-being. Feist et al. (1995) argued for taking a state/trait approach to subjective well-being, namely, that we can experience well-being *at the moment* even as we might or might not generally believe ourselves to be relatively happy or content with our lives (or vice versa).

Harter's (1986b) work is, in fact, a top-down approach, using global self-worth as the organizing principle and functioning much like a "trait" in terms of its influence on subjective well-being. She has also empirically looked at the developmental antecedents of self-worth found in social support, positive regard, and judgments of competence in domains important to the self. Thus, developmentally, there appear to be some facets of daily living that might over time contribute to having a general positive appraisal style, which Harter would probably argue is largely influenced by a positive regard for the self. More recently, Nurmi, Berzonsky, Tammi, and Kinney (1997) proposed that it is how we go about constructing an *identity* for ourselves that may be relevant to how self-worth contributes to subjective well-being. They conducted a study with Finnish and American college students in which they looked at how these young adults made use of an identity information processing style for themselves. They hypothesized that identity styles could be looked at from three perspectives: (1) an information-seeking orientation in which individuals seek out self-relevant information, regardless of whether it is confirming or discrepant with what they believe about themselves, and the implication is that they attempt to integrate varied sources of information about themselves in their construction of an identity; (2) a normative orientation, in which individuals seek out stereotyped or conventional definitions for themselves, and (3) a diffuse/avoidant orientation in which individuals rely on the environmental demands of the moment to produce a definition of who they are. Based on their results from a variety of self-report measures, the authors concluded that the approach used by people to forge a sense of self-identity was highly associated with a perceived sense of well-being. Specifically, the diffuse/avoidant subjects were more likely to report that they felt depressed and self-*in*efficacious (e.g., delaying choices and acting indecisively), the normative identity subjects had the most stable self-concepts over time (i.e., it may be difficult "to rock the boat" of an identity definition that everyone agrees on), and the information-seeking subjects had the highest level of self-esteem, perhaps due to their more frequent experience of success and positive feedback when they competently engaged in challenging situations (as opposed to conventional or predictable ones). The authors argued that subjective well-being was indeed reflective of one's self-concept but that self-concept influenced subjective well-being through the cognitive strategies relied on to construct one's identity.

Although Nurmi et al. (1997) confirmed that subjective well-being goes hand in hand with a self-concept, their study was only over a 4-month period and used young adult subjects. I think that a self-concept that is diversified into a system may best reconcile the research undertaken by social psychologists on the phenomenon of subjective well-being. Recall the argument in Chapter 2 about the sense of efficacy gained by an infant when it learns to control contingencies; such learning requires a self that becomes aware of that which is not-self, but the infant also becomes capable of influencing that which is not-self to do its bidding, so to speak. Recall also Neisser's (1988) topology of the self-system: the ecological self, the extended self, and the evaluated self. Without a construct such as the ecological self, it becomes difficult to entertain a concept of subjective well-being that has its roots simultaneously in the individual and in the *context* experienced by that individual. The notion of an extended self is necessary for the development of schemata and scripts; it allows us to anticipate the future: We do expect to survive the truly terrible day of car breakdowns, leaky washing machines, rude panhandlers, our smelly shoes, and endless phone messages. Our evaluative self facilitates our goal-directed action: We try to figure out the best ways to get what is advantageous to us (this begins to sound like the information-seeking identity negotiation style). These constructs about the self provide conceptual anchorage for subjective well-being. If this notion of a self-system is integrated with emotional experience, I see emotional self-efficacy as highly related to subjective well-being. However, I will still argue that emotional self-efficacy goes beyond subjective well-being insofar as negative emotions, including eccentric appraisals leading to unconventional emotional responses and the recognition of dignity within melancholy, are not typically considered under the rubric of well-being. Such emotional experience may reflect what an individual views as a *morally justified* response; that is, we may experience these difficult feelings because of our commitment to our moral code in conjunction with our relationships with others. Recall from the discussion of moral disposition in Chapter 1 that Colby and Damon (1992) found, in their study of individuals who had led morally exemplary lives, that an emotional responsiveness to others was very much a part of their personal integrity. When we are involved deeply with others in caring relationships, it is inevitable that we will feel pain. It probably goes without saying that this area needs further research.

DEVELOPMENTAL RESEARCH RELATED
TO EMOTIONAL SELF-EFFICACY

From a developmental standpoint, I am intrigued by the idea of how children recognize that some sort of integration or *balance* is important in their emotional life: Both negative and positive feelings have their place in emotional self-efficacy, as does the expression of both genuine and dissembled emotional displays in interpersonal exchanges. I do not mean that this idea of balance should convey that we feel an "equal amount" of positive and negative feelings; rather, I wish to emphasize that emotional self-efficacy entails an acceptance of ups and downs in our emotional experience. We would not judge ourselves negatively for feeling sad, angry, tense, or afraid; nor would we distort our self-awareness by putting a false positive gloss on our emotional experience. However, emotional self-efficacy would include a clear recognition of *what* we feel and *why* we feel this way, including the fact that we can have multiple feelings that can be quite contradictory because we are facing a complex emotional dilemma. Thus, with emotional self-efficacy we have a good idea of how our emotions serve us as cues for effective problem solving, including those situations that are subtle and consist of multiple challenges. It is with the effective reaching of our goals that we experience emotional self-efficacy: Our emotions worked for us.

If we think of emotional self-efficacy from the standpoint of recognizing that we can have both positive and negative feelings and strike a balance between the two different emotional valences as we plot our course of action, we would not get mired down in seemingly unsolvable inner conflict. This idea of getting stuck in a resistant inner conflict with our mixed feelings is related to the issues examined in a few developmental studies. I briefly discuss a couple of these studies, but they are more suggestive than definitive in terms of what I would like to see investigated about children's real-life attempts to integrate efficaciously their feelings with their values and goal-directed behavior.

Opposite-Valence Feelings

Harter and Whitesell (1989) interviewed children 9 to 12 years old about whether experiencing two opposite-valence feelings (i.e., happy/sad or happy/mad combinations) created an internal conflict for the children. They found that only about 50% of the children (across ages) reported any internal conflict. Children who said there was little or no conflict made statements such as the following: "If I am really happy, the mad feeling just sort of fades and gets covered up by the happy," or "The sad feeling is there, but it's not really controlling how I feel." In these statements, we can see how subjective well-being operated as a background buffer for the children to absorb the downside of emotional experience. They reported feeling in charge of their emotions as opposed to their emotions overwhelming them. They did not deny their negative feelings, but they were not immobilized by them and could presumably continue to pursue goal-relevant action.

On the other hand, half the children did report an internal conflict, and what appeared to be a major contributor was the relative intensity of the two opposite-valence emotions. If the two feelings (e.g., mad and happy) were reported as having relatively the same intensity, then internal conflict was more likely to be reported. Conflict was infrequently mentioned if happiness was experienced as the more intense feeling. *Interpersonal* conflict appeared to result from predominantly negative feelings. Harter and Whitesell suggested that negative emotions would be rated as highly intense (and therefore would "overpower" positive emotions) if they occurred within a close relationship, such as between parent and child, and particularly if an expectancy had been contradicted. The child would then feel a severe sense of betrayal or loss, leading to intense anger or sadness, respectively. There would be no *inner* conflict over how one felt; the negative feeling simply surpassed any positive emotion the child may have also felt toward the parent. Consider the following examples as to how they illustrate these patterns:

No Conflict: Positive Emotion More Intense than Negative Emotion

Dan had recently started middle school and like many of his peers, he loved to hang out with his skateboard. He had been practicing some pretty amazing jumps and thought he was ready to show his skill to some other guys who hung out at the mall. There was a fountain there with stone benches and stuff that he thought he could jump over with his board. He got his board all prepped and ready to go.

Dan was spectacular! All the guys seemed to think he was really good. They were maybe a little envious and so one of them dared him to jump the fountain. He wasn't sure he could do it, but why not try? He sailed toward it, pushing off at the right moment, was airborne, and came down with a horrible thud. One of the wheels of his board broke! Everything seemed to go black. The next thing Dan knew was that his head and body hurt like hell, his board was broken, but all the guys were exclaiming that they had never seen anything like his jump. He felt pretty proud, even though he hurt, and he wondered what he'd do about his busted skateboard.

NO CONFLICT: NEGATIVE FEELING OVERPOWERS POSITIVE EMOTION

Sandy's parents were divorced, and she spent most of her time with her mom. She missed her dad a lot, and she saw less of him now that he had remarried and had moved to Honolulu. Her grandmother told her she'd double the money Sandy earned at odd jobs so that she could buy an airplane ticket to visit her dad over the holidays. Sandy worked hard and saved her money; her dad said it would be great for her to come for a visit.

Sandy bought her ticket with pride and looked forward eagerly to seeing her dad and to exploring Hawaii. Two days before her departure, her dad left a message on the answering machine saying it wasn't a good time to come after all, with no further explanation. Sandy was crushed.

CONFLICT: SIMILAR INTENSITIES OF POSITIVE AND NEGATIVE EMOTION

Martin was 12 when he went to live with his dad; fortunately, his mom lived in the same city, so he could see her and his sister as often as he wanted to. But he much preferred to stay with his dad, because his dad wasn't always ragging on him like his mom usually did. He felt more grown-up with his dad, more independent compared to how his mom treated him.

For his 13th birthday Martin's mom was going to put on a real nice dinner, and she hinted that she had a really neat gift for him too. He suspected it was a ticket to the play-offs game for his favorite hockey team, the San Jose Sharks. His mom didn't have much money, and he knew that to get one of those tickets was really hard for her. On the day of the birthday dinner, his mom called to say there would be a special guest at the dinner. He briefly wondered who it was, but didn't think anything more about it until he got to her apartment that evening. There was some guy there named Antonio. Martin's mom handed him an envelope, he opened it, and there were two tickets! He was really pleased and grateful, thinking now he could take his friend, Sergio, and he turned to hug his mom, but she gestured him aside, and said he should thank Antonio, who was going to be his new Dad. Martin slumped into his chair, weakly thanked Antonio without looking at him, and thought to himself, "Oh great, I get to go to the game, but with him?"

Emotional balance in Harter and Whitesell's work appears to refer to having a mixture of feelings, generated by multiple appraisals about complex and unfolding circumstances, but overall the positive ones predominate in the long run. How children come to be able to regulate their internal emotional experience so that they can reliably produce more positive than negative emotional states over time is related to their developmental histories (e.g., the contributors to self-worth) and to their ability to cope with aversive emotions and challenging circumstances as discussed in Chapter 9. The connection to emotional self-efficacy is evident both in the balancing of negative and positive emotions and in the general movement toward subjective well-being, despite periodic upsets and emotional conflicts with others. I turn next to a study that looks specifically at how we engage with others and the effects it has on our view of ourselves.

Self-Presentation and Self-Worth

Harter and Lee (1989) examined what they called "true" and "not true" selves in adolescence as related to youths' global self-worth. The youth described "true selves" as "acting naturally, being who one really is inside" as opposed to false selves, described as acting to please others, make positive impressions, or generally fulfill what others expect rather than one's own desires for self-definition. This latter view of the false self seems a lot like the maneuvers we might undertake to create self-presentations that gain advantages for ourselves, yet the majority of Harter and Lee's subjects did not much like having to adopt a not true self. Whereas the actual adoption of true self behavior was only minimally correlated with self-worth, *knowing* one's true self was highly correlated with self-worth. In short, having a sense of self-definition and accepting it as valid for oneself went hand in hand with positive self-regard. However, how one *acted* with another person was more dependent on the relationship context rather than on one's self-worth.

Harter and Lee (1989) asked the youth to respond how they would evaluate true and false selves within different kinds of relationships: mother, father, romantic partner, and friend. This context, namely, close relationships, is usually defined by the occurrence of mutual exchanges of genuine and often vulnerable emotion-laden disclosures about the self (see Chapters 8 and 10). Thus, it is not especially surprising that when adolescents are asked whether they like their false self in the context of a close relationship, they generally answer no. On some level, it violates the premise of close relationships. Indeed, among the reasons the youth gave for not liking their false selves was the anticipation of being rejected for who they really were. For example, relative to their mothers, if they felt that her support was conditional on their meeting her high expectations, they were less likely to present a vulnerable (but genuine) self that might fail in her eyes. In the case of their romantic partners, they experienced anxiety about not having their real selves understood and accepted. Such responses suggest that these close relationships have some degree of ambivalence embedded in them for those youth who gave such reasons. For those youth who said their false selves were acceptable, the reason provided was most often because the false self allowed them to impress or please others. Whether this was framed as simply observing etiquette or as trying to put themselves in a good light from a strategic standpoint to gain advantages and avoid disadvantages was unknown in this study.

Harter and her colleagues followed up this study with a more recent one (Harter, Marold, Whitesell, & Cobbs, 1996) in which they investigated adolescents' expectations about receiving support from peers and parents. Consistent with the earlier study, they found that youth who experienced their parents and peers as conditional in giving their support were more likely to believe that they presented false selves under these circumstances. However, if they stated that their motive in presenting a false self was *because they felt themselves devalued*, they also tended to exhibit the most distressed psychological health profile and reported engaging the most often in false portrayals of themselves. In contrast, those youth who simply said they adopted false-self behavior to impress or please their parents or peers obtained higher psychological health scores, reported that they more often expressed their true selves, and believed that they had more knowledge of who they really were. Their false self presentations apparently were acknowledged by the youth as socially expedient and as not detracting from their sense of themselves as unique individuals. The adolescents who viewed themselves as devalued appeared to be at risk for depression, and they reported feeling little hope for gaining acceptance and support; fortunately, they were in a distinct minority in the sample.

The preceding two studies have implications for the construct emotional self-efficacy. It appears that emotional self-efficacy requires (1) an informed self-awareness of when we adopt either "true" or dissembled emotional–expressive *behavior,* (2) an understanding that both "true" and dissembled behavior can *coexist* within ourselves (i.e., adoption of dissembled behavior does not somehow cancel out our true self), and (3) the ability to distinguish between strategic social–emotional behavior and the self-representations we hold about ourselves (see Harter, 1998). Engaging in a self-presentation to others in which we put "our best foot forward," so to speak, does not constitute a violation of our true selves. However, it is also likely that such a social exchange is probably not characterized by mutual responsivity and intimate support. What Harter et al.'s (1996) research indicates is that those adolescents who perceive themselves as *generally* unlikely to receive genuine support from either peers or parents are also those who hold representations of themselves that are globally negative. Given their futile beliefs about receiving supportive responses from others, I would guess that they are likely isolated as well. In considering what sort of adolescent might be at risk for being characterized as self-devaluing, anticipating little or no social support, experiencing some degree of social isolation (perhaps self-imposed), and prone to projecting a false self, the following case of a gay teen appears, regrettably, to fit the profile (see also Unks, 1995).

> Gene, 16 years old, had recently realized he was much more attracted to his male peers and adult men than to girls or women, although, once when drunk, he had lost his virginity with a girl. He had become terrified that his buddies could see through to his thoughts of attraction to them. He found it very stressful to act like "Joe cool" around his friends, yet tried desperately to act like one of them. Increasingly Gene stayed at home. His grades suffered, and he couldn't seem to concentrate anymore. But staying at home was painful too, for his stressed-out mother, emotionally unavailable father, and hyper-critical older sister made life miserable for Gene as well. They too "required" phony games from him. He was certain that everyone could see what a loser and a freak he was. Insomnia, suicidal fantasies, homophobic judgments about himself, somatic complaints, and a general sense of hopelessness descended on Gene like a thick dank cloud.

Fortunately for Gene, a sensitive teacher became concerned about him after reading some of his fatalistic poetry for her English literature class. She referred him to a local adolescent outreach organization that ran various kinds of support groups for youth. Gene did agree to par-

ticipate in a group for gay, lesbian, and bisexual youth, and the validation he received there for his "true self" quickly helped him to
renegotiate how he thought about himself and how he presented himself to others. With increasing awareness he was able to choose consciously whether to reveal himself as gay or not, and he could begin to
appraise under what conditions and with what sorts of people he was
willing to present a genuine self or a socially expedient role.

Gene's growth in self-awareness is a prominent feature of emotional self-efficacy, and like Gene's experience, this self-awareness is
pivotally related to the sorts of emotional–expressive behavior we use
communicatively with others. Specifically, understanding emotional
communication within relationships is critical to figuring out how our
emotional–expressive behavior will be perceived by others and the reciprocal, how to understand the complex emotional metacommunications others send to us. Chapter 10 addressed just these issues.
Indeed, mature emotional self-efficacy assumes that the individual has
developed to a reasonable degree the preceding emotional competencies described so far in this volume. However, to make the point
clearer, I describe another study with younger preadolescent children
(Saarni, 1988).

Balance between Dissembled and Genuine Emotional-Expressive Behavior

As part of the study described earlier in Chapter 8 in which I examined
children's beliefs about the interpersonal consequences of dissemblance (Saarni, 1988), I also asked the children how they thought they
achieved a sense of *balance* between when to express their genuine feelings and when to dissemble how they felt. I am using the word "balance" here to try to get at the idea that adopting extreme or rigid
stances in our emotional–expressive self-presentations is likely to be
maladaptive; more moderate and flexible adoption of emotional–
expressive behavior strategies is likelier to facilitate our social goals.

The children's responses were coded according to five categories
that ranged from saying something utterly tangential to answering with
a concrete example (e.g., "One time I fell off my bike, and I didn't cry")
to providing what we called "integration-plus" responses. This last category was reserved for explanations that connected both an elaborated
context (e.g., "It would depend on whether it was someone I knew well
or if there was a whole group of people around") *and* consideration of
the emotion itself (e.g., "If I felt very strongly, and it was really important to me"). Not surprisingly, age differences were pronounced, with
the big jump occurring around 10 to 11 years in terms of giving elabo-

rated contextual responses. However, the 13- to 14-year-old girls were most likely to give integration-plus responses. Thus, these young teenage girls were aware of how their relationships affected whether they would reveal their true selves or not, yet at the same time they were willing to risk some degree of social rejection if they felt very invested in their emotional response and deemed it justified. Interestingly, in Harter and Lee's (1989) research it was also the adolescent girls who reported significantly more often that they displayed more true-self behavior than boys did.

Balance in this study, and perhaps in a parallel fashion in the Harter and Lee (1989) study, had to do with coming to terms both with how one felt and with how one perceived the interpersonal situation. The oldest girls seemed to be saying that one has to respect one's feelings *if they were important* and therefore express them, even if the interpersonal consequences were less than desirable. From the standpoint of emotional self-efficacy, regard for our emotional experience may begin to overlap with an ethical evaluation of what gave rise to these important feelings such that they are perceived as having a morally sanctioned quality to their expression. I pursue this idea further, but we must return to the beginning of childhood to examine it.

Infant Reactivity and Expressiveness

This notion, that emotional self-efficacy also reflects regard for emotional experience, even if it flies in the face of social approval, may have its origins in the infant's attachment relationship. An intriguing speculation that bears repeating here is Cassidy's (1994) consideration that infant temperament may have more to do with the infant's emotional *reactivity* to events, and that it is within the context of the attachment relationship that the infant's *expressiveness* may be understood. The infant's emotional–expressive behavior *is* its communicative repertoire for signaling its caregivers to interact with it. The caregivers, in turn, differentially respond to the infant's emotional–expressive behavior, socializing it according to their beliefs and conscious or unconscious needs (e.g., Saarni, 1985; Malatesta, Culver, Tesman, & Shepard, 1989; Thompson, 1990). Thus, the infant's emotional–expressive behavior, over time, may well become more reflective of the dynamics within its close relationships rather than of its temperament-linked emotional reactivity. Cassidy suggests this possibility as a way of further understanding why insecure-avoidantly attached infants appear to be vigilantly suppressing negative emotional–expressive behavior around their parents. To maintain parental attachment, such infants learn to minimize negative emotion when around their parents (see also my discussion of her argument about the links between attachment and emotion regulation in Chapter 9, in this volume). In contrast, securely attached infants display the *greatest variability* of emotional–expressive behavior. Cassidy wonders whether "parents of secure infants are more willing to accept the temperamental proclivities of the infant whereas parents of insecure infants more strongly attempt to influence their children's expressiveness to suit their own preferences" (p. 247). This query may eventually be linked to developmental precursors to emotional self-efficacy: Children mature with a sense of *parental* acceptance of their emotional experience, which becomes internalized as their own acceptance of their emotional responsiveness (e.g., Saarni, 1985). As they venture forth beyond the family, they can explore "from a secure base" strategies for self-presentation with others with whom their relationship is more contingently defined, such as peers, teachers, and the like. Children's secure base may also allow them to acknowledge their feelings and express them in these more contingent relationships, if they so choose, for what they have also internalized is respect for their emotional experience, even if it is unconventional or risks social disapproval (for related arguments, see also Crittenden, 1992; Davies & Cummings, 1994).

Lastly, Walker and Taylor (1991) found that those children who demonstrated the most mature ethical understanding in a moral dilemmas assessment enjoyed emotionally supportive relationships with their parents, characterized by the parents' encouragement, humor, and willingness to listen to their children as they worked through the moral dilemmas. We may only speculate that such children, as they mature, are better prepared for the challenges to their self-efficacy that occur during adolescence. Hopefully, their personal respect for themselves and compassion toward others, in conjunction with their families' supportive scaffolding, will facilitate their effective negotiation of both moral and emotional stressors. Forging a sense of emotional self-efficacy that is coordinated with a budding personal integrity is no easy task when you are 14!

INDIVIDUAL DIFFERENCES IN EMOTIONAL SELF-EFFICACY

Given that emotional self-efficacy is a broad construct and it does not have a readily identified operational definition or measure associated with it, there is no body of research that clearly describes individual differences in it. However, in this section I describe research that further illuminates emotional self-efficacy relative to gender, social maturity, and cultural influence.

Gender and Emotional Self-Efficacy

I consider only one study here, but it is a significant one for considering how gender may influence the "dance" between self-esteem and personality, both of which appear highly linked to emotional self-efficacy. This investigation was based on the longitudinal sample studied by Block and Block (1980); the present study examined changes in self-esteem and personality in adolescents from ages 14 to 23 (Block & Robins, 1993).

Block and Robins used Q-sort instruments for both the self-esteem and personality assessments at age 14 and repeated these assessments at ages 18 and 23. Their correlational analyses, aggregated and corrected for various statistical purposes, yielded the following patterns: At age 14, girls with high self-esteem tended to have the following personality characteristics, which stayed with them to age 18 and predicted a continuing rise in self-esteem: They were protective, generous, sympathetic, and humorous. In contrast, girls at age 14 who were critical, hostile, irritable, and negative tended to show a decrease in self-esteem as they matured. Boys who at age 14 were calm, relaxed, not socially anxious, and relatively self-satisfied tended also to increase in self-esteem when reassessed at age 18, whereas those boys who were anxious and fantasized a lot tended to decrease in self-esteem. However, the personality pattern of the girls tended to be much more consistent across these two ages, whereas the boys at age 18, despite having high self-esteem, did not necessarily possess the same personality patterns as they did at age 14. Because of this personality variability in the adolescent boys, Block and Robins (1993) conclude that boys' personality characteristics do not consolidate as readily or as early as the adolescent girls' personalities.

By the time the subjects were age 23, high-self-esteem young men and women began to converge in personality characteristics, obtaining a rather impressive $r = .76$. The characteristics they tended to have most in common were assertiveness, satisfaction with self, cheerful and happy mood state, being sought out by others for advice/reassurance, being socially at ease, and having a sense of productivity. Those 23-year-old men and women with low self-esteem were most likely to have as their personality characteristics the following: reluctance to commit self or demonstration of indecisiveness, lack of meaning in life, withdrawal from frustration, and doubting of adequacy of self, and they were more likely to be self-defeating, generally fearful and anxious, maladaptive when stressed, and self-pitying. High self-esteem men and women differed from one another at age 23 in that the women were more likely to demonstrate greater interpersonal warmth, talkativeness, generosity, and demonstration of capacity for close relationships than were the men. The high-self-esteem men were more likely to view themselves as physically attractive, as not wanting others to be dependent on them, or as not wanting to seek reassurance from others, whereas these characteristics were not present in the women's profile. In other words, the young adult man with high self-esteem is similar to his female peer with high self-esteem in many ways, but he differs from her in that she is more concerned with interpersonal connection and he with interpersonal independence. He also freely that admits he likes his good looks, whereas her view of her physical attractiveness is *unrelated* to her self-esteem. This research (Block & Robins, 1993) led me to speculate that if young adolescent girls can resist media and peer pressure about body-image ideals, they may be more able to sustain their self-esteem through adolescence and launch themselves into adulthood with considerable ego strength (see also Ruble & Martin, 1998).

How does emotional self-efficacy fit here? I think it is noteworthy that it appears to be the link between high self-esteem and comfort with relationships that persists across all three age points (e.g., warmth, assertiveness, and feeling socially at ease). Low self-esteem seems linked with deficits in subjective well-being: Those adolescents and young adults who reported low self-esteem felt more often anxious, critical, irritable, hostile, fearful, and generally negative. Harter's (1986b) model of self-worth as mediating affect, which in turn mediates motivation, would seem to apply to Block and Robins's data as well. The conviction in one's self-efficacy also seems to fit with some of the personality descriptors at age 23: assertive, productive, satisfied with oneself, and socially at ease. These are people who expect they will generally get what they want and feel the way they expect to. They do not act in self-defeating ways or doubt their self-adequacy. Their subjective well-being seems captured in the description of them as generally cheerful and happy. What we see here is that emotional self-efficacy is a dynamic construct that reflects emotional experience, self-worth, personality, and history of interpersonal relationships. It is truly a *contextualized* skill of emotional competence.

Social Maturity and Emotional Self-Efficacy

Aldwin's (1994) analysis of how coping strategies change with age in adulthood is relevant to examining the relations between social maturity and emotional self-efficacy. She found that among adults (ages 20 to 70), the older they became, the more likely they disavowed responsibility for having caused problems for themselves, yet they more often undertook problem-solving efforts to solve the problems they did have.

For example, the older adults in her sample would generally have not viewed themselves as having caused their own health problems. However, they would have approached physical limitations as problems to be solved; indeed, she found no age differences in perceived efficacy across this age span.

If we can generalize from her results, then social maturity would be served if we perceived interpersonal differences and conflicts as problems to be solved, regardless of whether or not we thought we had caused the conflict. We may not have controlled, in a *causal* sense, the onset of an interpersonal problem, but its ultimate outcome might well be under our control. In such circumstances, active problem-solving coping is adaptive. In stressful situations in which we have no control over the outcome (e.g., aversive medical procedures), emotion-focused strategies may be our only option for efficacious coping (see also Chapter 9). However, in my opinion, it would be rather rare in interpersonal conflict situations that one would have no control over the outcome, and thus problem-solving approaches would generally be viewed as more socially mature than simply trying to defuse social anxiety. Of course, there are exceptions wherein our control over a social outcome might be nil, and these exceptions might well be found in extreme physical assault situations (child abuse, bullying, gang attacks, criminal victimization, etc.). Compas et al. (1988) reported that children believed they had relatively little control over stressful social encounters and thus would presumably rely on emotion-focused coping strategies such as distraction, distancing, and denial. Yet my own research (described in greater detail in Chapter 9) suggested that children prefer by large margins problem-solving approaches to social situations involving emotions as diverse as shame, fear, anger, hurt feelings, and sadness (Saarni, 1997). However, they also appreciated that avoidance of escalation of conflict might also be an effective strategy when angered or hurt. In a sense, avoiding escalation of interpersonal conflict *is* a problem-solving strategy in that it reduces the likelihood of aggression and retaliation.

Intentional Coping

Laux and Weber (1991) contend that whether a coping effort is judged adaptive or maladaptive depends on what the individual's goal or intention was vis-à-vis the stressful situation and what emotions the individual experienced (i.e., anger vs. anxiety), with anger likely eliciting confrontive social coping strategies and anxiety more face-saving social strategies. This idea that coping is *intentional* implies that if it is successful for the individual, it tends to enhance feelings of mastery and thus validates self-esteem. The implications for social maturity seem evident, for mastery and resilient self-esteem are generally associated with more effective social negotiation (e.g., Selman & Demorest, 1984) and satisfaction with interpersonal relations (e.g., Harter, 1987, 1998).

In my study of children's expectations of what would be the best and worst ways of coping with the aversive feelings, noted earlier (Saarni, 1997), it was consistent with Laux and Weber's view on intentional coping that virtually all the children, younger and older, saw coping as purposeful and anchored in both emotion and the social context. Justifications for the "best" coping strategy often suggested motives for improving the social relations between protagonist and interactant, and the children most often expected the protagonist's subsequent feelings to be positive. "Bad" coping strategies from the children's perspectives were those that resulted in interpersonal aggression and escalation of conflict; they also expected such coping choices to result in feeling even worse.

It was intriguing that while aggressive externalizing responses were by far most often chosen as the "worst" thing to do when coping in a social situation, a number of children, albeit a small minority, said they would feel happy, victorious, relieved, or just somehow "better" after they had behaved in this aggressive fashion. In other words, even though these few children believed this was not a desirable way to act (they typically justified it as the worst way because it would get the protagonist in trouble or rejected by others), still the emotional reinforcement of feeling good afterward was a salient incentive for some children. Not surprisingly, this anticipated positive emotional experience after acting aggressively was often cited for the anger story but interestingly also for the shame story in which the protagonist was teased on the playground for her or his underwear showing through a tear in her or his pants.

An interpretation of these findings is suggested by Kernis (1993), who found that individuals with *unstable but also high* self-esteem may be especially prone to hostile and aggressive acts toward those who threaten their self-image. The reason they act angrily and aggressively may be to restore their fragile self-esteem or to defend in a preemptive fashion their threatened self-image. Having then acted in this attacking fashion and momentarily having shored up their self-esteem, they experience a positive emotional boost. This would appear to be what is happening in the responses given by those children in my study who reported that the protagonist would feel happy after attacking someone. Unfortunately, such a coping strategy may appear to be emotionally self-efficacious in the short run (i.e., enhanced self-esteem and positive emotional state are experienced). In the long run, however, bullies and other hostile individuals do not effectively solve their interpersonal conflicts, nor do they adequately develop the more stable subjective well-being that might otherwise buffer them from threats to their self-esteem. Kernis also found that individuals with *stable and high* self-esteem reported the lowest incidence of anger and hostility relative to all other combinations of stable/unstable and high/low self-esteem.

Regrettably, Kernis's (1993) work was with adults, and we lack research that extends Kernis's results to school-age children and which can then be evaluated relative to children's interpersonal coping behavior. However, my study showed that children can articulate how coping with the feelings they have in interpersonal contexts can serve adaptive goals. An intriguing question remains: If they know what should work well for themselves and will make them feel better, why do so many children in their own lives persist in coping in self-defeating ways? Perhaps one answer is that emotional self-efficacy still eludes many children: It is more likely to be achieved in adolescence and assumes that the other emotional competency skills have also be acquired.

Culture and Emotional Self-Efficacy

Different cultural conceptualizations of emotion and of the self obviously influence how emotional self-efficacy might be construed. Potter (1988), in her discussion of the cultural construction of emotion among rural Chinese, describes a viewpoint that is different from Western notions of self and emotion. A summary of her essay illustrates how emotional self-efficacy plays a much different role in that society than in ours.

Potter begins by highlighting Western societies' views of the assumption that our social relationships are based on exchanges of emotions and sentiments (see also Berscheid, 1986, for a parallel analysis of western emotional *investment* in relationships). Given that our culture is individualistic in orientation, we emphasize the significance of the self when we see relationships as *defined, created, and legitimized* by the individual's expression of emotion. Indeed, much of Chapter 10 described just this process. Potter contends that this is a cultural construction and need not be universal in application. She describes Chinese beliefs about emotion in ways that are different from Western notions: In village life, a range of emotions is readily expressed, but these emotions are negligible for the definition of social institutions and formal relationships. They do not define symbolically the relationship structure between two individuals nor between an individual and a group. To quote Potter (1988): "A person whose emotions have no significance for the social order experiences social reality differently. In many important contexts, such a person has no need to manipulate emotions in order to serve social ends since emotional experience is not thought to have a significant role in the *symbolization* of relationship" (p. 194; emphasis added). For the rural Chinese, emotions are most definitely expressed interpersonally. The expression of emotion, be it with smiles or with tears, informs the interactant what someone is feeling, but to say that those smiles and tears are more likely to be genuine emotional expressions *because* one is in a close relationship with this particular interactant would not occur in rural China. To illustrate, a wrenching scene in the 1994 movie *Ju Dou,* whose story was supposed to occur in the 1920s, shows the protagonist trying to say a toast at a birthday party for his young son, yet this son's birth is attributed to another man, his uncle, who is much more powerful and wealthy. The protagonist must conceal his paternity for fear of punishment (he has obviously cuckolded his rich uncle), yet he openly weeps and expresses nonverbally great anguish as he toasts his ostensible nephew. The others at the party look at his tears, say he is drunk, and point out that he too should acquire a wife so that he can have a son. The point here is that relationships per se, such as between father and son, are not symbolically defined by particular kinds of emotional expressions or exchange of emotions but rather by cultural tradition. In the early decades of this century in China, it was important to have a son to carry on the family ancestral line.

To give another related example, Chinese society values filial piety. If we asked a Chinese youth to tell us what an optimal relationship between a parent and child would be like, he or she would emphasize the child's filial piety, consisting of the child's obedience and respect toward the parent. If we then asked a North American "mainstream" adolescent to describe an optimal relationship between parent and child, he or she might use such words as "caring," "affection," and "love" to describe the *mutual* relationship between child and parent. To use Berscheid's term, American parents and children are typically "emotionally invested" in one another, and the nature of that emotional investment plays a major role in defining the relationship. In many non-Western societies having children serves different functions, many of them economic and lineage related, than those commonly endorsed in North America as the "right" reasons for having children. Americans give great weight to love for a child and having a family (based on mutual affection, Pederson & Gilby, 1986) as appropriate reasons for bearing or adopting children. However, this reflects our Western cultural values and beliefs, and there is considerable variation among societies in the degree to which mutual exchange of love and affection between parent and child is emphasized.

Where does this leave us with our construct of emotional self-efficacy? According to Potter's (1988) thought-provoking essay, emotional self-efficacy can be applied to other cultural emotion meaning systems, but it takes on different nuances according to the culture in question. The individual in a Chinese village who is emotionally self-efficacious views her emotional experience as justified and appropriate to the eliciting circumstances (e.g., she takes pleasure in an artistic creation; she weeps in sorrow over a familial loss), but she will not use her emotional experience to define her relationships with others. Recall the beautiful Chinese poem at the end of Chapter 6, in which no emotion words were used, but the imagery was highly evocative of intense emotion, and there would be no mistaking the poet's description of grief and sorrow. Emotional experience is clearly validated in Chinese culture by such a poem, but the symbolic expression of emotion (in this case, verbal expression) may take other forms than what we in Western societies are accustomed to (and Potter gives a number of examples in her essay). Indeed, we have no problem in comprehending the emotional message of the poet's words. It is also interesting to note that he uses only two phrases that describe specific somatic experience, that is, a reference to his tears ("My eyes are not allowed a dry season.") and his chest ("My chest tightens against me."). It is our recognition of these somatic feelings that confirms for us the poet's experience of sadness, but without the remaining imagery contained in the poem we might not understand the connotations of despair, futility, and loneliness that are also suggested in the poet's emotional experience. Perhaps in China not only would emotional self-efficacy entail a sense of justification for the feelings one experiences, but also when discussing one's emotions with others, one would communicate indirectly about one's emotions (which is in accord with what Potter also reports about her informants), for it would be in this form that one's goals would be best served.

CONCLUSION

Emotional self-efficacy may ultimately reflect one's personal theory of emotion (cf. Thompson, 1990). Recall the discussion of folk theories of emotion in Chapter 3: They are open-ended and fluid "working models" for making sense of one's emotional experience in different situations and relationships. They can also change with development and with experience. As children acquire their culture's beliefs about how emotions "work," they also reveal at different ages their changing expectations as to what they will feel, how they will express their feeling, and what they will do to cope. Much of this development is described in this book as the acquisition of skills of emotional competence. These expectations can also be looked at as coalescing into scripts, which have some degree of social consensus about their meaning and predictability but which also contain some degree of unique personal "flavor" in how they are applied to particular situations at a given time. For example, if a child develops a positive appraisal style (Lazarus, 1991), her script for anger, for example, will have a rather different quality to it than that of the child who develops a defensive appraisal style. The former child will likely experience fewer episodes of anger: She will be less vigilant about threats to her self and will be less likely to attribute hostile intent to others. When she does become angry, her anger is more likely to be approved of by others because a moral or social obligation was clearly violated. The child with a defensive appraisal style is likely to have more frequent anger episodes because of her tendency to see hostile intent in others and to experience more readily threats to her self. Her anger is more apt to be judged by others as overreactive, hypersensitive, or outright paranoid. The former child is more likely to be emotionally self-efficacious, because as she matures, she receives validation from others that her emotional experience is justified, her self-regard is well-buffered, and overall the hedonic tone of her day-in, day-out living feels more positive due to her appraisal style (i.e., she experiences subjective well-being). On the other hand, the latter child will likely view herself as often not wanting to be feeling the way she does. Her emotional experience drains her: She has to be on guard so much of the time. Her self-regard is fragile, and subjective well-being is elusive for her.

Emotional self-efficacy is more than a collection of emotion scripts, for as the previous comparison illustrates, the construct also includes personal traits and styles of "being in the world." It also seems to me that emotional self-efficacy is dynamic. We may find ourselves at times in our lives to be going through a period of living *in*efficaciously: Our emotions then become a significant cue for us to change something about the direction or meaning in our lives to restore emotional self-efficacy. Often this is the impetus for people to begin personal therapy, to leave relationships, or to change careers. In some ways, I see the struggles of adolescence as a personal renegotiation of how to restore emotional self-efficacy in the context of major changes in one's body, peer relations, values, and social expectations. Thus, emotional self-efficacy may be more fluid than socially agreed on emotion scripts, and this fluidity may be completely normal and expectable. However, the fact that girls, for example, in our society are more likely to experience depression in adolescence than are boys also suggests that our cultural context can make it harder for some to reconstruct their emotional self-efficacy in the face of significant change than for others. When there is this sort of systematic bias against a group striving for emotional self-efficacy, as would be the case in oppression of ethnic and social minorities, larger questions of justice and access to social rights need to be raised. It is no accident that our society has as one of its basic tenets the pursuit of happiness. Indeed, Markus and Kitayama (1994) identify this as one of the core ideas in American culture, and that it is further embedded in the belief that the pursuit of happiness is one of the inalienable rights of the individual (i.e., the Declaration of Independence and the Bill of Rights).

Finally, I want to reemphasize that emotional self-efficacy is more than the pursuit of simple happiness. The construct is also useful for its inclusion of negative emotions as appropriate, justified, and adaptive. Earlier I alluded to the experience of dignity within melancholy. (I avoid using the term "depression" here because of its connotation of self-*dis*regard.) Individuals may feel melancholy, but their sense of a strong self is not impaired; they retain their dignity even as they reflect on their circumstances as deeply grievous or agonizing. I believe we need a construct that recognizes differences among people in terms of what they view as desirable emotional experiences. Some of those differences might reflect eccentricities, and some may reflect highly sensitive responses to certain emotion-eliciting circumstances. But these differences in view of what constitutes desirable and valued emotional responsiveness are all experienced in the context of individuals who see themselves as feeling generally the way they want to, even if it is morose.

Chapter 12

Emotional Incompetence and Dysfunction

A view long held in Western culture has been that madness—or psychopathology more generally—was due to an excess of emotion. Passion, emotional intensity, unrestrained ardor, uncontrolled feelings of grief or fury, and so forth were thought to lead to a downward spiral of self-destruction. The solution was to suppress emotionality and replace it with reason and stoicism. A more contemporary version of this perspective portrays reason as a check system on one's emotions, particularly if they are elicited by "faulty" or irrational appraisals (e.g., Ellis, 1993). Recently considerable attention has been given to the role of emotions in the *development* of psychopathology, with this view emphasizing the systemic or organizational role played by emotions (Cicchetti, Ackerman, & Izard, 1995). Cicchetti et al. (1995) believe that most instances of childhood psychopathology involve problems in emotional regulation, whether these come about due to impairments in neurophysiological functioning or stem from traumatic maltreatment. Although I do not wholly agree with this perspective, I do agree with their view that the construct emotion regulation is too inclusive, with the result that we are far from recognizing the exact processes that converge to produce psychopathology.

Because I appreciate the crucial role played by context, I see problematic emotional regulation as a product of the interaction of particular children with particular circumstances. A contextual view would not locate *in the child* the problem of "dysfunctional" emotional regulation; instead, I would want to examine closely the interface of that unique child and his or her world of peer relations, of family and school contexts, with pets, in the world of nature, at play, and when involved in creative activities. I would also want to take into account how cultural context may or may not facilitate a welcoming niche for that particular child. In short, a child may function maladaptively, even pathologically, in some or even most contexts, but often there is a relationship or a setting in which that child does not exhibit dysfunction. Probing those instances of relatively adaptive and efficacious behavior when demonstrated by an otherwise deeply troubled child may yield intriguing ideas not only for therapeutic intervention but also in how the emotion system works *with* context (see also Lewis, 1997, for similar arguments).

Recall also the research described in Chapter 9 on temperament and coping (e.g., Eisenberg et al., 1994). In that study, negative emotionality was associated with some problem behaviors as *rated by the teacher*, whereas the child's emotional reactions were not linked to problem behaviors when *rated by the mother*. Similarly, the pattern of problem behaviors and negative emotionality varied by gender. Thus, school and home contexts elicited different social judgments as to whether a behavior was problematic or not, and discernible associations of negative emotionality with socially *in*effective behavior were primarily found for boys. Gender role has a rather profound impact on social contexts, and our sex may indeed be one of the contributing agents to the interface between emotional response and eliciting circumstances (see Golombok & Fivush, 1994, for a similar argument regarding the prevalence of depression in adolescent girls).

Given my emphasis throughout this text on the inseparability of emotional and social experience in human development, it should not come as a surprise that the same close association between emotions and social interaction should also figure prominently in cases of emotional "incompetence." I argue that distortions in emotional communication in close relationships (and thereby within cultural context) are most often implicated in maladaptive emotional functioning. However, those distortions in emotional exchanges between people can have their origin in biology; for example, the flat affective expressive style of some Down syndrome babies can adversely influence their parents, who, in turn, reduce their interaction with their Down syndrome infants (Emde, Katz, & Thorpe, 1978; Kasari & Sigman, 1996). When we have to relate to others our *dys*function becomes most apparent. In other words, an individual could live as a hermit and his or her relative "deficits" in emotional competence might go unnoticed because the social context is not present. But when hermits emerge from their solitude and have to go into town for their supplies, their ineptitude at dealing with social transactions becomes apparent to all.

I am reminded of the notorious Unabomber Theodore Kaczynski, once a brilliant mathematician. Kaczynski lived pretty much as a hermit in the wilds of Montana, but interpersonally he was clearly a very destructive and violent man with very extensive maladaptive distortions in his emotional functioning ("The Mind of the Unabomber," 1996; Taylor, 1997). Kaczyncski apparently was systematic about building his bombs but quite vague or even unconcerned about his victims (Salladay, 1997). It was as though the destructiveness of the bomb was the critical event, not the suffering of the victim, or, for that matter, even the victim's identity. In this juxtaposition of emotional detachment from people with obsessive investment in the particulars of bomb making, we can see profound emotional *in*competence: Kaczynski's emotional preoccupation was not with any real people of his everyday existence, for he was largely alone. His emotional "connection," as it were, was with material objects, albeit with potent social consequences. An anonymously delivered bomb is perhaps the ultimate in remote aggression against others; it is also the "stuff" of paranoia and delusions, and Kaczynski is alleged to have both. I would be hard pressed to suggest which of the skills of emotional competence he had developed, if any.

Kaczynski's emotional functioning was not simply immature; it was profoundly dysfunctional and incompetent with very tragic consequences. But this raises the important question as to the difference between immature emotional functioning and incompetent emotional functioning. If by immature we mean that a preschooler simply has not yet acquired the requisite cognitive and social skills to be able, for example, to recognize that her facial expression need not be congruent with her emotional experience, then her immaturity is simply due to development not yet having taken place in the cognitive and social–behavioral domains. If she is an 8-year-old and still is fully unable to dissociate her facial expression from her emotional state as the situation may call for it (e.g., she does not try to look somewhat agreeable when her grandmother gives her a disappointing birthday gift but instead clearly shows her aggravation), we would call her behavior immature relative to our expectations of 8-year-olds' ability to demonstrate some degree of compliance with etiquette (and cultural display rules). If this sort of emotional immaturity is relatively isolated or sporadic, it can probably be remedied by parental guidance. But what if the pattern of emotionally immature behaviors is more extensive and the child is now

12 years old and still does not show evidence of monitoring her emotional–expressive behavior relative to social contexts and demands? Such a youngster undoubtedly has already had a history of difficult peer relations and may also have serious behavioral problems in school. We would probably not be surprised to find out that she is impulsive and copes poorly when stressed. Deficits in emotional competence relative to one's age group and cultural context are often accompanied by other behavioral, social, and cognitive problems such as excessive impulsivity, short attention spans, and maladaptive strategies for engaging socially with others. When this sort of profile of problematic qualities characterizes a child (or adult, for that matter), the social context for that individual also changes its affective tone. Such a child is more likely to be rejected, punished, avoided, and reviled. Clearly a vicious cycle is likely to be in place for such a child, and effective interventions must address both what the child is doing, feeling, and thinking, and how the social context (e.g., family and school) responds to the child. To sum up, emotional incompetence is largely *a systemic* problem.

For the most part, I focus in this chapter on school-age children and adolescents, as it is by these ages that many of the skills of emotional competence should have normally been acquired, assuming a healthy neurophysiological system and a supportive and favorable environment that fosters their development. The dilemma facing many children and youth is that their social and physical environment is not supportive and, indeed, we are amazed at the resilience of some children when we come to realize what ordeals they have experienced. When young children are immersed in negative environments with little hope of those circumstances improving or have the misfortune of being born with maladaptive biopsychological functioning, emotional development may deviate from its expected course, and the first few skills of emotional competence may not be adequately established. If this occurs, there are likely to be serious impairments in acquiring the other emotional competencies, again assuming that the harshly negative environments persist and the biopsychological systems remain vulnerable. If such children have only limited awareness of their own feelings and of others' feelings, major hurdles are in their way for developing the other skills of emotional competence: sharing in discourse about emotion, feeling sympathetic with another's plight, managing their emotional–expressive behavior in interpersonal contexts, coping with stressful circumstances, recognizing how emotional communication and experience define relationships, and achieving emotional self-efficacy.

Relative to this idea of awareness of our own and others' feelings, I must mention several critical issues raised by Southam-Gerow and Kendall (1997) in their excellent review about the role of understanding emotional experience in psychopathology:

1. Children's understanding of emotion may *moderate* their susceptibility to pathological functioning. To illustrate, if two teens are equally at risk for depression or adjustment disorders but one has greater sophistication of insight into problem-solving strategies for coping with stressful situations, that enhanced understanding may lessen the likelihood of his or her vulnerability to depression or extreme anxiety.

2. Children's understanding of emotion may *mediate* their propensity for psychological problems with the result that deficits in understanding function as precursors to psychopathology. For example, it is possible that deficits in capacity for empathic understanding of others' emotional experience would potentiate the development of antisocial personality disorder.

3. Finally and perhaps most important, deficits in emotion understanding may *result* from psychopathological processes. For example, impaired emotion understanding may be a consequence of dissociation, a defense associated with experiencing traumatic abuse.

In the cases presented in this chapter, I make use of all three ways of examining how psychopathological processes affect emotional functioning and vice versa. Given the intersecting nature of the skills of emotional competence with one another and with interpersonal contexts, I fully anticipate that moderating and mediating roles are also present in the relations between emotional *in*competence and maladaptive functioning relative to specific contexts. Exploring those relations has yet to be investigated in a systematic fashion.

This concluding chapter is organized by examining some of the likely effects of serious limitations or deficits in the eight skills of emotional competence. I assume that the contexts in which these limitations are demonstrated also tend to be inadequate or not in synchrony with the needs of the developing child. Indeed, these inadequate contexts may be the reason why these limitations come about. I highlight some interesting research related to maladaptive emotional functioning and include case descriptions and vignettes to illustrate the impairments in emotional functioning that emerge when the skills of emotional competence are compromised. On occasion I refer to some categories of emotional disturbance (e.g., internalizing and externalizing problems) or diagnostic disorders (e.g., posttraumatic stress disorder), but I do not intend the discussion of limitations in skills of emotional competence to refer to diagnostic criteria for these clinical phenomena. Framing the potential deficits in emotional competencies as questions yields the following list:

1. What happens if awareness of one's emotions is inadequate?
2. What happens if understanding others' emotional experience is limited?
3. What happens when there is an impoverished emotional lexicon?
4. What happens if one is either overwhelmed by others' emotional experience or the other extreme, unable to vicariously respond to another's feelings?
5. What happens if one cannot dissociate expression from feeling or if one's ability to do this is rigidly applied across situations and relationships?
6. What happens if one's coping strategies are limited or one's ability to regulate one's emotions is deficient?
7. What happens when emotional communication in relationships is impaired or distorted?
8. What happens when emotional self-efficacy is rarely experienced?

I turn next to a consideration of the issues raised by each of these questions and begin with a case example of a severely neglected infant to illustrate the dire impact when awareness of one's own feeling states is inadequate; the rest of the illustrations are based on older children.

DEFICITS IN AWARENESS OF ONE'S OWN EMOTIONS

Larry had not had an easy entry into his life. He had been born 4 weeks early with low birthweight to a 16-year-old mother, Cathy. Cathy had a history of drug abuse and violent victimization by her boyfriend. When Larry was 6 months of age, Pat, a social worker with Child Protective Services, began her investigation of reports of neglect and possible abuse regarding little Larry. Subsequently, Larry was removed from Cathy's care and diagnosed as exhibiting the effects of acute neglect and failure to thrive. He was placed with a foster family. Cathy visited infrequently, and Larry was unresponsive to both her arrival and her departure. Three months later, when he was age 9 months, Larry became a subject in a research study examining the effects of neglect on infants, and Doris, his foster mother, was a supportive participant as well.

During the research project's observational sessions, Larry alternated between a flat, unresponsive emotional style and irritable, incessant crying. He showed little interest in exploring toys and tended to play in a haphazard fashion, picking up an object, dropping it, looking around, touching another object, sucking on the side of his hand, grabbing his foot, and so forth. He did not babble at all except for a repetitive sound that seemed to be a blend between a grunt and a mournful moan. He did not look at Doris's eyes but instead seemed to look at her chin or mouth region when she tried to engage him. But if she got up from her chair, he followed her with his eyes. He had learned to scrunch around a bit on his stomach but could not properly crawl.

Doris reported to the research team that Larry rarely showed that he was happy, afraid, curious, or even especially sad. His irritable crying sounded odd to her, as though it wasn't really a distress cry that was intended to attract anyone's attention to help him. She still had hopes for Larry, because she was quite convinced that she had felt a gradual softening of his body in her arms when she held him to give him his bottle, as though he were learning to relax next to her body's warmth. She also thought that the fact that he tracked her with his eyes might mean she was beginning to be important to him. But she confessed that it was draining to be around an infant who didn't respond emotionally to her.

The case of Larry could have come out of the early work done by Gaensbauer and his associates (Gaensbauer, Mrazek, & Harmon, 1981; Gaensbauer & Sands, 1979). They identified several subgroups of maltreated children, among them a developmentally and emotionally impaired group of infants and toddlers who showed emotion blunting and lack of responsiveness; a second group who were inhibited, withdrawn, and appeared very sad; a third group who were very labile and irritable in their emotional expressions; and a fourth group who were prone to angry temper tantrums and played in a disorganized fashion. Larry demonstrated aspects of each of these groups. Gaensbauer's work has been replicated descriptively in others' investigations of infant maltreatment, and the distorted caregiver–infant communication system (e.g., Aber & Cicchetti, 1984) seems to be central. Indeed, maltreated infants are likely to be categorized as insecurely attached or as disorganized/disoriented in their attachment, and these dysfunctional attachment patterns appear to be paralleled by declines in their assessed mental age scores (reviewed in Cicchetti, 1987). Thus, psychologically unavailable or overtly abusive caregivers deliver literal and figurative blows to their infants' development, handicapping them in their future trajectory of emotional, social, cognitive, and behavioral functioning (for a comprehensive review, see Cicchetti & Carlson,

1989). When prenatal substance abuse is also present, the infant's functioning is compromised further by the interactive effects of drugs, alcohol, poor nutrition, and maternal stress, frequently resulting in premature birth and/or low birthweights (e.g., Beeghly & Tronick, 1994; Lewis & Bendersky, 1995).

INADEQUATE UNDERSTANDING OF OTHERS' EMOTIONAL EXPERIENCE

Traumatic abuse by caregivers also impairs children's ability to understand others' feelings (e.g., Camras & Rappaport, 1993; Klimes-Dougan & Kistner, 1990; Parker & Herrera, 1996), but in this section I briefly look at the interesting puzzle presented by children affected by autism or pervasive developmental disorder. I start with a brief adaptation of an interview with Susan, mother of an autistic 5-year-old.

INTERVIEWER: When and what did you first notice that suggested to you that something was different about your daughter, Anne?

SUSAN: She was about 4 or 5 months old, and my older boy [Danny] by that age would try to grab at things, including my nose, my fingers, my jewelry. And when he'd grab at some part of me, I'd play around with him or pretend I was going to eat up his fingers when he'd try to grab my mouth. Anne didn't grab. She looked at things a lot but didn't reach out much and never to me. So we didn't have those kind of goofy play times together. She had some mobiles over her crib, and she learned to kick the bars of her crib to make them jiggle. She'd do that a lot, but didn't get much of anything out of peek-a-boo games or throw-your-toy-out-of-the-playpen-and-watch-mommy-fetch.

INTERVIEWER: Does Anne express emotions?

SUSAN: Yes, a general sort of upset, sometimes an irritated sort of fearfulness—or maybe it's a fearful irritation, I'm not sure; an expression that looks "sour," I'm not sure how to describe it, but it's as though she is disgusted and disappointed at the same time, and finally what I call her "dreaming" expression. It's fairly calm looking, she's usually absorbed in a rhythmic activity at the time, and it's about the closest she looks to "happy."

INTERVIEWER: How does Anne show her responsiveness to you now?

SUSAN: As a toddler she started following me if I left a room, even though she may not directly engage with me in the room, she doesn't like to be left. She does seem attached to me and likes to have me next to her on her bedside when she goes to sleep. She'll touch me and call me Mama.

INTERVIEWER: This may sound like an odd question, but have you ever accidentally injured yourself in front of Anne? Did she respond to your being hurt?

SUSAN: Yes, I got a terrible splinter a month or so ago and was obviously in pain as I tried to pull it out. She just looked at me with that irritated/scared face of hers. Danny was in the next room and heard me and came right in; he was all concerned. But we've noticed that about Anne: She seems to *react* to our more vocal and obvious emotions, but she does not make any overture to help or comfort, and although she can talk some, she does not say anything about us having feelings.

INTERVIEWER: Does Anne show any fantasy in her play, like with action figures, dolls, or dress-up?

SUSAN: No. It was very obvious from an early age that her way of playing had nothing to do with imagination or pretend. I'm not sure she even imitates any of our actions, but then we use pretty behavioral methods to guide her in things like eating. She makes objects move or her own body move. She has some little plastic ponies, but she doesn't make them "talk" or interact together; they're just objects to hold up against the light and move back and forth. She watches cartoons on TV, but listening to me read a book to her is pretty useless.

As Susan's comments indicate, little Anne's behavior shows many of the deficits in pervasive developmental disorder, in particular in emotional responsiveness toward others. Her understanding of her mother's feeling hurt appeared to be limited; her capacity for fantasy play with feelings, wants, and dislikes attributed to favorite toy objects was absent; and the meaning of her own expressed emotions was somewhat hard to decipher, even for her mother, although the expressions were almost all negative (see also Yirmiya, Kasari, Sigman, & Mundy, 1989). Harris (1989) has suggested that autistic children's emotion-related difficulties may have to do with their inability to recognize that other people have feelings. He thinks that not only do autistic children have deficits in recognizing the meaning of others' emotional signals, including facial expressions, gestures, and vocalization (see Hobson's 1986 research), but they do not recognize that other people have motives and expectations. He found in research with autistic children matched with mental age-equivalent normal children that the autistic children did not appear to conceptualize that others have *minds*, and as a result they could not comprehend how people could have desires, anticipations, motives, and beliefs. Thus, autistic children cannot *share* in ordinary interpersonal exchanges if they have no appreciation of how others function in an emotion-laden and goal-directed way. This presents a considerable problem for parents trying to interact with such children, for the children tend not to demonstrate even something as elementary as "shared joint attention." Their gaze does not follow their caregivers' response to some stimulus, as in social referencing, or even when parents pick up a toy, pretend to offer it to their child but then teasingly withdraw it (usually a toddler makes eye contact with the parent after the toy withdrawal) (e.g., Charman et al., 1997). Similarly, Baron-Cohen (1987) found that even high-functioning autistic children (with language skills) did not demonstrate imaginative pretend play, although the vast majority of the retarded Down syndrome children did. Thus, the intellectual deficits of autistic children have a unique pattern, for they can understand physical causality (e.g., a pushed rock rolls downhill) but cannot understand psychological emotional causality (e.g., another's distress over a disappointment).

Kasari and Sigman (1996) reviewed research on emotional functioning in autistic children and in children with Down syndrome. With regard to how mentally retarded, normal, and autistic children responded to emotion in others, they found that among their developmentally matched 3- to 6-year-old children, only the autistic children ignored their mother's feigned distress in three different contexts (Sigman, Kasari, Kwon, & Yirmiya, 1992). A sample of autistic children was also followed for 5 years, and there appeared to be some stability in the degree to which a given child attended to emotion in others, but noticing an emotional expression in another person does not necessarily mean an empathic response (e.g., looking concerned when another is visibly distressed or hurt).

Finally, several studies have been done with autistic and other emotionally disturbed children and recognition of facial expressions. Weeks and Hobson (1987) found that whereas normal and mentally retarded children sorted photos of people's faces on the basis of facial expression, the autistic children sorted by the type of hat worn! (Other sorting schemes that the children could use included age and gender as well as facial expression and type of hat.) If facial expressions simply are not salient information for many autistic children, then it is not surprising that they also show little empathy toward others' expressions of distress. Other investigators have examined children who have serious emotional problems or have been abused and have found that these children also show deficits in their understanding of links between facial expression and emotion, in their producing facial expressions, and in their discriminating emotion expressions (Camras et al., 1983; Feldman, White, & Lobato, 1982; Walker, 1981). However, in contrast to autistic children, these maltreated and disturbed children can, depending on the context, produce, discriminate, and understand the meaning of others' emotional–expressive behavior.

IMPOVERISHED EMOTIONAL LEXICON

We may be aware of our own emotions and recognize that others have feelings, motives, and expectations. But if our language is limited in being able to articulate emotional experience, we will have difficulty in communicating to others what we have felt if we are not in the immediate emotion-provoking situation (where others could see our expressions, yelps of dismay, gestures of aggravation, etc.) Similarly, others may try to talk to us about their emotional experience, but if our lexicon and concurrent skills at representing emotion are impoverished, we may only comprehend a rather global sense of their emotional experience and not obtain a detailed picture of what they felt. A rather facetious example may be found in adults' reactions to rap music: A father says to his teenage son, "I can tell they [rap singers] are mad about something, but their vocabulary is limited to 10 words, most of which consist of 4 letters." Exasperatedly, the son retorts, "The message is more than just the words; it's the rage of the streets; you're just not listening to the music." The father leaves the room dumbfounded, "What music???" Neither understands the other's "language," as it were.

Serious compromises in acquisition of emotion-descriptive language are found in children enduring profound trauma. Sometimes a traumatic episode is psychologically encapsulated and repressed; thus it is simply not available for verbal discourse or "reality testing" (see an excellent discussion of this process in Breger, 1974). Other traumas are repeated, as in many cases of physical and sexual abuse, and although the abuse is not necessarily repressed from consciousness, it is *emotionally dissociated* from the self. Van der Kolk and Fisler (1994) reviewed the psychological aftermath of trauma and its effects on symbolic representation. In some of their own clinical work they found that adolescents with histories of early and severe abuse were remarkably alienated from their emotions such that they claimed that their abuse had no effect on them, and they saw no relationship between their history of abuse and their current involvement in abusive relationships with peers, high-risk activities, and substance abuse. In van der Kolk and Fisler's words, "They have difficulty putting feelings into words and instead act out their feelings without being able to resort to intervening symbolic representations that would allow for flexible response strategies" (p. 157). If our construal of our own traumatic experience is somehow short-circuited (often seen in posttraumatic stress disorder), it becomes difficult indeed to learn from that experience, to understand how it has affected us, and how to avoid its recurrence. We continue to bang our head on the same old proverbial brick wall instead of going around it or getting something to help us climb over it. Along similar lines, Cicchetti and White (1990) have hypothesized that traumatically abused children have problems with verbalizing emotions because their neurophysiological systems have altered in reaction to the trauma. They appear to be unable to delay their responses to stimuli and thus impulsively react, especially to stress-inducing stimuli. Aggression and self-destructive behavior are the outcome. The following case captures this representational deficit about emotional experience and the concurrent inability to use an emotion lexicon to make sense of experience.

Ten-year-old Rashid had recently been placed in a group home for emotionally disturbed children. He had been removed from his grandfather's care after he set a fire in a nearby apartment building's basement that resulted in serious burns to the building's custodian. The grandfather said he could not control Rashid anymore. Rashid had a documented history of fire setting (which had until now been minor), had already been identified by the school system as disturbed and been placed in special education classes, and had been placed with his grandfather after being removed from his parents' care because they sexually and physically victimized Rashid. His parents were addicts and had "sold" him for pornography purposes to make money to buy drugs.

At the group home Rashid's behavior appeared to have two extremes: withdrawal or near-seizure-like temper tantrums, brought on by seemingly trivial provocations. Rashid admitted to his counselor that he had set the fire, but he appeared to have no inkling of being able to look into himself and consider what led up to his doing so. He had placed paint-soaked rags near the central heating system and had gone to some bother to sneak into the basement. His counselor thought that with this much planning, Rashid must have had some awareness of what he was thinking at the time, but all he could get from Rashid was "I just did it."

During his art therapy sessions, Rashid drew elaborate fire scenes with people running from fires, people burning in fires, and fire engines coming to the rescue. His counselor, Ben, one day asked him to draw how a fire got started, and Rashid drew a stick figure holding a torch to the side of a house with another figure inside. Ben asked, "Who is in the house?" and Rashid answered softly, "A kid." Ben continued, "Is he alone?" and the response was affirmative. Ben asked him, "Who will save him from the fire?" Rashid responded, "No one; he'll get burned up." Ben probed further, "Why is that guy setting the house on fire? Is he trying to hurt the boy inside?" Rashid said, "That guy doesn't like him; he wants him to burn up." At that moment, Rashid swept the paper and markers to the floor and started screaming. Rashid calmed a bit, and in a near-whisper, said, "That guy in the basement was at my parents', and I knew him." It then hit Ben: The building's caretaker might have been involved in Rashid's abuse. But Rashid could not or would not talk further; it was as though whatever moment of access he had to his experience had been erased.

Young Rashid illustrates the construct of alexithymia (Krystal, 1988), mentioned in Chapter 6 as a deficiency in using emotion-descriptive language due to severe trauma. Although it is common for victimized children and youth to deny the *impact* of their abuse (e.g., Trepper & Niedner, 1996; van der Kolk & Fisler, 1994), Rashid demonstrated a near amnesiac quality to being able to describe his inner experience. When he was under stress, he either resorted to tantrums or used the fire setting as a way to release the tension that built up in him; using words "to vent" was not an available strategy. But Rashid was not without recognizing that others have emotions: In the group home he could be sympathetic to others and on occasion used simple emotion-descriptive words for some of the other boys' experiences. But when it came to his own emotional *vulnerability*, Rashid did not have the language to represent what he may have felt. Thus, he was limited in what he could get from others in the way of sympathetic understanding. In the end, it tended to isolate him as well, for the other boys in the group home characterized him as "the glass door: someone whom you looked right through, but if you ran into it, it'd shatter." Rashid's personhood was experienced by the boys as both fragile and invisible, and in that sense, he was unknowable, for they were unable to grasp how he felt because he could not communicate about himself emotionally. Rashid was, in a sense, emotionally tone-deaf: He could not hear his own plaintive emotional song.

PROBLEMS IN EMPATHIC RESPONSIVITY

Empathy allows us to share in others' emotional experiences, and with our ability to take another's perspective comes our capacity for sympathy for the other. In sympathy we offer a helpful hand, an understanding ear, a shoulder to lean on. It is noteworthy that these idiomatic phrases of sympathetic "body parts" are used to support and assist another; these phrases quite literally put our body next to another in distress to comfort and help directly. But what happens if empathic responsivity is excessive and a person feels overaroused? Chapter 7 mentioned personal distress reactions as problematic responses to empathy-eliciting situations: Some individuals became more preoccupied with their own intensely distressed empathic reaction and short-circuited the sympathy loop, as it were. They then dealt with their own upset feelings, and thus the focus was no longer on the person experiencing the original misfortune. Eisenberg et al. (1991) found in their research that parents who restricted their children's vulnerable emotional expressions had children who were more inclined to experience personal distress rather than sympathy when faced with another person's distress. Reproaching or chiding a youngster for revealing his or her hurt or anxious feelings apparently produces a child who worries about not living up to some standard of emotional stoicism. Then, when confronted with an intense emotional situation in which another needs help, such a child does not emotionally engage and indeed avoids the stricken individual. Children whose parents allow the expression of vulnerable feelings, especially in their sons, appear to be more likely to experience sympathy with another's misfortune and are more likely to comfort or provide assistance. As mentioned in Chapter 7, research by Cassidy and Asher (1992) also found that children who were rejected by their peers were rated by their teachers as less prosocial in their behavior, and, not surprisingly, they also felt more lonely. Social deficits as well as reduced prosocial behavior seem to go hand in hand.

Another group that demonstrates deficits in empathic responsiveness are those who have grown up in harsh homes in which physical and psychological battering are commonplace (e.g., Klimes-Dougan & Kistner, 1990). Children witnessing domestic violence are also at risk for having a blunted sense of empathy, although empirical research has not explicitly confirmed this deficit. Instead, we see that children from battering homes tend to be quite aggressive with their peers, and thus we infer that they are not especially empathic toward the victims of their bullying and assaults. Violent adolescents are also likely to come from violent homes, but, as Straus (1994) reminds us, not all teens from violent homes are violent themselves; the ones who are violent are most likely also from problem-ridden *communities* that have been abandoned by social policy in that funds for prevention, education, and employment have been cut off. If parental warmth, involvement, and emotional sensitivity to their children's emotional experience are critical for the development of empathy, it comes as no surprise that longitudinal research shows that parents who are cold, neglectful, and uninvolved are more likely to have children who become delinquent, especially in communities that provide little in the way of options (Pulkkinen, 1983).

DIFFICULTIES IN MANAGING
EMOTIONAL–EXPRESSIVE BEHAVIOR

As described in Chapter 8, children with externalizing problems (e.g., oppositional behavior and excessive aggression) were less likely to mask their disappointment in front of the gift-giver when they received something they did not like (Cole et al., 1994). Indeed, these children showed their anger, became disruptive, and were generally quite obviously negative about the whole exchange. Most of these acting-out children were boys in the Cole et al. (1994) research, and smooth self-presentation or impression management is not something impulsive, acting-out children do well. The at-risk girls in the Cole et al. (1994) study tended to have attention-deficit problems, and they expressed a rather flat affect. It also appears that this paradigm does not elicit the same meaning for many girls, who relate to the situation as primarily a social one (e.g., Josephs, 1993).

One group of girls who may not reliably or effectively manage their emotional–expressive behavior and thus have difficulties as they mature with their self-presentation may be those who are risk for becoming adolescent parents. These girls may also develop physically earlier than their peers, thus appearing older than their psychological immaturity would suggest. Recent research by Underwood, Kupersmidt, and Coie (1996) on girls who become adolescent mothers was the stimulus for this notion, and the following composite case provides a window into these dynamics of emotional–expressive behavior, self-presentation, and risk.

> Thirteen-year-old Eva enjoyed being taller and more developed than the other kids her age, and her agility on the volleyball court made her a popular teammate. By the time she turned 14, Eva was on her own a lot due to stressful family circumstances. She sported several earrings in both ears, dressed provocatively, and waved languorously her red-alternating-with-black fingernails in the face of anyone half-interested in looking. Her grades had slipped from junior high as she had become inconsistent in studying. Although Eva tried to present herself as older (including trying to buy cigarettes as an alleged 18-year-old), her poses were often punctuated by a young teen's giggles.
> The next year, Eva, now 15, was identified with a group of

girls who were much attended to by the other kids: They were a source of excitement and envy for their flaunting of conventions but also scandal and wariness for their recklessness. Eva's mom despaired of trying to control her; in any case, she was too exhausted much of the time to keep track of what Eva was doing. Eva started to go out with a 22-year-old man, and she smoked marijuana regularly. Eva was also suspended for vandalizing some lockers at school and was subsequently grounded by her mother.

But things started to unravel when Eva repeatedly sneaked out to stay with her boyfriend in his trailer. She impulsively agreed to unprotected sex, and not long after, the boyfriend disappeared. Three months later, to Eva's horror, she still hadn't gotten her period. Too late to terminate the pregnancy, Eva eventually delivered a healthy little girl, and she had a glimmer of realization that her life was ambiguously but forever transformed, whether she liked it or not.

Eva would have been characterized as one of the "controversial" girls in the study by Underwood et al. (1996). She was both liked and disliked by her peers, and she was known for being a member of a group of girls who in another age might have been described as "wild" (or as a "deviant group" in social science jargon). Underwood et al. (1996) describe the characteristics of girls who become teen parents as including a willingness to "break rules," to be part of a deviant group, to engage in early sexual activity, to behave aggressively, yet also to be capable of social leadership and enjoy some degree of support even as they take risks that endanger their position. However, their really extraordinary finding is that they were able to substantially predict adolescent motherhood from *fourth-grade* (9 years old) sociometric ratings: 50% of girls identified as controversial or as aggressive in the fourth grade in the working-class sample they studied had become parents in adolescence, a proportion twice as high as the base rate in the sample.

Earlier research by Block, Block, and Keyes (1988) also found that marijuana usage in young adolescent girls (14-year-olds) correlated with such personality characteristics as rebelliousness, unconventional thinking, rejection of conservative values, difficulty delaying gratification, and stretching limits, similar to the profile of controversial children described in the preceding study. Eva appears to demonstrate some of these characteristics, and were we to have access to early preschool data on Eva and her family, we might find, as the Block et al. (1988) longitudinal study did, that marijuana usage in young adolescent girls was correlated with a number of preschool emotional behaviors such as "immature in behavior when under stress, sulky, emotionally labile, unrecognizing of the feelings of others, inconsiderate, not calm, feeling deprived, and cries easily" (p. 343), among others. At age 6, the mothers of such girls were described as frequently angry and disappointed with their daughters, had few expectations of their daughters, and felt that they had given up their own personal interests on the daughter's behalf. Fathers were lax, also had few achievement expectations for their daughters, and were permissive of daughters' negative emotionality (crying, negative remarks). The homes of these girls were also characterized as disorganized. The investigators concluded that the pattern evidenced by the young girls who later used marijuana was one of *ego undercontrol* and *compromised ego resiliency*. The stage was set for them to succumb to peer pressure even as they already had difficulty in directing themselves toward a healthy autonomy.

Admittedly speculative, I wonder whether some of the personality or character structure problems associated with ego undercontrol and inadequate ego resiliency found in the preceding study by Block et al. (1988) would be associated with (1) deficits in realizing how we are perceived by diverse social audiences and (2) limitations in recognizing that multiple social goals require multiple and flexible ways of presenting ourselves. Such a pattern of personality and restricted sensitivity might well contribute to a constriction within the self of possible roles or even identities. In adolescence, rehearsal of possible roles and potential identities is a significant developmental activity. If our limitations preclude us from perceiving "affordances" in our social environment for rehearsal of these options for self-definition, then we have effectively entrapped ourselves in a well-worn rut. We may get stuck in a premature foreclosure of identity (Erikson, 1968) or yield to social pressures to engage in activities that put us at risk (illicit drug use, unprotected sex, gang violence, etc.).

Different from the preceding speculation dynamically but perhaps having the same rigid developmental outcome are those youngsters who suffer from internalizing disorders characterized by severe anxiety such that they present an emotional front that is as brittle as it is unchanging. Recall Chapter 8, in which I described a study about what children thought about other kids who almost never showed their real feelings (Saarni, 1988). Such children were viewed as possibly emotionally maladjusted and hard to get to know, and they were simply disliked. As one child put it, "You wouldn't be able to trust a kid like that—because you'd never know what [the kid was] feeling," and another child said, "Then one day she'd explode. . . . " A hidden self and a potential for volatility seem to be among the problems suspected by the peers of youngsters presenting a chronic emotional facade. Ostracism, loneliness, and loss of opportunities to develop socially are additional liabilities when children seek to manage their emotional experience by adopting rigid emotional–expressive behavior for their self-presentations with others.

A fairly substantial research literature has emerged about lonely and rejected children (e.g., Asher & Coie, 1990; Cassidy & Asher, 1992; Parkhurst & Asher, 1992). Not surprisingly, lonely children are perceived as shy, but in addition there appear to be at least a couple of subgroups of lonely children: Some are aggressive and demonstrate minimal prosocial behavior and others are submissive and withdrawn (e.g., Parkhurst & Asher, 1992). Boys may be overrepresented in the former group (Cassidy & Asher, 1992), and children in the aggressive subgroup appear to be more often also rejected by their peers. From the standpoint of emotion management, I infer that lonely, rejected children do not have the skills to be able to maneuver their self-presentations to achieve more effective impressions on their peers. They may be using faulty social cognition in how they appraise what would be effective impression management, or they have an idea of what to do but have difficulty implementing it behaviorally. The latter may occur as a result of anticipatory anxiety about possible rejection. If their shyness is characterized by general cautiousness, such a wary inhibited style may contribute to delays in emotional responsiveness toward others, and poor timing may impair their entry into social interaction. The fact that a low prosocial orientation has been found in a significant number of lonely children also suggests possible deficits in empathic understanding of others or deficits in comprehending the emotional communicative behavior of others. Thus, lonely (and rejected) children may have deficits both at the *encoding* level of sending emotional–expressive signals as well as at the *decoding* level of receiving and comprehending others' emotional–expressive communicative behavior (see also Underwood, 1997).

DIFFICULTIES IN COPING AND EMOTION REGULATION

In Chapter 9 I discussed some of the serious dilemmas faced by sexually abused children relative to developing healthy coping and emotion regulation strategies. One study on college-age women's retrospective reports (Long & Jackson, 1993) stated that those women who used almost exclusively *emotion-focused* coping strategies (e.g., "I went on as if nothing happened") reported more psychiatric and psychosomatic symptoms, including depression, anxiety, and hypersensitivity, than did those who sought support by telling someone or who more actively attempted to stop the molestation using problem-solving coping strategies. It would seem that using emotion-focused coping strategies might allow the molestation to continue, and thus the sheer duration of traumatization for the child is longer. Stigmatizing may occur if individuals view themselves with shame as a result of sexual abuse; by so doing, they may also put themselves at greater risk for a poor outcome (Feiring et al., 1996).

Recall that emotion-focused coping strategies are most useful when we do not have control over the circumstances; the dilemma for maltreated children is that they may feel helpless and thus do not see options for controlling the negative circumstances surrounding their maltreatment, even though such options might exist (e.g., telling someone about their victimization). Not surprisingly, the most prominent advice in abuse prevention programs given to children is "tell someone" because the reality of children's lives is such that they may have relatively little control, other than to get help from others who are not involved in the maltreatment. To sum up, one of the ways that incompetent coping may show itself is an overreliance on any one strategy to deal with a wide variety of circumstances and feelings. Diversity and flexibility in using coping and emotion regulation strategies are clearly more effectively adaptive for the self.

Another way that traumatic abuse negatively affects children's coping and emotion regulation was mentioned earlier with regard to deficits in having access to an emotion lexicon. If traumatically abused children's impulsive aggression and self-destructive behavior are responses to stress (Cicchetti & White, 1990), these children are seriously impaired when it comes to being able to regulate their emotional upheaval if they have difficulty in representing to themselves what their emotional experience is. As a consequence, their subsequent coping efforts are ineffectual and often contribute to a worsening of the stressful circumstances. In addition, what might be a mild stressor for nontraumatized children may set off a severely maltreated child. The following case, adapted from a recent research project (Saarni, 1997), illustrates how a seemingly innocuous situation may prove to be too destabilizing for a child who has been sexually abused.

> K, age 7, had been removed from her home due to severe sexual abuse by her stepfather and because her mother was unwilling or unable to protect the child. She was living with her guardian when she was interviewed in a research project about how kids might cope with various feelings and problematic situations, using hypothetical stories accompanied by cartoons. Several features of the interview situation would have been considered demand characteristics in other studies and analyzed as such, but for K, these situational aspects became profoundly stressful, and her ability to cope began to deteriorate rapidly.
>
> The first obvious stressor was being taken from the play ther-

apy room at the agency where she was being treated to a different room, accompanied by the interviewer, a "familiar stranger." In this room was a video camera on one side of a low table and a mirror on the other side of the table (no concealed taping was permitted). K couldn't decide which was more fascinating (or distracting, as the case may be): the camera or the mirror. She appeared to disregard the presence of the interviewer, a woman she had met a couple of times at the agency, as she began an unusually energetic clowning routine in front of the mirror and then whirled around to do the routine in front of the camera. Her physical activity level was high and intense.

After many patient attempts, the interviewer succeeded in getting K to sit down at the table and begin to look at the cartoons. However, K almost immediately became agitated and started to gnaw on her hands, eventually asking the interviewer, "Are you going to ask me those things again. . . . I don't want to talk about it." The interviewer knew that it was customary in the county to video children's depositions about their abuse so that repeated interviews would be unnecessary, and so she sought to reassure K that they would not talk about "those things." They had barely completed the first story and questions about coping with feeling angry and were beginning the next story about feeling afraid of a fiercely barking dog when K bounced out of her seat and started to "bark" vociferously and turned to the mirror behind her to pretend to bite her own image.

After that, the next two stories also elicited from K an extremely intense and active enactment of the emotion combined with some element of trying to pretend-hurt herself, the interviewer, or an object. Although she did answer the interview questions, she also appeared to be getting more and more wound up. The fifth and final story was about a girl whose pants tore during recess and she felt embarrassed. K became clearly overwhelmed: She started grabbing at the interviewer's clothing and became almost hysterical. The interviewer took K to her therapist down the hall, who was able to calm her down, but the interviewer realized that the interview process presented K with too much arousal and stress, and she discontinued K's participation in the rest of the study.

Whereas K may have also had a temperamental disposition to emotional reactivity and hyperactivity that contributed to her vulnerability to stress, a destructive and abusive family would have exacerbated how that emotionally reactive disposition manifested itself. Interestingly, among the frequently reported sequelae of sexual abuse of children is impulsivity (e.g., Cole & Putnam, 1992), and whereas boys are overrepresented in diagnoses of attention-deficit/hyperactivity disorder (ADHD) in general, when girls are diagnosed with ADHD, it may be functionally related to a history of sexual abuse (Trickett & Putnam, 1991). This theme of dysfunctional family processes is continued in the next section, which examines how family conflict and violence affect children's emotional adaptation.

IMPAIRED EMOTIONAL COMMUNICATION WITHIN RELATIONSHIPS

Aggressive, oppositional, and defiant children may develop emotionally maladaptive behaviors as a function of being embedded within maladaptive patterns of emotional communication, especially intense conflict, in their families (e.g., Cummings & Owens, 1994; Grych & Fincham, 1990; Katz & Gottman, 1993; Mann & MacKenzie, 1996). Similarly, depressed and suicidal children also report their families as being conflict-ridden and stressful, accompanied by parental negativity (criticism, humiliation) toward the child (Asarnow et al., 1987; Messer & Gross, 1995). When children demonstrate emotional incompetence in their peer relationships, they may simply be mirroring their families' impaired emotional communication. For example, Katz and Gottman (1993) found that mutually hostile interaction between parents was associated with their children behaving at school in an antisocial manner, a link also found by Jenkins and Smith (1993). However, Katz and Gottman (1993) found that when parents demonstrated a marital interaction pattern characterized by the husband experiencing anger but demonstrating emotional withdrawal, the children were more likely to show social withdrawal at school. Parenthetically, in that study the researchers ruled out the influence of children's temperament as a factor in their maladaptive emotional functioning at school. In another study examining the effects on children when they witness prolonged and unresolved conflicts between adults, Cummings, Ballard, El-Sheikh, and Lake (1991) noted that such children were more likely to show persistent negative affect and less effective coping. Gottman and Katz (1989) also found that children's peer relations and health were adversely affected by their parents' chronic discord, confirmed by Graham-Bermann (1997) who found that children from violent homes worried significantly more about their own and family members' safety.

In addition to these patterns of parental conflict negatively affecting children's emotional and social functioning, a number of investigations indicate that parental discipline, characterized by escalating aggression and coercion of their children, is also thought to contribute to child psychopathology (e.g., Patterson, DeBaryshe, & Ramsey, 1989;

Weiss, Dodge, Bates, & Pettit, 1990). Thus, aggressive punishment as a so-called disciplinary strategy, rejection and/or shaming of the child (Asarnow et al., 1987; Mann & MacKenzie, 1996), and verbal and physical conflict between parents all combine to produce an assortment of externalizing and internalizing problems in children. Whether it is aggressive and oppositional behavior or withdrawn and depressed behavior in children, the emotional lives of these children reflect *systemic* family problems rather than their affective behavior being uniquely attributable to their temperament alone (Alexander & Pugh, 1996; but compare with Wootton, Frick, Shelton, & Silverthorn, 1997). In short, their difficult negative behavior is multiply determined and intertwined with relationship deficits in their families.

The following composite case description captures this wasteland of family emotion communication patterns, ranging from ineffectual to truly destructive. In this case we might see the child's attempt to deal with this context as a survival strategy of sorts, but in the rest of the child's social world, such behavior is emotionally incompetent.

Fred, age 8, lived with his mother, 3-year-old sister, and stepfather, Rudy. Rudy was an alcoholic; the mother was economically dependent on Rudy as some years earlier she had experienced a severe head injury that resulted in a variety of disabilities. The police had been called a few times to the apartment where they lived, but Mom would not file charges. Rudy's battering of Mom was preceded by his binge drinking, and Mom was not the sole target of his violence; the family dog was routinely beaten, and Rudy used emotional violence (threats, insults) to tyrannize the children. Because the children often witnessed what Rudy did to their mother and their pet, his threats seemed likely and vividly real.

Fred protected his little sister as much as possible and would lie about both her and the dog's minor messes and the like to distract the stepfather's wrath from being directed at her or the dog. His hypervigilance may have contributed to his also developing assorted dermatitis problems, asthma, allergic reactions to various foods, and respiratory infections. As a result, Fred missed a lot of school (but was thus at home to intervene in his sister's, the dog's, and mother's behalf). His academic progress suffered, and the family was told he would have to repeat the second grade. School personnel had no knowledge of the family's chaotic home life. His teacher thought he was immature for his age, and she was particularly harshly judgmental about his "constant" lying, unpredictable aggression toward his peers, and distractibility in the classroom. Little did she know that these emotionally "incompetent" behaviors had parallels in the "strategic" behavior Fred used at home. There his deception served prosocial purposes, and his hypervigilance, while appropriate at home, translated into seeming distractibility in the classroom. His witnessing the outbursts of aggression at home by a man who controlled his family in this fashion led to Fred's using this method as well as a way to deal with peer conflicts at school.[1]

Fortunately for Fred and his little sister, the maternal grandparents offered to take the children (and the dog) for a while until Mom "could get her life back on track." Ultimately she left her husband, and with her parents' help and supportive counseling she worked hard to provide a more secure family life for her children.

Fred's response to family violence is consistent with that described by McCloskey et al. (1995). They found a wide range of both internalizing and externalizing problem behaviors in children living in violent homes, and no particular type of partner abuse was associated with specific problematic behavior in the children. These authors also speculate that it is the anticipatory fear of violence that disrupts children's functioning: "It is also likely that the abusive acts within these families are the visible crest of a pervasive wave of terror. The dread of violence might disrupt psychosocial development more than the event itself" (p. 1258). In their complex analyses they were also able to rule out the mothers' reduced warmth toward her children as a significant factor in their children's psychopathology; it was being trapped in the family "war" that correlated most highly with the general patterns of pathology found in the children.

Interestingly, the fact that Fred's pet dog was also subjected to abuse has been found as an indicator of domestic violence. Ascione (1998) found that fully 71% of battered women seeking safe shelters reported past or current threats to injure or kill the family pet by their abusive partner, and actual (as opposed to threatened) pet abuse was reported by 57% of his sample. In about 30% of the households, the children were also reported to have abused family pets, perhaps in emulation of their violent fathers (see also Ascione, 1993, 1997).

Clinical anecdote and empirical research suggests that children who grow up in conflict-laden and violent families are at risk for reproducing these patterns of maladaptive emotional communication and impaired social problem-solving skills within their own relationships (Rosenberg, 1987), such as in their friendships (Parker & Herrera, 1996) and their future spousal relationships (e.g., Dutton, 1998; Sonkin, 1988). Katz and Gottman (1997) provide some reassuring data that despite marital discord, if the parents can continue to be warm, praising, and supportive and have an emotional coaching approach *toward their children,* their children will function with greater competence than those children whose parents lack these skills. However, even these buffered children still continued to demonstrate some degree of behavior problems. Ideally children can begin to mend their emotional scars and learn more adaptive ways of emotionally communicating within relationships if the family "war" ceases and is replaced by supportive and consistent family relationships. Unfortunately, the "war" often continues after divorce and the custodial parent, typically the mother, is also likely to be further stressed by poverty and inadequate support (e.g., Koss et al., 1994).

INADEQUATE EMOTIONAL SELF-EFFICACY

Recall from the preceding chapter that emotional self-efficacy refers to feeling relatively in control of one's emotional experience from the standpoint of mastery and positive self-regard. If emotional self-efficacy is rarely experienced, then both self-esteem and a sense of mastery are likely to be fragile or fleeting. Inadequate emotional self-efficacy can leave an individual feeling the gnawing doubts of diminished self-confidence, a general sense of dysphoria, and in more extreme cases, depression. I illustrate impaired emotional self-efficacy by examining childhood dysphoria and depression.

Cole and Kaslow (1988) suggested in their review of developmental issues in childhood depression that the newly emerging cognitive skill in middle childhood of being able to reflect on one's internal experience (thoughts, feelings, beliefs, etc.) leads to the capacity for self-evaluation. Self-monitoring and self-reinforcing thoughts and behaviors also become evident at this time, as does increased likelihood of comparing oneself to others on an ever-widening number of dimensions (physical attractiveness, athletic prowess, popularity, etc.; see Ruble, Boggiano, Feldman, & Loebl, 1980). Together, these self-related cognitive skills facilitate the child's construction of a more consolidated and integrated identity (Selman, 1981), but these same cognitive skills may also be used by the child to construct an identity that is premised on a negative self-evaluation with attributions of helplessness and futility that persist over time (e.g., Seligman et al., 1984). Depressed children also hold more negative self-expectancies—even as they simultaneously are more likely to endorse more strict standards for their behavior and believe they should be punished when they do not meet these standards (Kaslow, Rehm, & Siegel, 1984). As reviewed by Cole and Kaslow (1988), depressed children's school performance is lower than that of nondepressed children, and they are more often lonely and rejected by their peers. Their home life is also unhappy and stress-laden (e.g.,

Asarnow et al., 1987; Messer & Gross, 1995). The picture that emerges of such depressed children is one of demoralization, sad and/or anxious affect, distressed and unsupportive families, and a self-defeating approach to coping with stressful circumstances. Indeed, the threshold for experiencing stress may also be lower for depressed children and youth, given their frequently ineffectual coping efforts (e.g., Garber et al., 1995). The composite case of the 11-year-old girl presented next illustrates many of these features, yet ambiguities remained in this case, suggesting a subclinical depression.

> Laura was referred for counseling by her mother, who felt that her daughter was not dealing well with her parents' divorce and subsequent remarriage to other spouses. She was the only child of her parents, although her mother had a toddler from her second husband. Laura presented herself as an odd child. She wore peculiar and rather dirty hats, did not appear to bathe very frequently, and expressed her feelings in a brittle fashion. She reported spending most of her time at home in her bedroom watching television, even eating her supper in her room. In her therapy sessions her approach to using art materials was constricted; she did not want to play games with her therapist or join in other shared projects, but she responded well to going outside into the garden and swinging on a swing hanging from a tree.
>
> While swinging, Laura talked. She hated all the kids in her class, and she believed they all hated her. She hated her stepfather and appeared to barely tolerate her little brother. She hated her stepmother, and she thought she probably hated her mother too, but not so much. The person she adored and missed terribly was her father. As it turned out, Laura's father may have been the only adult in her life who accepted her for who she was and readily showed her affection. Her mother's recent move to California meant that Laura saw her father in Oregon only during school vacations, and she was not permitted "to run up big phone bills calling him." His new wife was resistant to Laura's living with them, and not surprisingly, Laura felt unwanted by everyone because she perceived her father as having sided with his wife against her.
>
> Family counseling with the mother, stepfather, and Laura revealed communication patterns of contempt, shaming, and invalidation of others' perspectives and wishes. Laura felt alone, hopeless, and helpless about doing anything to improve her situation. Avoidance, escape, and withdrawal were her coping strategies, and she applied them to both home and school contexts. The more she behaved in this fashion, the fewer social rewards she experienced, although before the divorce she had been a good student and had enjoyed having a few friends. It was as though a filter had come down over her way of seeing herself and her world, and

nothing could remove this biased view that clouded how she experienced herself. Deprecatory comments about herself and everyone around her were repeated again and again, but Laura never cried about her losses. She resigned herself to wait until summer vacation, or in her words, "when I come to life again."

Laura's and her family's experience could be characterized as mutually aversive and yet curiously stable. Laura's solitary behavior was reinforced by the mother's and stepfather's relatively disengaged behavior with one another and with Laura, and thus no one seemed to respond warmly or positively to any other family member with the exception of the baby. This pattern of family interaction was also found by Messer and Gross (1995) in their observations of families with school-age children who were assessed as having subclinical depression. They argued that family uninvolvement may lead to children's developing both dysphoria and anxiety, resulting in internalizing symptoms of withdrawal as well as irritability. What was most noteworthy in their research, in my opinion, was the sheer absence of anything positive or rewarding in these families vis-à-vis their children. A chronic "blandness" of disengagement characterized the families in Messer and Gross's sample, which may have been the quality that contributed to the seeming stability of Laura's family's interaction pattern; it never got so bad that either adult did anything to change it.

Perhaps it is not so surprising that Laura felt defeated in trying to change anything about how she viewed herself while living in this family context, given the unrelenting flatness of interpersonal exchange within her family. The next summer I received several postcards from Laura after she had returned to Oregon. She candidly wrote that she hoped her stepmother would be abducted by aliens, but she was having a good time with her dad. He was negotiating with both Laura's mother and with his wife to have Laura live with them, and this family's "interpersonal exchanges" appeared to be anything but "flat."

In returning to the idea of what the emotional quality of our lives would be like if we rarely experienced emotional self-efficacy, I think it would be more like an endless barren landscape than a life characterized by melancholy. Granted, depression may well yield an internal emotional landscape that is indeed arid, but clinically we also see despair or melancholy that is a reaction to circumstances that appear hopeless to the individual enveloped in them. Changing those circumstances often leads to emotional renewal and a lifting of the melancholy or despair (as in Laura's case). Thus, I also include in diminished emotional self-efficacy a leaden, flat, and alienated quality of living, as suggested by the protagonist in Camus's (1954) *The Stranger*.

Rereading that novel a couple of years ago provoked me to think about emotional self-efficacy as a skill of emotional competence that might be particularly applicable to late adolescence and adulthood when we are more likely to have choices about the contexts in which we live and the people with whom we become involved. Anthony (1987) also examined Camus's protagonist, whose name was Meursault, and saw the character as having a false invulnerability premised on being "a passive, detached observer of life who will not involve himself or engage himself in the world around him" (p. 6). Anthony referred to this "Meursault phenomenon" as a possible form of psychological immunization against trauma, albeit at considerable psychological cost (e.g., inability to form intimate relationships). Such detachment may well allow individuals to cope with stressors, but it is by rendering much of experience relatively distant and meaningless. Genuine emotional resilience eludes such disengaged individuals, as does intimacy and mature emotional mutuality with others. With emotional self-efficacy we retain a meaningful connection with our experience and our relationships (see also Hermans & Kempen, 1993). When emotionally self-efficacious, we can sustain our self-confidence and self-regard even in the face of serious setbacks and losses, for we have developed a buffering social support system. Relative to the case described previously, choices had been made for young Laura by the adults in her life, but they were not choices she felt were supportive of her needs and developing identity. However, we must give Laura credit: With time, she managed to enlist support (most importantly from her father but also from her therapist) so that changes did come about that were more beneficial for her. As for Camus's Meursault, he lost access to choice, for he spent his last days in prison awaiting his execution.

Extreme existential "angst," severe social alienation such as evidenced by the Unabomber, Theodore Kaczynski ("The Mind of the Unabomber," 1996), and possibly some personality disorders (e.g., borderline and narcissistic) might be additional instances of seriously impaired emotional self-efficacy that are not likely to change much when one's life circumstances are altered. When faced with the inevitable stresses of living in a complex world, these emotionally inefficacious individuals respond with brittle, repetitive, and frequently inflexible strategies for regulating themselves, their feelings, and the circumstances in which they live. Just as biologically induced vulnerability may predispose a person to deficiencies in emotional development and thus make the acquisition of emotional competence problematic, so too might unrelenting emotional adversity contribute to an adult personality pattern that is resistant to change. Emotional self-efficacy, if experienced, may prove to be evanescent for these individuals.

The connection between emotional self-efficacy and capacity for emotional mutuality with others that was noted earlier may have its origins in healthy attachment relationships in childhood or in healthy nonfamilial relationships that compensated for less than adequate family bonds. Perhaps it comes as no surprise that researchers have found emotionally responsive caregiving to be one of the most significant protective factors in helping children to develop the resilience they needed to overcome the adverse effects of poverty, maltreatment, and family stress (Egeland, Carlson, & Sroufe, 1993). In addition, adaptable ego strength and an intact well-functioning intelligence also seem to aid a child in weathering harsh circumstances and even in overcoming the aftermath of trauma (e.g., Cicchetti & Garmezy, 1993; Felsman & Vaillant, 1987; Garmezy, 1993).

CONCLUSION

I began this chapter with the idea that emotional *incompetence* reflected systemic problems. Biogenetic problems in the individual may well disrupt "normal" emotional development, thus making it all the more difficult for emotional competence to be acquired. Given that a person has a well-functioning nervous system and has grown up in a "good enough" social environment, deficits in emotional competence would not be found "inside" the person; they are *transactional* deficiencies. They cannot be separated from the contextual demands with which an individual is engaged. The present circumstances in which we live can be "sick," render us vulnerable, and put us at risk, depending on our strengths and vulnerabilities. In this sense, I propose here both a functionalist position (e.g., Campos et al., 1994) and a relatively radical contextual position (e.g., Lewis, 1997). Yet I find myself loathe to give up the idea that who we are emotionally also reflects our cumulative emotional *history*. I admit to being in something of a theoretical bind: To what extent is emotional competence (or incompetence) a matter of destructive and defeating circumstances (the contextual position), a function of transactional demands (the functionalist position), or an outcome of past learned associations? I suspect that just as much in human development is multiply determined, so too are the skills of emotional competence (or their deficiencies). We all demonstrate at one time or another sporadic behavior that someone or even ourselves would probably label as maladaptive, maladjusted, inappropriate, nonsensical, or just plain stupid. Does this mean that we are characterologically emotionally incompetent? Not at all. It just means that in this transaction we demonstrated an emotionally incompetent response and that we had better remember some humility relative to notions of "emotional intelligence" and emotional competence; they are not global and enduring characteristics of the person. We will, on occasion, have our "comeuppance," given the right combination of taxing circumstances.

My thoughts lean toward emotional *in*competence as more reflective of contexts in which we are at odds as to how to promote our *healthy* self-interests. The latter, by definition as healthy, will also have integrated with them the concerns and well-being of others. Another way to describe this predicament is to say that our otherwise adaptable ego strength is hindered from asserting itself. Some of the time, we function emotionally at a less than optimal level, but this is not to say that something pathological about ourselves has occurred. Instead, we need to take stock of what eludes us, what challenges our resilience or ego strength, what leaves us in a undifferentiated muddle as to what will be an adaptive course of action to take and how to make sense of the *ambiguous* feelings we experience. Thus, we are thrown back to the most elemental skill of emotional competence: Do we know what we are feeling? And it may well be complex, filled with subtlety and nuance and ordinary confusion.

At this point, we should return to moral character as also part of emotional competence. Without a sense of what is the right thing to do relative to our subculture, we are cast adrift, rudderless, and without a current or wind to provide direction. Confusion is often a result of perplexing experience: We do not know the meaning of the circumstances in which we find ourselves; we do not have a map for guidance. Fortunately, culture provides us with a way, namely, values. They are an indispensable part of what gives meaning to emotional experience, and they drive what become the goals of motivated behavior. When personal integrity or moral character is conjoined with emotional experience, such motivated behavior itself stems from having experienced emotions in conjunction with contexts that are interpreted in light of moral meaning systems. Such moral meaning systems may well reflect the Aristotelian virtues of courage, temperance, justice, and wisdom or Wilson's (1993) sympathy, self-control, fairness, and a sense of obligation. How we represent our world, our action in it and with others, is intimately embedded in our emotional life. Moral character is part of that representation, and deficits in moral character reveal themselves in emotional life. This is also the transactional and functionalist model of emotion, as well as our past experiential learning that leads us to associate, for example, pleasure with mutual responsiveness and aversion with coercion. Perhaps it is in this way that functionalist, contextualist, and social learning positions can be integrated in emotional development. The common threads provided by culture allow us to find consensual meaning with others in emotional experience. Those common threads also reflect moral meaning in emotionally competent action.

The distinction between emotional development and emotional competence needs further clarification. I think the latter has to do with self-efficacy, and it is also relative: In comparison with our peers, do we appear to reach our goals more often? Do we seem to bounce back from stress in a way that enriches our coping repertoire rather than depleting it? Can we communicate with greater flexibility, depending on our social "affordances," what it is that we feel? Can we step into the shoes of another and share, in part, what they feel and yet not become so overwhelmed by their experience that we cannot assist them? Relative to our peers, can we more readily see the bigger picture of our emotions and yet simultaneously conceptualize our emotional experience with individualized hue, texture, and weave? Can we also on occasion ignore our peers and feel justified in how we feel, even if it is an unconventional response? In short, can we strive for emotional self-efficacy even if it is not "popular?" To the extent that we can answer these questions affirmatively *and* with regard to personal integrity, I would argue that we are demonstrating emotional competence, which by definition must build on emotional development and self-development, as well as on a supportive set of circumstances in which we live. The question for social scientists remains, of course, how to understand just what those circumstances realistically are and how to nurture the individual whose development is transactionally intertwined with his or her context.

NOTE

1. Graham-Bermann (1997) found that the intense degree of worrying found in children exposed to domestic violence was associated with externalizing behavior, suggesting that aggression and acting out by these children may be related to their constant anxiety.

References

Abelson, R. (1981). Psychological status of the script concept. *American Psychologist, 36,* 715–729.

Aber, J., & Cicchetti, D. (1984). Socioemotional development in maltreated children: An empirical and theoretical analysis. In H. Fitzgerald, B. Lester, & M. Yogman (Eds.), *Theory and research in behavioral pediatrics* (Vol. 2, pp. 147–205). New York: Plenum.

Achenbach, T., & Edelbrock, C. (1982). *Manual for the Child Behavior Checklist and Child Behavior Profile.* Burlington: University of Vermont Press.

Ackerman, R. J. (1983). *Children of alcoholics: A guidebook for educators, therapists, and parents* (2nd ed.). Holmes Beach, FL: Learning Publications.

Adams-Tucker, C. (1985). Defense mechanisms used by sexually abused children. *Children Today, 14,* 8–12.

Adlam-Hill, S., & Harris, P. L. (1988). *Understanding of display rules for emotion by normal and maladjusted children.* Unpublished manuscript, Department of Experimental Psychology, University of Oxford, Oxford, UK.

Aldwin, C. (1994). *Stress, coping, and development.* New York: Guilford Press.

Alexander, J., & Pugh, C. (1996). Oppositional behavior and conduct disorders of children and youth. In F. Kaslow (Ed.), *Handbook of relational diagnosis and dysfunctional family patterns* (pp. 210–224). New York: Wiley.

Alexander, P. C. (1992). Application of attachment theory to the study of sexual abuse. *Journal of Consulting and Clinical Psychology, 60,* 185–195.

Allen, J. P., Leadbeater, B., & Aber, J. L. (1987, April). *The relationship of adolescents' expectations and values to delinquency, hard drug use, and unprotected sexual intercourse.* Paper presented at the meeting of the Society for Research in Child Development, Baltimore.

Allessandri, S., & Lewis, M. (1996). Development of the self-conscious emotions in maltreated children. In M. Lewis & M. W. Sullivan (Eds.), *Emotional development in atypical children* (pp. 185–201). Mahwah, NJ: Erlbaum.

Altshuler, J., & Ruble, D. (1989). Developmental changes in children's awareness of strategies for coping with uncontrollable stress. *Child Development, 60,* 1337–1349.

Anderson, S., & Messick, S. (1974). Social competency in young children. *Developmental Psychology, 10,* 282–293.

Anthony, E. J. (1987). Risk, vulnerability, and resilience: An overview. In E. J. Anthony & B. Cohler (Eds.), *The invulnerable child* (pp. 3–48). New York: Guilford Press.

Anthony, E. J., & Cohler, B. (Eds.). (1987). *The invulnerable child.* New York: Guilford Press.

Aristotle. (trans. 1985). *Nichomachean ethics* (T. Irwin, Trans.). Indianapolis: Hackett.

Armon-Jones, C. (1986). The thesis of constructionism. In R. Harre (Ed.), *The social construction of emotions* (pp. 32–56). Oxford, UK: Basil Blackwell.

Asarnow, J., Carlson, G., & Guthrie, D. (1987). Coping strategies, self-perceptions, hopelessness, and perceived family environments in depressed and suicidal children. *Journal of Consulting and Clinical Psychology, 55,* 361–366.

Ascione, F. (1993). Children who are cruel to animals: A review of research and implications for developmental psychopathology. *Anthrozoos, 6*(4), 226–247.

Ascione, F. (1997). The abuse of animals and domestic violence: A national survey of shelters for women who are battered. *Society and Animals, 5,* 1–14.

Ascione, F. (1998). Battered women's reports of their partners' and their children's cruelty to animals. *Journal of Emotional Abuse, 1,* 119–133.

Asher, S., & Coie, J. D. (Eds.). (1990). *Peer rejection in childhood.* New York: Cambridge University Press.

Asher, S., Hymel, S., & Renshaw, P. (1984). Loneliness in children. *Child Development, 55,* 1456–1464.

Asher, S., Parker, J., & Walker, D. (1996). Distinguishing friendship from acceptance: Implications for intervention and assessment. In W. Bukowski, A. Newcomb, & W. Hartup (Eds.), *The company they keep: Friendship during childhood and adolescence* (pp. 366–405). New York: Cambridge University Press.

Asher, S., Parkhurst, J., Hymel, S., & Williams, G. (1990). Peer rejection and loneliness in childhood. In S. Asher & J. Coie (Eds.), *Peer rejection in childhood* (pp. 253–273). New York: Cambridge University Press.

Asher, S., & Rose, A. (1997). Promoting children's social–emotional adjustment with peers. In P. Salovey & D. Sluyter (Eds.), *Emotional development and emotional intelligence* (pp. 196–224). New York: Basic Books.

Asher, S., & Wheeler, V. (1985). Children's loneliness: A comparison of rejected and neglected peer status. *Journal of Consulting and Clinical Psychology, 53,* 500–505.

Astington, J., Harris, P. L., & Olson, D. R. (Eds.). (1988). *Developing theories of mind.* Cambridge, UK: Cambridge University Press.

Attie, I., Brooks-Gunn, J., & Petersen, A. (1990). A developmental perspective on eating disorders and eating problems. In M. Lewis & S. Miller (Eds.), *Handbook of developmental psychopathology* (pp. 409–420). New York: Plenum.

Band, E., & Weisz, J. (1988). How to feel better when it feels bad: Children's perspectives on coping with everyday stress. *Developmental Psychology, 24,* 247–253.

Bandura, A. (1977). Self-efficacy: Toward a unifying theory of behavioral change. *Psychological Review, 84,* 191–215.

Bandura, A. (1989). Human agency in social cognitive theory. *American Psychologist, 44,* 1175–1184.

Bandura, A. (1991). Social cognitive theory of moral thought and action. In W. Kurtines & J. Gewirtz (Eds.), *Handbook of moral behavior and development* (Vol. 1, pp. 45–103). Hillsdale, NJ: Erlbaum.

Barden, R. C., Zelko, F., Duncan, S. W., & Masters, J. C. (1980). Children's consensual knowledge about the experiential determinants of emotion. *Journal of Personality and Social Psychology, 39,* 968–976.

Baron-Cohen, S. (1987). Autism and symbolic play. *British Journal of Developmental Psychology, 5,* 139–148.

Barrett, K. C. (1995). A functionalist approach to shame and guilt. In J. P. Tangney & K. W. Fischer (Eds.), *Self-conscious emotions: The psychology of shame, guilt, embarrassment, and pride* (pp. 25–63). New York: Guilford Press.

Barrett, K. C., Zahn-Waxler, C., & Cole, P. M. (1993). Avoiders versus amenders: Implications for the investigation of guilt and shame during toddlerhood? *Cognition and Emotion, 7,* 481–505.

Barth, J., & Bastiani, A. (1997). A longitudinal study of emotion recognition and preschool children's social behavior. *Merrill–Palmer Quarterly, 43,* 107–128.

Bates, J. (1976). Effects of children's nonverbal behavior upon adults. *Child Development, 47,* 1079–1088.

Batson, C., Sager, K., Garst, E., Kang, M., Rubchinsky, K., & Dawson, K. (1997). Is empathy-induced helping due to self–other merging? *Journal of Personality and Social Psychology, 73,* 495–509.

Baumeister, R. F. (1982). A self-presentational view of social phenomena. *Psychological Bulletin, 91,* 3–26.

Baumeister, R. F. (Ed.). (1993a). *Self-esteem: The puzzle of low self-regard.* New York: Plenum.

Baumeister, R. F. (1993b). Lying to yourself: The enigma of self-deception. In M. Lewis & C. Saarni (Eds.), *Lying and deception in everyday life* (pp. 166–183). New York: Guilford Press.

Beeghly, M., Bretherton, I., & Mervis, C. (1986). Mothers' internal state language to toddlers: The socialization of psychological understanding. *British Journal of Developmental Psychology, 4,* 247–260.

Beeghly, M., & Tronick, E. (1994). Effects of prenatal exposure to cocaine in early infancy: Toxic effects on the process of mutual regulation. *Infant Mental Health Journal, 15,* 158–175.

Bell, R. Q. (1974). Contributions of human infants to caregiving and social interaction. In M. Lewis & L. Rosenblum (Eds.), *The effect of the infant on its caregiver* (pp. 1–19). New York: Wiley.

Bem, S. L. (1981). Gender schema theory: A cognitive account of sex typing. *Psychological Review, 88,* 354–364.

Berscheid, E. (1986). Emotional experience in close relationships: Some implications for child development. In W. Hartup & Z. Rubin (Eds.), *Relationships and development* (pp. 135–166). Hillsdale, NJ: Erlbaum.

Blasi, A. (1983). Moral cognition and moral action: A theoretical perspective. *Developmental Review, 3,* 178–210.

Block, J., & Block, J. (1980). The role of ego-control and ego-resiliency in the organization of behavior. In W. A. Collins (Ed.), *Minnesota Symposia on Child Psychology: Vol. 13. Development of cognition, affect, and social relations* (pp. 39–101). Hillsdale, NJ: Erlbaum.

Block, J., Block, J., & Keyes, S. (1988). Longitudinally foretelling drug usage in adolescence: Early childhood personality and environmental precursors. *Child Development, 59,* 336–355.

Block, J., & Robins, R. (1993). A longitudinal study of consistency and change in self-esteem from early adolescence to early adulthood. *Child Development, 64,* 909–923.

Blurton-Jones, N. (1967). An ethological study of some aspects of social behaviour of children in nursery school. In D. Morris (Ed.), *Primate ethology* (pp. 347–368). London: Weidenfeld & Nicolson.

Bond, M. H. (1993). Emotions and their expression in Chinese culture. *Journal of Nonverbal Behavior, 17,* 245–262.

Bond, M. H. (Ed.). (1996). *The handbook of Chinese psychology.* New York: Oxford University Press.

Bowlby, J. (1979). *The making and breaking of affectional bonds.* London: Tavistock.

Breger, L. (1974). *From instinct to identity.* Englewood Cliffs, NJ: Prentice-Hall.

Brenner, E., & Salovey, P. (1997). Emotion regulation during childhood: Developmental, interpersonal, and individual considerations. In P. Salovey & D. Sluyter (Eds.), *Emotional development and emotional intelligence* (pp. 168–192). New York: Basic Books.

Bretherton, I. (1995). Attachment theory and developmental psychopathology. In D. Cicchetti & S. Toth (Eds.), *Rochester Symposium on Developmental Psychopathology: Vol. 6. Emotion, cognition, and representation* (pp. 231–260). Rochester, NY: University of Rochester Press.

Bretherton, I., Fritz, J., Zahn-Waxler, C., & Ridgeway, D. (1986). Learning to talk about emotions: A functionalist perspective. *Child Development, 57,* 529–548.

Briere, J., Evans, D., Runtz, M., & Wall, T. (1988). Symptomatology in men who were molested as children: A comparison study. *American Journal of Orthopsychiatry, 58,* 457–461.

Brislin, R. (1993). *Understanding culture's influence on behavior.* Orlando, FL: Harcourt Brace.

Brody, L., & Hall, J. A. (1993). Gender and emotion. In M. Lewis & J. Haviland (Eds.), *Handbook of emotions* (pp. 447–460). New York: Guilford Press.

Brothers, L. (1989). A biological perspective on empathy. *American Journal of Psychiatry, 146,* 10–19.

Brown, J. R., & Dunn, J. (1991). "You can cry, mum": The social and developmental implications of talk about internal states. *British Journal of Developmental Psychology, 9,* 237–256.

Brown, L. M., & Gilligan, C. (1992). *Meeting at the crossroads: Women's psychology and girls' development.* Cambridge, MA: Harvard University Press.

Bryant, B. K., (1982). An index of empathy for children and adolescents. *Child Development*, *53*, 413–425.

Buck, R., Miller, R. E., & Caul, W. (1974). Sex, personality, and physiological variables in the communication of emotion via facial expression. *Journal of Personality and Social Psychology*, *30*, 125–133.

Bugental, D. B. (1986). Unmasking the "polite smile": Situational and personal determinants of managed affect in adult–child interaction. *Personality and Social Psychology Bulletin*, *12*, 7–16.

Bugental, D. B., Blue, J., & Lewis, J. (1990). Caregiver beliefs and dysphoric affect directed to difficult children. *Developmental Psychology*, *26*, 631–638.

Bugental, D. B., Cortez, V., & Blue, J. (1992). Children's affective responses to the expressive cues of others. In N. Eisenberg & R. Fabes (Eds.), *New directions for child development: Vol. 55. Emotion and its regulation in early development* (pp. 75–89). San Francisco: Jossey-Bass.

Bugental, D. B., & Goodnow, J. (1998). Socialization processes. In N. Eisenberg (Ed.), *Handbook of child psychology* (5th ed.): *Vol. 3. Social, emotional and personality development* (pp. 389–462). New York: Wiley.

Bugental, D. B., Love, L., & Gianetto, R. (1971). Perfidious feminine faces. *Journal of Personality and Social Psychology*, *17*, 314–318.

Bugental, D. B., & Shennum, W. (1984). "Difficult" children as elicitors and targets of adult communication patterns: An attributional–behavioral transactional analysis. *Monographs of the Society for Research in Child Development*, *49*(1, Serial No. 205, whole issue).

Cairns, R. B. (1979). *Social development: The origins and plasticity of interchanges.* San Francisco: Freeman.

Calverley, R., Fischer, K., & Ayoub, C. (in press). Complex splitting of self-representations in sexually abused adolescent girls. *Development and Psychopathology.*

Campbell, R. L., & Christopher, J. C. (1996). Moral development theory: A critique of its Kantian presuppositions. *Developmental Review*, *16*, 1–47.

Campos, J. (1994, Spring). The new functionalism in emotion. *SRCD Newsletter.*

Campos, J., & Barrett, K. C. (1984). Toward a new understanding of emotions and their development. In C. Izard, J. Kagan, & R. Zajonc (Eds.), *Emotions, cognition, and behavior* (pp. 229–263). New York: Cambridge University Press.

Campos, J., Campos, R., & Barrett, K. (1989). Emergent themes in the study of emotional development and emotion regulation. *Developmental Psychology*, *25*, 394–402.

Campos, J., Mumme, D., Kermoian, R., & Campos, R. G. (1994). A functionalist perspective on the nature of emotion. In N. Fox (Ed.), The development of emotion regulation: Behavioral and biological considerations. *Monographs of the Society for Research in Child Development*, *59* (2–3, Serial No. 240), 284–303.

Camras, L. A. (1985). Socialization of affect communication. In M. Lewis & C. Saarni (Eds.), *The socialization of emotions* (pp. 141–160). New York: Plenum.

Camras, L. A. (1992). Expressive development and basic emotions. *Cognition and Emotion*, *6*, 269–283.

Camras, L. A., Grow, G., & Ribordy, S. C. (1983). Recognition of emotional expressions by abused children. *Journal of Clinical and Child Psychology, 12,* 325–328.

Camras, L. A., & Rappaport, S. (1993). Conflict behaviors of maltreated and nonmaltreated children. *Child Abuse and Neglect, 17,* 455–464.

Camras, L. A., Sachs-Alter, E., & Ribordy, S. (1996). Emotion understanding in maltreated children: Recognition of facial expressions and integration with other emotion cues. In M. Lewis & M. W. Sullivan (Eds.), *Emotional development in atypical children* (pp. 203–225). Mahwah, NJ: Erlbaum.

Camus, A. (1954). *The stranger.* New York: Random House.

Cappella, J. (1981). Mutual influence in expressive behavior: Adult–adult and infant–adult dyadic interaction. *Psychological Bulletin, 89,* 101–132.

Carlson, C., Felleman, E., & Masters, J. C. (1983). Influence of children's emotional states on the recognition of emotion in peers and social motives to change another's emotional state. *Motivation and Emotion, 7,* 61–79.

Carroll, J., & Steward, M. (1984). The role of cognitive development in children's understanding of their own feelings. *Child Development, 55,* 1486–1492.

Carson, D., Swanson, D., Cooney, M., Gillum, B., & Cunningham, D. (1992). Stress and coping as predictors of young children's development and adjustment. *Child Study Journal, 22,* 273–302.

Carson, J., & Parke, R. D. (1996). Reciprocal negative affect in parent–child interactions and children's peer competency. *Child Development, 67,* 2217–2226.

Case, R., Hayward, S., Lewis, M., & Hurst, P. (1988). Toward a neo-Piagetian theory of affective and cognitive development. *Developmental Review, 8,* 1–51.

Casey, R. (1993). Children's emotional experience: Relations among expression, self-report, and understanding. *Developmental Psychology, 29,* 119–129.

Casey, R. (1996). Emotional competence in children with externalizing and internalizing disorders. In M. Lewis & M. W. Sullivan (Eds.), *Emotional development in atypical children* (pp. 161–183). Mahwah, NJ: Erlbaum.

Cassidy, J. (1994). Emotion regulation: Influences of attachment relationships. In N. Fox (Ed.), The development of emotion regulation: Behavioral and biological considerations. *Monographs of the Society for Research in Child Development, 59*(2–3, Serial No. 240), 228–249.

Cassidy, J., & Asher, S. (1992). Loneliness and peer relations in young children. *Child Development, 63,* 350–365.

Cassidy, J., Parke, R., Butovsky, L., & Braungart, J. (1992). Family–peer connections: The roles of emotional expressiveness within the family and children's understanding of emotions. *Child Development, 63,* 603–618.

Cervantes, C., & Callanan, M. (1998). Labels and explanations in mother–child emotion talk: Age and gender differentiation. *Developmental Psychology, 34,* 88–98.

Chandler, M., Fritz, A., & Hala, S. (1989). Small-scale deceit: Deception as a marker of two-, three-, and four-year-olds' early theories of mind. *Child Development, 60,* 1263–1277.

Chapman, M. (1981). Isolating causal effects through experimental changes in parent–child interaction. *Journal of Abnormal Child Psychology, 9,* 321–327.

Chapman, M., Zahn-Waxler, C., Cooperman, G., & Iannotti, R. (1987). Empathy and responsibility in the motivation of children's helping. *Developmental Psychology, 23,* 140–145.

Charman, T., Swettenham, J., Baron-Cohen, S., Cox, A., Baird, G., & Drew, A. (1997). Infants with autism: An investigation of empathy, pretend play, joint attention, and imitation. *Developmental Psychology, 33,* 781–789.

Ch'en, M. Y. (1965). Sorrow. In K. Rexroth (Trans.), *One-hundred poems from the Chinese* (p. 42). New York: New Directions.

Chen, X., Dong, Q., & Zhou, H. (1997). Authoritative and authoritarian parenting practices and social and school performance in Chinese children. *International Journal of Behavioral Development, 21,* 855–873.

Chen, X., Rubin, K., Li, B., & Li, D. (in press). Adolescent outcomes of social functioning in Chinese children. *International Journal of Behavioral Development.*

Cialdini, R., Brown, S., Lewis, B., Luce, C., & Neuberg, S. (1997). Reinterpreting the empathy–altruism relationship: When one into one equals oneness. *Journal of Personality and Social Psychology, 73,* 481–494.

Cicchetti, D. (1987). Developmental psychopathology in infancy: Illustration from the study of maltreated youngsters. *Journal of Consulting and Clinical Psychology, 55,* 837–345.

Cicchetti, D., Ackerman, B., & Izard, C. (1995). Emotions and emotion regulation in developmental psychopathology. *Development and Psychopathology, 7,* 1–10.

Cicchetti, D., & Carlson, V. (Eds.). (1989). *Child maltreatment: Theory and research on the causes and consequences of child abuse and neglect.* New York: Cambridge University Press.

Cicchetti, C., & Garmezy, N. (1993). Prospects and promises in the study of resilience. *Development and Psychopathology, 5,* 497–502.

Cicchetti, D., & Toth, S. (Eds.). (1993). *Rochester Symposium on Developmental Psychopathology: Vol. 5. Disorders and dysfunctions of the self.* Rochester, NY: University of Rochester Press.

Cicchetti, D., & White, J. (1990). Emotion and developmental psychopathology. In N. Stein, B. Leventhal, & T. Trabasso (Eds.), *Psychological and biological approaches to emotion* (pp. 359–382). Hillsdale, NJ: Erlbaum.

Colby, A., & Damon, W. (1992). *Some do care: Contemporary lives of moral commitment.* New York: Free Press.

Cole, P. M. (1986). Children's spontaneous control of facial expression. *Child Development, 57,* 1309–1321.

Cole, P. M., Jenkins, P., & Shott, C. (1989). Spontaneous expressive control in blind and sighted children. *Child Development, 60,* 683–688.

Cole, P. M., & Kaslow, N. (1988). Interactional and cognitive strategies for affect regulation: Developmental perspective on childhood depression. In L. Alloy (Ed.), *Cognitive processes in depression* (pp. 310–343). New York: Guilford Press.

Cole, P. M., & Putnam, F. (1992). Effect of incest on self and social functioning: A developmental psychopathology perspective. *Journal of Consulting and Clinical Psychology, 60,* 174–184.

Cole, P. M., & Tamang, B. L. (1998). Nepali children's ideas about emotional displays in hypothetical challenges. *Developmental Psychology, 34,* 640–652.

Cole, P. M., Woolger, C., Power, T., & Smith, K. (1992). Parenting difficulties among adult survivors of father–daughter incest. *Child Abuse and Neglect, 16,* 239–249.

Cole, P. M., Zahn-Waxler, C., & Smith, K. D. (1994). Expressive control during a disappointment: Variations related to preschoolers' behavior problems. *Developmental Psychology, 30,* 835–846.

Compas, B., Malcarne, V., & Fondacaro, K. (1988). Coping with stressful events in older children and young adolescents. *Journal of Consulting and Clinical Psychology, 56,* 405–411.

Compas, B., Phares, V., & Ledoux, N. (1989). Stress and coping preventive interventions for children and adolescents. In L. Bond & B. Compas (Eds.), *Primary prevention and promotion in the schools* (pp. 319–340). London: Sage.

Compas, B., Worsham, N., & Ey, S. (1992). Conceptual and developmental issues in children's coping with stress. In A. La Greca, L. Siegel, J. Wallander, & C. Walker (Eds.), *Stress and coping in child health* (pp. 7–24). New York: Guilford Press.

Conger, R., Conger, C., Elder, G., Lorenz, F., Simons, R., & Whitbeck, L. (1993). Family economic stress and adjustment of early adolescent girls. *Developmental Psychology, 29,* 206–219.

Conroy, M., Hess, R. D., Azuma, H., & Kashiwagi, K. (1980). Maternal strategies for regulating children's behavior: Japanese and American families. *Journal of Cross-Cultural Psychology, 11,* 153–172.

Conte, J., & Schuerman, J. (1987). Factors associated with an increased impact of child sexual abuse. *Child Abuse and Neglect, 11,* 201–211.

Cook, W., Kenny, D., & Goldstein, M. (1991). Parental affective style risk and the family system: A social relations model analysis. *Journal of Abnormal Psychology, 100,* 492–501.

Cooley, C. H. (1902). *Human nature and the social order.* New York: Charles Scribner's Sons.

Cooper, C. R., & Carlson, C. I. (1989, July). *Individuation in family and peer relations in adolescence.* Paper presented at the meeting of the International Society for the Study of Behavioral Development, Jyvaskyla, Finland.

Cooper, C. R., & Cooper, R. G. (1992). Links between adolescents' relationships with their parents and peers: Models, evidence, and mechanisms. In R. Parke & G. Ladd (Eds.), *Family–peer relationships: Modes of linkage* (pp. 135–158). Hillsdale, NJ: Erlbaum.

Copans, S. (1989). The invisible family member: Children in families with alcohol abuse. In L. Combrinck-Graham (Ed.), *Children in family contexts: Perspectives on treatment* (pp. 277–298). New York: Guilford Press.

Covell, K., & Abramovitch, R. (1987). Understanding emotion in the family: Children's and parents' attributions of happiness, sadness, and anger. *Child Development, 58,* 985–991.

Cramer, P. (1991). *The development of defense mechanisms.* New York: Springer Verlag.

Crick, N., & Dodge, K. (1994). A review of social-information processing mechanisms in children's social adjustment. *Psychological Bulletin, 115,* 74–101.

Crittenden, P. (1992). Quality of attachment in the preschool years. *Development and Psychopathology, 4,* 209–241.

Crockenberg, S. (1985). Toddlers' reactions to maternal anger. *Merrill–Palmer Quarterly, 31,* 361–373.

Cummings, E. M., Ballard, M., & El-Sheikh, M. (1991). Responses of children and adolescents to interadult anger as a function of gender, age, and mode of expression. *Merrill–Palmer Quarterly, 37,* 543–560.

Cummings, E. M., Ballard, M., El-Sheikh, M., & Lake, M. (1991). Resolution and children's responses to interadult anger. *Developmental Psychology, 27,* 462–470.

Cummings, E. M., & Davies, P. (1994). *Children and marital conflict.* New York: Guilford Press.

Cummings, E. M., Vogel, D., Cummings, J. S., & El-Sheikh, M. (1989). Children's responses to different forms of expression of anger between adults. *Child Development, 60,* 1392–1404.

Custrini, R., & Feldman, R. S. (1989). Children's social competence and nonverbal encoding and decoding of emotion. *Journal of Child Clinical Psychology, 18,* 336–342.

D'Andrade, R. (1987). A folk model of the mind. In D. Holland & B. N. Quinn (Eds.), *Cultural models inlanguage and thought* (pp. 112–148). New York: Cambridge University Press.

Davies, P., & Cummings, E. M. (1994). Marital conflict and child adjustment: An emotional security hypothesis. *Psychological Bulletin, 116,* 387–411.

Davis, T. (1995). Gender differences in masking negative emotions: Ability or motivation? *Developmental Psychology, 31,* 660–667.

de Lissovoy, V. (1979). Toward the definition of "abuse-provoking child." *Child Abuse and Neglect, 3,* 341–350.

Denham, S., & Auerbach, S. (1995, April). *Mother–child dialogue about emotions and preschoolers' emotional competence.* Paper presented at the biennial meeting of the Society for Research in Child Development, Indianapolis, IN.

Denham, S., & Grout, L. (1993). Socialization of emotion: Pathway to preschoolers' affect regulation. *Journal of Nonverbal Behavior, 17,* 215–227.

Denham, S., McKinley, M., Couchoud, E., & Holt, R. (1990). Emotional and behavioral predictors of preschool peer ratings. *Child Development, 61,* 1145–1152.

Denham, S., Mitchell-Copeland, J., Strandberg, K., Auerbach, S., & Blair, K. (1997). Parental contributions to preschoolers' emotion competence: Direct and indirect effects. *Motivation and Emotion, 21,* 65–86.

Denham, S., Zoller, D., & Couchoud, E. (1994). Preschoolers' causal understanding of emotion and its socialization. *Developmental Psychology, 30,* 928–936.

DePaulo, B. (1991). Nonverbal behavior and self-presentation: A developmental perspective. In R. S. Feldman & B. Rimé (Eds.), *Fundamentals of nonverbal behavior* (pp. 351–397). New York: Cambridge University Press.

DePaulo, B., Kashy, D., Kirkendol, S., Wyer, M., & Epstein, J. (1996). Lying in everyday life. *Journal of Personality and Social Psychology, 70,* 979–995.

Derryberry, D., & Rothbart, M. (1988). Arousal, affect, and attention as components of temperament. *Journal of Personality and Social Psychology, 55,* 958–966.

Dix, T. (1991). The affective organization of parenting: Adaptive and maladaptive processes. *Psychological Bulletin, 110,* 3–25.

Dodge, K. (1986). A social information processing model of social competence in children. In M. Perlmutter (Ed.), *Minnesota Symposium on Child Psychology* (Vol. 18, pp. 77–125). Hillsdale, NJ: Erlbaum.

Dodge, K. (1989). Problems in social relationships. In E. Mash & R. Barkley (Eds.), *Treatment of childhood disorders* (pp. 222–247). New York: Guilford Press.

Donaldson, S., & Westerman, M. (1986). Development of children's understanding of ambivalence and causal theories of emotion. *Developmental Psychology, 22,* 655–662.

Downey, G., & Coyne, J. C. (1990). Children of depressed parents: An integrative review. *Psychological Bulletin, 108,* 50–76.

Dryfoos, J. (1990). *Adolescents at risk: Prevalence and prevention.* New York: Oxford University Press.

Dunn, J. (1988). *The beginnings of social understanding.* Oxford, UK: Basil Blackwell.

Dunn, J., Bretherton, I., & Munn, P. (1987). Conversations about feeling states between mothers and their young children. *Developmental Psychology, 23,* 132–139.

Dunn, J., Brown, J. R., & Beardsall, L. (1991). Family talk about feeling states and children's later understanding of others' emotions. *Developmental Psychology, 27,* 448–455.

Dunn, J., & Brown, J. R. (1991). Relationships, talk about feelings, and the development of affect regulation in early childhood. In J. Garber & K. Dodge (Eds.), *The development of emotion regulation and dysregulation* (pp. 89–108). Cambridge, UK: Cambridge University Press.

Dunn, J., & Brown, J. R. (1994). Affect expression in the family, children's understanding of emotions, and their interactions with others. *Merrill–Palmer Quarterly, 40,* 120–137.

During, S., & McMahon, R. (1991). Recognition of emotional facial expressions by abusive mothers and their children. *Journal of Clinical Child Psychology, 20,* 132–139.

Dutton, D. G. (1998). *The abusive personality: Violence and control in intimate relationships.* New York: Guilford Press.

Eagly, A., & Crowley, M. (1986). Gender and helping behavior: A meta-analytic review of the social psychological literature. *Psychological Bulletin, 100,* 283–308.

Eagly, A., & Steffen, V. (1986). Gender and aggressive behavior: A meta-analytic review of the social–psychological literature. *Psychological Bulletin, 100,* 309–330.

Eder, R. (1994). Comments on children's self-narratives. In U. Neisser & R. Fivush (Eds.), *Emory Symposia in Cognition: Vol. 6. The remembering self: Construction and accuracy in the self-narrative* (pp. 180–190). New York: Cambridge University Press.

Edinger, J., & Patterson, M. L. (1983). Nonverbal involvement and social control. *Psychological Bulletin, 93,* 30–56.

Egeland, B., Carlson, E., & Sroufe, L. A. (1993). Resilience as process. *Development and Psychopathology, 5,* 517–528.

Egeland, B., Jacobvitz, D., & Sroufe, A. (1988). Breaking the cycle of abuse. *Child Development, 59,* 1080–1088.

Edwards, R., Manstead, A., & MacDonald, C. (1984). The relationship between children's sociometric status and ability to recognize facial expressions of emotion. *European Journal of Social Psychology, 14,* 235–238.

Eisenberg, A. R. (1986). Teasing: Verbal play in two Mexicano homes. In B. B. Schieffelin & E. Ochs (Eds.), *Language socialization across cultures* (pp. 182–198). Cambridge, UK: Cambridge University Press.

Eisenberg, N. (Ed.). (1982). *The development of prosocial behavior.* New York: Academic Press.

Eisenberg, N., & Fabes, R. (1991). Prosocial behavior and empathy: A multimethod, developmental perspective. In P. Clark (Ed.), *Review of personality and social psychology* (Vol. 12, pp. 34–61). Newbury Park, CA: Sage.

Eisenberg, N., & Fabes, R. (1992). Emotion, regulation, and the development of social competence. In M. S. Clark (Ed.), *Review of personality and social psychology: Vol. 14. Emotion and social behavior* (pp. 119–150). Newbury Park: CA: Sage.

Eisenberg, N., & Fabes, R. (1998). Prosocial development. In N. Eisenberg (Ed.), *Handbook of child psychology* (5th ed.). *Vol. 3. Social, emotional, and personality development* (pp. 701–778). New York: Wiley.

Eisenberg, N., Fabes, R., Bernzweig, J., Karbon, M., Poulin, R., & Hanish, L. (1993). The relations of emotionality and regulation to preschoolers' social skills and sociometric status. *Child Development, 64,* 1418–1438.

Eisenberg, N., Fabes, R., Carlo, G., & Karbon, M. (1992). Emotional responsivity to others: Behavioral correlates and socialization antecedents. *New Directions for Child Development, 55,* 57–73.

Eisenberg, N., Fabes, R., Carlo, G., Troyer, D., Speer, A., Karbon, M., & Switzer, G. (1992). The relations of maternal practices and characteristics to children's vicarious emotional responsiveness. *Child Development, 63,* 583–602.

Eisenberg, N., Fabes, R., Miller, P. A., Fultz, J., Shell, R., Mathy, R., & Reno, R. (1989). Relation of sympathy and personal distress to prosocial behavior: A multi-method study. *Journal of Personality and Social Psychology, 58,* 55–66.

Eisenberg, N., Fabes, R., Nyman, M., Bernzweig, J., & Pinuelas, A. (1994). The relations of emotionality and regulation to children's anger-related reactions. *Child Development, 65,* 109–128.

Eisenberg, N., Fabes, R., Schaller, M., Carlo, G., & Miller, P. A. (1991). The relations of parental characteristics and practices to children's vicarious emotional responding. *Child Development, 62,* 1393–1408.

Eisenberg, N., & Lennon, R. (1983). Sex differences in empathy and related capacities. *Psychological Bulletin, 94,* 100–131.

Eisenberg, N., & McNally, S. (1993). Socialization and mothers' and adolescents' empathy-related characteristics. *Journal of Research on Adolescence, 3,* 171–191.

Eisenberg, N., & Miller, P. A. (1987). The relation of empathy to prosocial and related behaviors. *Psychological Bulletin, 101,* 91–119.

Eisenberg, N., & Strayer, J. (Eds.). (1987). *Empathy and its development.* New York: Cambridge University Press.

Ekman, P. (1984). Expression and the nature of emotion. In K. Scherer & P. Ekman (Eds.), *Approaches to emotion* (pp. 319–343). Hillsdale, NJ: Erlbaum.

Ekman, P. (1989). The argument and evidence about universals in facial expressions of emotion. In H. Wagner & A. Manstead (Eds.), *Handbook of social psychophysiology* (pp. 143–163). New York: Wiley.

Ekman, P., & Friesen, W. V. (1975). *Unmasking the face.* Englewood Cliffs, NJ: Prentice-Hall.

Ellis, A. (1993). Fundamentals of rational-emotive therapy for the 1990's. In W. Dryden & L. K. Hill (Eds.), *Innovations in rational-emotive therapy* (pp. 1–32). Thousand Oaks, CA: Sage.

Emde, R., Katz, E., & Thorpe, J. (1978). Emotional expression in infancy: II. Early deviations in down syndrome. In M. Lewis & L. Rosenblum (Eds.), *The development of affect* (pp. 352–360). New York: Plenum.

Emery, R. E. (1982). Interparental conflict and the children of discord and divorce. *Psychological Bulletin, 92,* 310–330.

Emery, R. E. (1988). *Marriage, divorce, and children's adjustment.* London: Sage.

Emery, R. E. (1989). Family violence. *American Psychologist, 44,* 321–328.

Erikson, E. H. (1968). *Identity, youth, and crisis.* New York: Norton.

Fabes, R., Eisenberg, N., & Miller, P. A. (1990). Maternal correlates of children's vicarious emotional responsiveness. *Developmental Psychology, 26,* 639–648.

Fabes, R., Eisenberg, N., Smith, M., & Murphy, B. (1996). Getting angry at peers: Associations with liking of the provocateur. *Child Development, 67,* 942–956.

Feinman, S. (1985). Emotional expression, social referencing, and preparedness for learning in early infancy—mother knows best, but sometimes I know better. In G. Zivin (Ed.), *The development of expressive behavior* (pp. 291–315). New York: Academic Press.

Feinman, S., & Lewis, M. (1983). Social referencing at ten months: A second order effect on infants' responses to strangers. *Child Development, 54,* 878–887.

Feiring, C., Taska, L., & Lewis, M. (1996). A process model for understanding adaptation to sexual abuse: The role of shame in defining stigmatization. *Child Abuse and Neglect, 20,* 767–782.

Feist, G., Bodner, T., Jacobs, J., Miles, M., & Tan, V. (1995). Integrating top-down and bottom-up structural models of subjective well-being: A longitudinal investigation. *Journal of Personality and Social Psychology, 68,* 138–150.

Feldman, R. S., Jenkins, L., & Popoola, O. (1979). Detection of deception in adults and children via facial expressions. *Child Development, 50,* 350–355.

Feldman, R. S., Philippot, P., & Custrini, R. (1991). Social competence and nonverbal behavior. In R. S. Feldman & B. Rimé (Eds.), *Fundamentals of nonverbal behavior* (pp. 329–350). New York: Cambridge University Press.

Feldman, R. S., White, J. B., & Lobato, D. (1982). Social skills and nonverbal behavior. In R. S. Feldman (Ed.), *Development of nonverbal behavior in children* (pp. 259–277). New York: Springer Verlag.

Felsman, J. K., & Vaillant, G. (1987). Resilient children as adults: A 40-year study. In E. J. Anthony & B. Cohler (Eds.), *The invulnerable child* (pp. 289–314). New York: Guilford Press.

Fendrich, M., Warner, V., & Weissman, M. M. (1990). Family risk factors, parental depression and childhood psychopathology. *Developmental Psychology, 26,* 40–50.

Ferguson, T., & Stegge, H. (1995). Emotional states and traits in children: The case of guilt and shame. In J. P. Tangney & K. W. Fischer (Eds.), *Self-conscious emotions: The psychology of shame, guilt, embarrassment, and pride* (pp. 174–197). New York: Guilford Press.

Ferguson, T., Stegge, H., & Damhuis, I. (1991). Children's understanding of guilt and shame. *Child Development, 62,* 827–839.

Fernald, A. (1993). Approval and disapproval: Infant responsiveness to vocal affect in familiar and unfamiliar languages. *Child Development, 64,* 657–674.

Feshbach, N. (1989). The construct of empathy and the phenomenon of physical maltreatment of children. In D. Cicchetti & V. Carlson (Eds.), *Child maltreatment* (pp. 349–373). New York: Cambridge University Press.

Fischer, K. W., & Ayoub, C. (1993). Affective splitting and dissociation in normal and maltreated children: Developmental pathways for self in relationships. In D. Cicchetti & S. Toth (Eds.), *Rochester Symposium on Developmental Psychopathology: Vol. 5. Disorders and dysfunctions of the self* (pp. 149–222). Rochester, NY: University of Rochester Press.

Fischer, K. W., Shaver, P., & Carnochan, P. (1989). From basic- to subordinate-category emotions: A skill approach to emotional development. In W. Damon (Ed.), *Child development today and tomorrow* (pp. 107–136). San Francisco: Jossey-Bass.

Fischer, K. W., Shaver, P., & Carnochan, P. (1990). How emotions develop and how they organize development. *Cognition and Emotion, 4,* 81–127.

Fivush, R. (1991). The social construction of personal narratives. *Merrill–Palmer Quarterly, 37,* 59–82.

Flanagan, O. (1991). *Varieties of moral personality: Ethics and psychological realism.* Cambridge, MA: Harvard University Press.

Fox, N., Sobel, A., Calkins, S., & Cole, P. (1996). Inhibited children talk about themselves: Self-reflection on personality development and change in 7-year-olds. In M. Lewis & M. W. Sullivan (Eds.), *Emotional development in atypical children* (pp. 131–14). Mahwah, NJ: Erlbaum.

Freud, A. (1965). *Normality and pathology in childhood: Assessments of development.* New York: International Universities Press.

Fridlund, A. (1991). Evolution and facial action in reflect, social motive, and paralanguage. *Biological Psychology, 32,* 3–100.

Friedrich, W., & Reams, R. (1987). Course of psychological symptoms in sexually abused young children. *Psychotherapy, 24,* 160–170.

Frijda, N. (1986). *The emotions.* Cambridge, UK: Cambridge University Press.

Frijda, N. (1987). Emotion, cognitive structure, and action tendency. *Cognition and Emotion, 1,* 115–143.

Frijda, N., & Mesquita, B. (1994). The social roles and functions of emotion. In S. Kitayama & H. Marcus (Eds.), *Emotion and culture* (pp. 51–87). Washington, DC: American Psychological Association.

Fruzzetti, A., & Jacobson, N. (1990). Toward a behavioral conceptualization of adult intimacy: Implications for marital therapy. In E. Blechman (Ed.), *Emotions and the family: For better or for worse* (pp. 117–135). Hillsdale, NJ: Erlbaum.

Fuchs, D., & Thelen, M. (1988). Children's expected interpersonal consequences of communicating their affective states and reported likelihood of expression. *Child Development, 59,* 1314–1322.

Gaensbauer, T., Mrazek, D., & Harmon, R. (1981). Emotional expression in abused and/or neglected infants. In N. Frude (Ed.), *Psychological approaches to child abuse* (pp. 120–135). Totowa, NJ: Rowman & Littlefield.

Gaensbauer, T., & Sands, K. (1979). Distorted affective communications in abused/neglected infants and their potential impact on caretakers. *American Journal of Child Psychiatry, 18,* 236–250.

Garbarino, J., Dubrow, N., Kostelny, K., & Pardo, C. (1992). *Children in danger.* San Francisco: Jossey-Bass.

Garber, J., Braafladt, N., & Weiss, B. (1995). Affect regulation in depressed and nondepressed children and young adolescents. *Development and Psychopathology, 7,* 93–115.

Garber, J., Braafladt, N., & Zeman, J. (1991). The regulation of sad affect: An information-processing perspective. In J. Garber & K. Dodge (Eds.), *The development of emotion regulation and dysregulation* (pp. 208–240). New York: Cambridge University Press.

Garber, J., & Dodge, K. (Eds.). (1991). *The development of emotion regulation and dysregulation.* New York: Cambridge University Press.

Gardner, D., Harris, P. L., Ohmoto, M., & Hamazaki, T. (1988). Japanese children's understanding of the distinction between real and apparent emotion. *International Journal of Behavioral Development, 11,* 203–218.

Garmezy, N. (1993). Children in poverty: Resilience despite risk. *Psychiatry, 56,* 127–136.

Garmezy, N., & Rutter, M. (Eds.). (1983). *Stress, coping, and development in children.* New York: McGraw-Hill.

Garner, P. (1996). The relations of emotional role taking, affective/moral attributions, and emotional display rule knowledge to low-income school-age children's social competence. *Journal of Applied Developmental Psychology, 17,* 19–36.

Gelinas, D. (1983). The persisting negative effects of incest. *Psychiatry, 46,* 312–332.

George, C., Kaplan, N., & Main, M. (1985). *The Attachment Interview for Adults.* Unpublished manuscript, University of California, Berkeley.

Gergen, K. J. (1990). Social understanding and the inscription of self. In J. Stigler, R. Shweder, & G. Herdt (Eds.), *Cultural psychology: Essays on comparative human development* (pp. 569–606). Cambridge, UK: Cambridge University Press.

Gibbs, J. C. (1991). Sociomoral developmental delay and cognitive distortion: Implications for the treatment of antisocial youth. In W. Kurtines & J. Gewirtz (Eds.), *Handbook of moral behavior and development* (Vol. 3, pp. 95–110). Hillsdale, NJ: Erlbaum.

Gibson, E. J. (1982). The concept of affordance in development: The renascence of functionalism. In A. W. Collins (Ed.), *Minnesota Symposium on Child Psychology: Vol. 13. Theoretical perspectives on development* (pp. 55–81). Hillsdale, NJ: Erlbaum.

Gilligan, C. (1982). *In a different voice: Psychological theory and women's development.* Cambridge, MA: Harvard University Press.

Glasberg, R., & Aboud, F. (1982). Keeping one's distance from sadness: Children's self-reports of emotional experience. *Developmental Psychology, 18,* 287–293.

Glass, L. (1992). *He says, she says: Closing the communication gap between the sexes.* New York: Putnam.

Gnepp, J. (1989a). Children's use of personal information to understand other people's feelings. In C. Saarni & P. L. Harris (Eds.), *Children's understanding of emotion* (pp. 151–180). New York: Cambridge University Press.

Gnepp, J. (1989b). Personalized inferences of emotions and appraisals: Component processes and correlates. *Developmental Psychology, 25,* 277–288.

Gnepp, J., & Chilamkurti, C. (1988). Children's use of personality attributions to predict other people's emotional and behavioral reactions. *Child Development, 59,* 743–754.

Gnepp, J., & Gould, M. E. (1985). The development of personalized inferences: Understanding other people's emotional reactions in light of their prior experiences. *Child Development, 56,* 1455–1464.

Goffman, E. (1967). *Interaction ritual.* Chicago: Aldine.

Goldsmith, H., & Campos, J. (1982). Toward a theory of infant temperament. In. R. Emde & R. Harmon (Eds.), *The development of attachment and affiliative systems: Psychobiological aspects* (pp. 161–193). New York: Plenum.

Goleman, D. (1995). *Emotional intelligence.* New York: Bantam.

Goleman, D. (1997). Foreword: Emotional intelligence in context. In P. Salovey & D. Sluyter (Eds.), *Emotional development and emotional intelligence* (pp. xiii–xvi). New York: Basic Books.

Gollwitzer, P., & Kinney, R. (1989). Effects of deliberative and implemental mindsets on illusion of control. *Journal of Personality and Social Psychology, 56,* 5331–542.

Golombok, S., & Fivush, R. (1994). *Gender development.* New York: Cambridge University Press.

Goodman, S., Brogan, D., Lynch, M., & Fielding, B. (1993). Social and emotional competence in children of depressed mothers. *Child Development, 64,* 516–531.

Goodwin, J., McCarthy, T., & DiVasto, P. (1981). Prior incest in mothers of sexually abused children. *Child Abuse and Neglect, 5,* 87–96.

Gordon, S. L. (1989). The socialization of children's emotions: Emotional culture, competence, and exposure. In C. Saarni & P. L. Harris (Eds.), *Children's understanding of emotion* (pp. 319–349). New York: Cambridge University Press.

Gottman, J. (1983). How children become friends. *Monographs of the Society for Research in Child Development, 44*(3, Serial No. 201), 1–72.

Gottman, J., & Katz, L. F. (1989). Effects of marital discord on young children's peer interaction and health. *Developmental Psychology, 25,* 373–381.

Gottman, J., Katz, L. F., & Hooven, C. (1997). *Meta-emotion.* Hillsdale, NJ: Erlbaum.

Gottman, J., & Levenson, R. W. (1992). Marital processes predictive of later dissolution: Behavior, physiological and health. *Journal of Personality and Social Psychology, 63,* 221–233.

Gottman, J., & Porterfield, A. (1981). Communicative competence in the nonverbal behavior of married couples. *Journal of Marriage and the Family, 43,* 817–824.

Graham, S., Doubleday, C., & Guarino, P. (1984). The development of relations between perceived controllability and the emotions pity, anger, and guilt. *Child Development, 55,* 561–565.

Graham, S., & Weiner, B. (1986). From an attributional theory of emotion to developmental psychology: A round-trip ticket? Special Issue: Developmental perspectives on social-cognitive theories. *Social Cognition, 4*(2), 152–179.

Graham-Bermann, S. (1997). Family worries: Assessment of interpersonal anxiety in children from violent and non-violent families. *Journal of Clinical Child Psychology, 25,* 280–287.

Gray, J. (1992). *Men are from Mars, women are from Venus: A practical guide for improving communication and getting what you want in your relationships.* New York: HarperCollins.

Greenberg, L., & Johnson, S. (1990). Emotional change processes in couples therapy. In E. Blechman (Ed.), *Emotions and the family: For better or for worse* (pp. 137–153). Hillsdale, NJ: Erlbaum.

Greenberg, M. T., & Snell, J. (1997). Brain development and emotional development: The role of teaching in organizing the frontal lobe. In P. Salovey & D. Sluyter (Eds.), *Emotional development and emotional intelligence* (pp. 93–119). New York: Basic Books.

Greenberg, M. T., & Kusché, C. (1993). *Promoting social and emotional development in deaf children: The PATHS project.* Seattle: University of Washington Press.

Greenberg, M. T., Kusché, C., Cook, E., & Quamma, J. (1995). Promoting emotional competence in school-aged children: The effects of the PATHS curriculum. *Development and Psychopathology, 7,* 117–136.

Gross, A. L., & Bailif, B. (1991). Children's understanding of emotion from facial expressions and situations: A review. *Developmental Review, 11,* 368–398.

Gross, D., & Harris, P. L. (1988). False beliefs about emotions: Children's understanding of misleading emotional displays. *International Journal of Behavioral Development, 11,* 475–488.

Gross, J. J. (1998). Antecedent and response-focused emotion regulation: Divergent consequences for expression, experience, and physiology. *Journal of Personality and Social Psychology, 74,* 224–237.

Gross, J. J., & John, O. P. (1997). Revealing feelings: Facets of emotional expressivity in self-reports, peer ratings, and behavior. *Journal of Personality and Social Psychology, 72,* 435–448.

Grynch, J., & Fincham, F. (1990). Marital conflict and children's adjustment: A cognitive–contextual framework. *Psychological Bulletin, 108,* 267–290.

Haan, N. (1991). Moral development and action from a social constructivist perspective. In W. Kurtines & J. Gewirtz (Eds.), *Handbook of moral behavior and development* (Vol. 1, pp. 251–273). Hillsdale, NJ: Erlbaum.

Haden, C., Haine, R., & Fivush, R. (1997). Developing narrative structure in parent–child reminiscing across the preschool years. *Developmental Psychology,* *33,* 295–307.

Halberstadt, A. G. (1991). Toward an ecology of expressiveness: Family Socialization in particular and a model in general. In R. S. Feldman & B. Rimé (Eds.), *Fundamentals of nonverbal behavior* (pp. 106–160). New York: Cambridge University Press.

Hall, J. A. (1984). *Nonverbal sex differences: Communication accuracy and expressive style.* Baltimore: Johns Hopkins University Press.

Hardy, D., Power, T., & Jaedicke, S. (1993). Examining the relation of parenting to children's coping with everyday stress. *Child Development, 64,* 1829–1841.

Harkness, S., & Super, C. (1985). Child-environment interactions in the socialization of affect. In M. Lewis & C. Saarni (Eds.), *The socialization of emotions* (pp. 21–36). New York: Plenum.

Harris, G. (1978). *Casting out anger.* Cambridge, UK: Cambridge University Press.

Harris, L. M., Gergen, K. J., & Lannamann, J. (1986). Aggression rituals. *Communication Monographs, 53,* 252–265.

Harris, P. L. (1985). What children know about the situations that provoke emotion. In M. Lewis & C. Saarni (Eds.), *The socialization of emotions* (pp. 161–185). New York: Plenum.

Harris, P. L. (1989). *Children and emotion: The development of psychological understanding.* Oxford, UK: Basil Blackwell.

Harris, P. L. (1995). Children's awareness and lack of awareness of mind and emotion. In D. Cicchetti & S. Toth (Eds.), *Rochester Symposium on Developmental Psychopathology: Vol. 6. Emotion, cognition, and representation* (pp. 35–57). Rochester, NY: University of Rochester Press.

Harris, P. L., & Gross, D. (1988). Children's understanding of real and apparent emotion. In J. W. Astington, P. L. Harris, & D. R. Olson (Eds.), *Developing theories of mind* (pp. 295–314). Cambridge, UK: Cambridge University Press.

Harris, P. L., Guz, G., & Lipian, M. S. (1985). *Thoughts and feelings. Insight into their time-course and mutual influence.* Unpublished manuscript, Department of Experimental Psychology, University of Oxford, Oxford, UK.

Harris, P. L., Guz, G., Lipian, M. S., & Man-Shu, Z. (1985). Insight into the time-course of emotion among Western and Chinese children. *Child Development, 56,* 972–988.

Harris, P. L., Johnson, C., Hutton, D., Andrews, G., & Cooke, T. (1989). Young children's theory of mind and emotion. *Cognition and Emotion, 3,* 379–401.

Harris, P. L., & Lipian, M. S. (1989). Understanding emotion and experiencing emotion. In C. Saarni & P. L. Harris (Eds.), *Children's understanding of emotion* (pp. 241–258). New York: Cambridge University Press.

Harris, P. L., & Olthof, T. (1982). The child's concept of emotion. In G. Butterworth & P. Light (Eds.), *Social cognition* (pp. 188–209). Brighton, Sussex, UK: Harvester Press.

Harris, P. L., Olthof, T., & Meerum Terwogt, M. (1981). Children's knowledge of emotion. *Journal of Child Psychology and Psychiatry and Allied Disciplines, 22,* 247–261.

Hart, C. H., Ladd, G., & Burleson, B. (1990). Children's expectations of the outcomes of social strategies: Relations with sociometric status and maternal disciplinary styles. *Child Development, 61,* 127–137.

Harter, S. (1978). Effectance motivation reconsidered: Toward a developmental model. *Human Development, 21,* 34–64.

Harter, S. (1982). Children's understanding of multiple emotions: A cognitive developmental approach. In W. Overton (Ed.), *The relationship between social and cognitive development* (pp. 147–194). Hillsdale, NJ: Erlbaum.

Harter, S. (1986a). Cognitive-developmental processes in the integration of concepts about emotions and the self. *Social Cognition, 4,* 119–151.

Harter, S. (1986b). Processes underlying the construction, maintenance, and enhancement of the self-concept in children. In J. Suls & A. Greenwald (Eds.), *Psychological perspectives on the self* (Vol. 3, pp. 137–181). Hillsdale, NJ: Erlbaum.

Harter, S. (1987). The determinants and mediational role of global self-worth in children. In N. Eisenberg (Ed.), *Contemporary issues in developmental psychology* (pp. 219–242). New York: Wiley.

Harter, S. (1990). Developmental differences in the nature of self-representations: Implications for the understanding, assessment, and treatment of maladaptive behavior. *Cognitive Therapy and Research, 14,* 113–142.

Harter, S. (1998). The development of self-representations. In N. Eisenberg (Ed.), *Handbook of child psychology* (5th ed.): *Vol. 3. Social, emotional, and personality development* (pp. 553–617). New York: Wiley.

Harter, S., & Buddin, B. (1987). Children's understanding of the simultaneity of two emotions: A five-stage developmental acquisition sequence. *Developmental Psychology, 23,* 388–399.

Harter, S., & Lee, L. (1989, April). *Manifestations of true and not true selves in adolescents.* Paper presented at the biennial meeting of the Society for Research in Child Development, Kansas City, MO.

Harter, S., Marold, D., Whitesell, N. R., & Cobbs, G. (1996). A model of the effects of parent and peer support on adolescent false self behavior. *Child Development, 67,* 360–374.

Harter, S., & Whitesell, N. R. (1989). Developmental changes in children's understanding of single, multiple, and blended emotion concepts. In C. Saarni & P. L. Harris (Eds.), *Children's understanding of emotion* (pp. 81–116). New York: Cambridge University Press.

Hartup, W., Laursen, B., Stewart, M. I., & Eastenson, A. (1988). Conflict and the friendship relations of young children. *Child Development, 59,* 1590–1600.

Hatfield, E., Cacioppo, J., & Rapson, R. (1994). *Emotional contagion.* Cambridge, UK: Cambridge University Press.

Haviland, J., & Lelwicka, M. (1987). The induced affect response: 10-week-old infants' responses to three emotional expressions. *Developmental Psychology, 23,* 97–104.

Hazan, C., & Shaver, P. (1994). Attachment as an organizational framework for research on close relationships. *Psychological Inquiry, 5,* 1–22.

Heckhausen, H. (1987). Emotional components of action: Their ontogeny as reflected in achievement behavior. In D. Gorlitz & J. Wohlwill (Eds.), *Curiosity, imagination, and play: On the development of spontaneous cognitive and motivational processes* (pp. 326–348). Hillsdale, NJ: Erlbaum.

Hermans, H., & Kempen, H. (1993). *The dialogical self.* San Diego, CA: Academic Press.

Herrera, C., & Dunn, J. (1997). Early experiences with family conflict: Implications for arguments with a close friend. *Developmental Psychology, 33,* 869–881.

Higgins, E. T. (1991). Development of self-regulatory and self- evaluative processes: Costs, benefits, and tradeoffs. In M. R. Gunnar & L. A. Sroufe (Eds.), *Minnesota Symposia on Child Psychology: Vol. 23. Self processes and development* (pp. 125–165). Hillsdale, NJ: Erlbaum.

Higgins, E. T., Loeb, I., & Moretti, M. (1995). Self- discrepancies and developmental shifts in vulnerability: Life transitions in the regulatory significance of others. In D. Cicchetti & S. Toth (Eds.), *Rochester Symposium on Developmental Psychopathology: Vol. 6. Emotion, cognition, and representation* (pp. 191–230). Rochester, NY: University of Rochester Press.

Hobson, R. (1986). The autistic child's appraisal of expressions of emotion. *Journal of Child Psychology and Psychiatry, 27,* 321–342.

Hochschild, A. (1983). *The managed heart: Commercialization of human feeling.* Berkeley: University of California Press.

Hoffman, M. L. (1977). Empathy: Its development and prosocial implications. In B. Keasey (Ed.), *Nebraska Symposium on Motivation* (Vol. 26). Lincoln: University of Nebraska Press.

Hoffman, M. L. (1978). Toward a theory of empathic arousal and development. In M. Lewis & L. Rosenblum (Eds.), *The development of affect* (pp. 227–256). New York: Plenum.

Hoffman, M. L. (1982). Development of prosocial motivation: Empathy and guilt. In N. Eisenberg (Ed.), *Development of prosocial behavior* (pp. 281–313). New York: Academic Press.

Hoffman-Plotkin, D., & Twentyman, C. (1984). A multimodal assessment of behavioral and cognitive deficits in abused and neglected preschoolers. *Child Development, 55,* 795–802.

Hoffner, C., & Badzinski, D. (1989). Children's integration of facial and situational cues to emotion. *Child Development, 60,* 411–422.

Hofstede, G. (1991). *Cultures and organization: Software of the mind.* London: McGraw-Hill.

Holderness, C., Brooks-Gunn, J., & Warren, M. (1994). Comorbidity of eating disorders and substance abuse: Review of the literature. *International Journal of Eating Disorders, 16,* 1–34.

Holland, D., & Kipnis, A. (1995). American cultural models of embarrassment. In J. A. Russell, J. Fernandez-Dols, A. Manstead, & J. Wellenkamp (Eds.), *Everyday conceptions of emotion: An introduction to the psychology, anthropology and linguistics of emotion* (pp. 181–202). Hingham, MA: Kluwer.

Horney, K. (1950). *Neurosis and human growth.* New York: Norton.

Hubbard, J. (1995, April). *Emotion expression, emotion awareness, and goal orientation: The role of sociometric status, aggression, and gender.* Paper presented at the biennial meeting of the Society for Research in Child Development, Indianapolis, IN.

Hubbard, J., & Coie, J. (1994). Emotional correlates of social competence in children's peer relationships. *Merrill–Palmer Quarterly, 40,* 1–20.

Hudson, J., Gebelt, J., Haviland, J., & Bentivegna, C. (1992). Emotion and narrative structure in young children's personal accounts. *Journal of Narrative and Life History, 2,* 129–150.

Hunt, J. McV. (1965). Intrinsic motivation and its role in psychological development. In D. Levine (Ed.), *Nebraska Symposium on Motivation* (pp. 189–282). Lincoln: University of Nebraska Press.

Hymel, S., Wagner, E., & Butler, L. (1990). Reputational bias: View from the peer group. In S. Asher & J. Coie (Eds.), *Peer rejection in childhood* (pp. 156–186). New York: Cambridge University Press.

Izard, C. (1993). Organizational and motivational functions of discrete emotions. In M. Lewis & J. Haviland (Eds.), *Handbook of emotions* (pp. 631–641). New York: Guilford Press.

Izard, C., & Malatesta, C. (1987). Perspectives on emotional development: I. Differential emotions theory of early emotional development. In J. Osofsky (Ed.), *Handbook of infant development* (2nd ed., pp. 494–554). New York: Wiley.

James, B. (1994). *Handbook for treatment of attachment–trauma problems in children.* New York: Lexington Books.

James, W. (1892). *Psychology: The briefer course.* New York: Holt, Rinehart & Winston.

Janoff-Bulman, R. (1979). Characterological versus behavioral self-blame: Inquiries into depression and rape. *Journal of Personality and Social Psychology, 37,* 1798–1809.

Jenkins, J. M., & Smith, M. A. (1993). A prospective study of behavioural disturbance in children who subsequently experience parental divorce: A research note. *Journal of Divorce and Remarriage, 19,* 143–160.

Jones, S., Collins, K., & Hong, H. (1991). An audience effect on smile productions in 10 month old infants. *Psychological Science, 2*(1), 45–49.

Josephs, I. (1993). *The regulation of emotional expression in preschool children.* Munster, Germany/New York: Waxmann.

Joshi, M. S., & MacLean, M. (1994). Indian and English children's understanding of the distinction between real and apparent emotion. *Child Development, 65,* 1372–1384.

Karasek, R., & Theorell, T. (1990). *Healthy work: Stress, productivity, and the reconstruction of working life.* New York: Basic Books.

Karniol, R., & Koren, L. (1987). How would you feel? Children's inferences regarding their own and others' affective reactions. *Cognitive Development, 2,* 271–278.

Kasari, C., & Sigman, M. (1996). Expression and understanding of emotion in atypical development: Autism and Down Syndrome. In M. Lewis & M. W. Sullivan (Eds.), *Emotional development in atypical children* (pp. 109–130). Mahwah, NJ: Erlbaum.

Kaslow, N., Rehm, L., & Siegel, A. (1984). Social cognitive and cognitive correlates of depression in children. *Journal of Child Psychology, 12,* 605–620.

Katz, L. F., & Gottman, J. (1993). Patterns of marital conflict predict children's internalizing and externalizing behaviors. *Developmental Psychology, 29,* 940–950.

Katz, L. F., & Gottman, J. (1997). Buffering children from marital conflict and dissolution. *Journal of Clinical Child Psychology, 26,* 157–171.

Kernis, M. (1993). The roles of stability and level of self-esteem in psychological functioning. In R. Baumeister (Ed.), *Self-esteem: The puzzle of low self-regard* (pp. 167–182). New York: Plenum.

Kitayama, S., & Markus, H. (1994). Introduction to cultural psychology and emotion research. In S. Kitayama & H. Markus (Eds.), *Emotion and culture* (pp. 1–19). Washington, DC: American Psychological Association.

Kitayama, S., Markus, H., & Matsumoto, H. (1995). Culture, self, and emotion: A cultural perspective on "self-conscious" emotions. In J. P. Tangney & K. W. Fischer (Eds.), *Self-conscious emotions: The psychology of shame, guilt, embarrassment, and pride* (pp. 439–464). New York: Guilford Press.

Kliewer, W. (1991). Coping in middle childhood: Relations to competence, Type A behavior, monitoring, blunting, and locus of control. *Developmental Psychology, 27,* 689–697.

Klimes-Dougan, B., & Kistner, J. (1990). Physically abused preschoolers' responses to peers' distress. *Developmental Psychology, 26,* 599–602.

Kobak, R., & Sceery, A. (1988). Attachment in late adolescence: Working models, affect regulation, and representations of self and others. *Child Development, 59,* 135–146.

Koestner, R., Franz, C., & Weinberger, J. (1990). The family origins of empathic concern: A 26-year longitudinal study. *Journal of Personality and Social Psychology, 58,* 709–717.

Konner, M. (1972). Aspects of the developmental ethology of a foraging people. In N. Blurton-Jones (Ed.), *Ethological studies of child behavior* (pp. 285–304). Cambridge, UK: Cambridge University Press.

Kopp, C. (1982). Antecedents of self-regulation: A developmental perspective. *Developmental Psychology, 18,* 199–214.

Kopp, C. (1989). Regulation of distress and negative emotions: A developmental view. *Developmental Psychology, 25,* 343–354.

Kopp, C. (1992). Emotional distress and control in young children. In N. Eisenberg & R. Fabes (Eds.), *New Directions for Child Development: Vol. 55. Emotion and its regulation in early development* (pp. 41–56). San Francisco: Jossey-Bass.

Kopp, C. (1997). Young children: Emotion management, instrumental control, and plans. In S. Friedman & E. Scholnick (Eds.), *The developmental psychology of planning: Why, now, and when do we plan* (pp. 103–124). Mahwah, NJ: Erlbaum.

Kopp, C., & Wyer, N. (1994). Self-regulation in normal and atypical development. In D. Cicchetti & S. Toth (Eds.), *Rochester Smposium on Developmental Psychopathology: Vol. 5. Disorders and dysfunctions of the self* (pp. 31–56). Rochester, NY: University of Rochester Press.

Koss, M., Goodman, L., Fitzgerald, L., Russo, N., Keita, G., & Browne, A. (1994).

No safe haven: Male violence against women at home, at work, and in the community. Washington, DC: American Psychological Association.

Kovacs, M. (1980). Rating scales to assess depression in school-aged children. *Acta Paedopsychiatrica, 46,* 305–315.

Kraut, R., & Johnson, R. (1979). Social and emotional messages of smiling: An ethological approach. *Journal of Personality and Social Psychology, 37,* 1539–1553.

Krevans, J., & Gibbs, J. (1996). Parents' use of inductive discipline: Relations to children's use of empathy and prosocial behavior. *Child Development, 67,* 3263–3277.

Krystal, H. (1988). *Integration and self-healing: Affect, trauma, alexithymia.* Hillsdale, NJ: Analytic Press.

Kurtines, W., & Gewirtz, J. (Eds.). (1991). *Handbook of moral behavior and development: Vol. 1. Theory; Vol. 2. Research; Vol. 3: Application.* Hillsdale, NJ: Erlbaum.

Kurtines, W., & Gewirtz, J. (Eds.). (1996). *Moral development: An introduction.* Boston: Allyn & Bacon.

Kusché, C. (1984). *The understanding of emotion concepts by deaf children: An assessment of an affective education curriculum.* Unpublished doctoral dissertation, University of Washington.

Ladd, G. W. (1992). Themes and theories: Perspectives on processes in family–peer relationships. In R. Parke & G. Ladd (Eds.), *Family–peer relationships: Modes of linkage* (pp. 3–34). Hillsdale, NJ: Erlbaum.

Ladd, G. W., & Le Sieur, K. (1995). Parents' and children's peer relationships. In M. Bornstein (Ed.), *Handbook of parenting* (pp. 377–409). Mahwah, NJ: Erlbaum.

Laux, L. (1986). A self-presentational view of coping with stress. In M. Trumbull & R. Appley (Eds.), *The dynamics of stress* (pp. 233–253). New York: Plenum.

Laux, L., & Weber, H. (1991). Presentation of self in coping with anger and anxiety: An intentional approach. *Anxiety Research, 3,* 233–255.

Lazarus, R. S. (1991). *Emotion and adaptation.* New York: Oxford University Press.

Lazarus, R. S., & Folkman, S. (1984). *Stress, appraisal, and coping.* New York: Springer Verlag.

Lazarus, R. S., & Launier, R. (1978). Stress-related transactions between person and environment. In L. A. Pervin & M. Lewis (Eds.), *Perspectives in interactional psychology* (pp. 287–327). New York: Plenum Press.

Lemerise, E., & Dodge, K. (1993). The development of anger and hostile interactions. In M. Lewis & J. Haviland (Eds.), *Handbook of emotions* (pp. 537–546). New York: Guilford Press.

Lennon, R., & Eisenberg, N. (1987). Gender and age differences in empathy and sympathy. In N. Eisenberg & J. Strayer (Eds.), *Empathy and its development* (pp. 195–217). New York: Cambridge University Press.

Levenson, R. W., Ekman, P., Friesen, W. V. (1990). Voluntary facial action generates emotion-specific autonomic nervous system activity. *Psychophysiology, 27,* 363–385.

Levine, L. (1995). Young children's understanding of the causes of anger and stress. *Child Development, 66,* 697–709.

Lewis, C. (1986). Children's social development in Japan: Research directions. In H. Stevenson, H. Azuma, & K. Hakuta (Eds.), *Child development and education in Japan* (pp. 186–200). New York: Freeman.

Lewis, M. (1989). Cultural differences in children's knowledge of emotional scripts. In C. Saarni & P. Harris (Eds.), *Children's understanding of emotion* (pp. 350–374). New York: Cambridge University Press.

Lewis, M. (1991). Ways of knowing: Objective self awareness or consciousness. *Developmental Review, 11,* 231–243.

Lewis, M. (1992a). The role of the self in social behavior. In F. Kessel, P. M. Cole, & D. Johnson (Eds.), *Self and consciousness: Multiple perspectives* (pp. 19–44).

Lewis, M. (1992b). *Shame: The exposed self.* New York: Free Press.

Lewis, M. (1993a). Self-conscious emotions: Embarrassment, pride, shame, and guilt. In M. Lewis & J. Haviland (Eds.), *Handbook of emotions* (pp. 563–573). New York: Guilford Press.

Lewis, M. (1993b). The emergence of human emotion. In M. Lewis & J. Haviland (Eds.), *Handbook of emotions* (pp. 223–235). New York: Guilford Press.

Lewis, M. (1995). Embarrassment: The emotion of self-exposure and evaluation. In J. P. Tangney & K. W. Fischer (Eds.), *Self-conscious emotions: The psychology of shame, guilt, embarrassment, and pride* (pp. 198–218). New York: Guilford Press.

Lewis, M. (1997). *Altering fate: Why the past does not predict the future.* New York: Guilford Press.

Lewis, M., Alessandri, S., & Sullivan, M. (1990). Expectancy, loss of control and anger in young infants. *Developmental Psychology, 25,* 745–751.

Lewis, M., Alessandri, S., & Sullivan, M. (1992). Differences in shame and pride as a function of children's gender and task difficulty. *Child Development, 63,* 630–638.

Lewis, M., & Bendersky, M. (Eds.). (1995). *Mothers, babies, and cocaine: The role of toxins in development.* Hillsdale, NJ: Erlbaum.

Lewis, M., & Brooks, J. (1978). Self-knowledge and emotional development. In M. Lewis & L. Rosenblum (Eds.), *The development of affect* (pp. 205–226). New York: Plenum.

Lewis, M., & Michalson, L. (1983). *Children's emotions and moods: Developmental theory and measurement.* New York: Plenum.

Lewis, M., & Michalson, L. (1985). Faces as signs and symbols. In G. Zivin (Ed.), *The development of expressive behavior: Biology–environment interactions* (pp. 153–180). New York: Academic Press.

Lewis, M., & Miller, S. M. (Eds.). (1990). *Handbook of developmental psychopathology.* New York: Plenum.

Lewis, M., & Saarni, C. (Eds.). (1985). *The socialization of emotions.* New York: Plenum Press.

Lewis, M., Stanger, C., & Sullivan, M. (1989). Deception in three-year-olds. *Developmental Psychology, 25,* 439–443.

Lewis, M., Sullivan, M., Stanger, C., & Weiss, M. (1989). Self-development and self-conscious emotions. *Child Development, 60,* 146–156.

Lewis, M., Sullivan, M., & Vasen, A. (1987). Making faces: Age and emotion differences in the posing of emotional expressions. *Developmental Psychology, 23,* 690–697.

Lindahl, K., & Markman, H. (1990). Communication and negative affect regulation in the family. In E. Blechman (Ed.), *Emotions and the family: For better or for worse* (pp. 99–115). Hillsdale, NJ: Erlbaum.

Long, P., & Jackson, J. (1993). Childhood coping strategies and the adult adjustment of female sexual abuse victims. *Journal of Child Sexual Abuse, 2,* 23–39.

Lutz, C. (1983). Parental goals, ethnopsychology, and the development of emotional meaning. *Ethos, 11,* 246–262.

Lutz, C. (1985). Cultural patterns and individual differences in the child's emotional meaning system. In M. Lewis & C. Saarni (Eds.), *The socialization of emotions* (pp. 37–53). New York: Plenum.

Lutz, C. (1987). Goals, events, and understanding in Ifaluk emotion theory. In D. Holland & N. Quinn (Eds.), *Cultural models in language and thought* (pp. 290–312). Cambridge, UK: Cambridge University Press.

Lutz, C. (1988). Ethnographic perspectives on the emotion lexicon. In V. Hamilton, G. H. Bower, & N. Frijda (Eds.), *Cognitive perspectives on emotion and motivation* (pp. 399–419). Norwell, MA: Kluwer Academic.

Lutz, C., & White, G. M. (1986). The anthropology of emotions. *Annual Review of Anthropology, 15,* 405–436.

MacIntyre, A. (1981). *After virtue: A study in moral theory.* Notre Dame, IN: University of Notre Dame Press.

MacLean, P. D. (1985). Brain evolution relating to family, play, and the separation call. *Archives of General Psychiatry, 42,* 405–417.

Mahler, M. S. (1968). *On human symbiosis and the vicissitudes of individuation: Vol. 1. Infantile psychosis.* New York: International Universities Press.

Main, M. (1990). Cross-cultural studies of attachment organization: Recent studies, changing methodologies, and the concept of conditional strategies. *Human Development, 33,* 48–61.

Main, M., & George, C. (1985). Responses of abused and disadvantaged toddlers to distress in agemates: A study in the day care setting. *Developmental Psychology, 21,* 407–412.

Main, M., Kaplan, N., & Cassidy, J. (1985). Security in infancy, childhood, and adulthood: A move to the level of representation. In I. Bretherton & E. Waters (Eds.), Growing points of attachment theory and research. *Monographs of the Society for Research in Child Development, 50*(1–2, Serial No. 209), 66–104.

Malatesta, C., Culver, C., Tesman, J., & Shepard, B. (1989). The development of emotion expression during the first two years of life. *Monographs of the Society for Research in Child Development, 54*(1–2, Serial No. 219), 1–136.

Manfredi, M. M. (1993). The emotional development of deaf children. In M. Marschark & M. D. Clark (Eds.), *Psychological perspectives on deafness* (pp. 49–63). Hillsdale, NJ: Erlbaum.

Mann, B., & MacKenzie, E. (1996). Pathways among marital functioning, parental behaviors, and child behavior problems in school-age boys. *Journal of Clinical child Psychology, 25,* 183–191.

Manstead, A. S. (1995). Children's understanding of emotion. In J. Russell, J. Fernandez-Dols, A. Manstead, & J. Wellenkamp (Eds.), *Everyday conceptions of emotion: An introduction to the psychology, anthropology, and linguistics of emotion* (pp. 315–331). Hingham, MA: Kluwer.

Manstead, A. S., Wagner, H. L., & MacDonald, C. J. (1984). Face, body, and speech as channels of communication in the detection of deception. *Basic and Applied Social Psychology, 5,* 317–332.

Markus, H., & Kitayama, S. (1991). Culture and the self: Implications for cognition, emotion, and motivation. *Psychological Review, 98,* 224–253.

Markus, H., & Kitayama, S. (1994a). The cultural construction of self and emotion: Implications for social behavior. In S. Kitayama & H. Markus (Eds.), *Emotion and culture* (pp. 89–130). Washington, DC: American Psychological Association.

Markus, H., & Kitayama, S. (1994b). The cultural shaping of emotion: A conceptual framework. In S. Kitayama & H. Markus (Eds.), *Emotion and culture* (pp. 339–351). Washington, DC: American Psychological Association.

Marschark, M. (1993). Origins and interactions in social, cognitive, and language development of deaf children. In M. Marschark & M. D. Clark (Eds.), *Psychological perspectives on deafness* (pp. 7–26). Hillsdale, NJ: Erlbaum.

Mascolo, M., & Fischer, K. W. (1995). Developmental transformations in appraisals for pride, shame, and guilt. In J. P. Tangney & K. W. Fischer (Eds.), *Self-conscious emotions: The psychology of shame, guilt, embarrassment, and pride* (pp. 64–113). New York: Guilford Press.

Mayer, J., & Salovey, P. (1997). What is emotional intelligence? In P. Salovey & D. Sluyter (Eds.), *Emotional development and emotional intelligence* (pp. 3–31). New York: Basic Books.

McCabe, A., & Peterson, C. (Eds.). (1991). *Developing narrative structure.* Hillsdale, NJ: Erlbaum.

McCloskey, L. A., Figueredo, A. J., & Koss, M. (1995). The effects of systemic family violence on children's mental health. *Child Development, 66,* 1239–1261.

McCoy, C., & Masters, J. (1985). The development of children's strategies for the social control of emotion. *Child Development, 56,* 1214–1222.

McGee, G., Feldman, R. S., & Chernin, L. (1991). A comparison of emotional facial display by children with autism and typical preschoolers. *Journal of Early Intervention, 15,* 237–245.

Mead, G. H. (1934). *Mind, self and society.* Chicago: University of Chicago Press.

Meerum Terwogt, M. (1989). Disordered children's acknowledgment of multiple emotions. *Journal of General Psychology, 117,* 59–69.

Meerum Terwogt, M., & Olthof, T. (1989). Awareness and self-regulation of emotion in young children. In C. Saarni & P. Harris (Eds.), *Children's understanding of emotion* (pp. 209–239). New York: Cambridge University Press.

Mehrabian, A. (1972). *Nonverbal communication.* New York: Aldeno Atherton.

Mendelson, R., & Peters, R. D. (1983). *The influence of relationship knowledge on children's interpretations of social behavior.* Paper presented at the meeting of the Society for Research in Child Development, Detroit, MI.

Mesquita, B., & Frijda, N. (1992). Cultural variations in emotions: A review. *Psychological Bulletin, 112,* 179–204.

Messer, S., & Gross, A. M. (1995). Childhood depression and family interaction: A naturalistic observation study. *Journal of Clinical Child Psychology, 24,* 77–88.

Michalson, L., & Lewis, M. (1985). What do children know about emotions and when do they know it? In M. Lewis & C. Saarni (Eds.), *The socialization of emotions* (pp. 117–139). New York: Plenum.

Miller, P. A., Eisenberg, N., Fabes, R., Shell, R., & Gular, S. (1989). Mothers' emotional arousal as a moderator in the socialization of children's empathy. In N. Eisenberg (Ed.), *New Directions for Child Development: No. 44. Empathy and related emotional responses* (pp. 65–83). San Francisco: Jossey-Bass.

Miller, P. J. (1994). Narrative practices: Their role in socialization and self-construction. In U. Neisser & R. Fivush (Eds.), *The remembering self: Construction and accuracy in the self-narrative* (Vol. 6, pp. 158–179). New York: Cambridge University Press.

Miller, P. J., Mintz, J., Hoogstra, L., Fung, H., & Potts, R. (1992). The narrated self: Young children's construction of self in relation to others in conversational stories of personal experience. *Merrill–Palmer Quarterly, 38,* 45–67.

Miller, P. J., Potts, R., Fung, H., Hoogstra, L., & Mintz, J. (1990). Narrative practices and the social construction of self in childhood. *American Ethnologist, 17*(2), 292–311.

Miller, P. J., & Sperry, L. L. (1987). The socialization of anger and aggression. *Merrill–Palmer Quarterly, 33,* 1–31.

Miller, S. M., & Green, M. L. (1985). Coping with stress and frustration: Origins, nature, and development. In M. Lewis & C. Saarni (Eds.), *The socialization of emotions* (pp. 263–314). New York: Plenum Press.

The mind of the Unabomber. (1996, April 15). *Newsweek,* pp. 30–36.

Mumme, D. L., Fernald, A., & Herrera, C. (1996). Infants' responses to facial and vocal emotional signals in a social referencing paradigm. *Child Development, 67,* 3219–3237.

Murphy, L. (1970). The problem of defense and the concept of coping. In J. Anthony & C. Koupernik (Eds.), *The child in his family.* New York: Wiley.

Murphy, L., & Moriarty, A. (1976). *Vulnerability, coping, and growth.* New Haven, CT: Yale University Press.

Murray, D. W. (1993). What is the Western concept of self? or forgetting David Hume. *Ethics, 21,* 2–3.

Neisser, U. (1988). Five kinds of self-knowledge. *Philosophical Psychology, 1,* 35–59.

Neisser, U. (1992). The development of consciousness and the acquisition of skill. In F. Kessel, P. M. Cole, & D. Johnson (Eds.), *Self and consciousness: Multiple perspectives* (pp. 1–18). Hillsdale, NJ: Erlbaum.

Neisser, U., & Fivush, R. (1994). *The remembering self: Construction and accuracy in the self-narrative.* New York: Cambridge University Press.

Nelson, K. (1996). *Language in cognitive development: Emergence of the mediated mind.* New York: Cambridge University Press.

Nurmi, J., Berzonsky, M., Tammi, K., & Kinney, A. (1997). Identity processing orientation, cognitive behavioural strategies and well-being. *International Journal of Behavioral Development, 21,* 555–570.

Ochs, E. (1986). From feelings to grammar: A Samoan case study. In B. B. Schieffelin & E. Ochs (Eds.), *Language socialization across cultures* (pp. 251–272). Cambridge, UK: Cambridge University Press.

Odom, R., & Lemond, C. (1972). Developmental differences in the perception and production of facial expressions. *Child Development, 43,* 359–369.

Oppenheim, D., Nir, A., Warren, S., & Emde, R. (1997). Emotion regulation in mother–child narrative co-construction: Associations with children's narratives and adaptation. *Developmental Psychology, 33,* 284–294.

Orley, J. H. (1973). *Culture and mental illness.* Nairobi, Kenya: East Africa.

Oswald, H., Krappmann, L., Chowdhuri, I., & von Salisch, M. (1987). Gaps and bridges: Interactions between girls and boys in elementary school. *Sociological Studies of Child Development, 2,* 205–223.

Panksepp, J. (1982). Toward a general psychobiological theory of emotions. With commentaries. *Behavioral and Brain Sciences, 5,* 407–467.

Parke, R. D. (1994). Progress, paradigms, and unresolved problems: A commentary on recent advances in our understanding of children's emotions. *Merrill–Palmer Quarterly, 40,* 157–169.

Parke, R. D., & Buriel, R. (1998). Socialization in the family: Ethnic and ecological perspectives. In N. Eisenberg (Ed.), *Handbook of child psychology* (5th ed.): *Social, emotional and personality development* (pp. 463–552). New York: Wiley.

Parke, R. D., Cassidy, J., Burks, V., Carson, J., & Boyum, L. (1992). Familial contribution to peer competence among young children: The role of interactive and affective processes. In R. Parke & G. Ladd (Eds.), *Family–peer relationships: Modes of linkage* (pp. 107–134). Hillsdale, NJ: Erlbaum.

Parker, J. G., & Asher, S. (1987). Peer relations and later personal adjustment: Are low-accepted children at risk? *Psychological Bulletin, 102,* 357–389.

Parker, J. G., & Herrera, C. (1996). Interpersonal processes in friendship: A comparison of abused and nonabused children's experiences. *Developmental Psychology, 32,* 1025–1038.

Parker, S. (Ed.). (1990). *"Language" and intelligence in monkeys and apes.* New York: Cambridge University Press.

Parkhurst, J. T., & Asher, S. (1992). Peer rejection in middle school: Sub-group differences in behavior, loneliness, and interpersonal concerns. *Developmental Psychology, 28,* 231–241.

Patterson, G. R., DeBaryshe, B., & Ramsey, E. (1989). A developmental perspective on antisocial behavior. *American Psychologist, 44,* 329–335.

Pederson, D., & Gilby, R. (1986). Children's concepts of the family. In R. Ashmore & D. Brodzinsky (Eds.), *Thinking about the family* (pp. 181–204). Hillsdale, NJ: Erlbaum.

Peng, M., Johnson, C., Pollock, J., Glasspool, R., & Harris, P. L. (1992). Training young children to acknowledge mixed emotions. *Cognition and Emotion, 6,* 387–401.

Perry, D., Perry, L., & Weiss, R. (1989). Sex differences in the consequences that children anticipate for aggression. *Developmental Psychology, 25,* 312–319.

Peskin, J. (1992). Ruse and representations: On children's ability to conceal information. *Developmental Psychology, 28,* 84–89.

Peters, S. D. (1988). Child sexual abuse and later psychological problems. In G. Wyatt & G. Powell (Eds.), *Lasting effects of child sexual abuse* (pp. 101–117). Newbury Park, CA: Sage.

Pettit, G., Harrist, A., Bates, J. E., & Dodge, K. (1991). Family interaction, social cognition, and children's subsequent relations with peers at kindergarten. *Journal of Social and Personal Relationships, 8,* 383–402.

Pittman, F. (1993). *Man enough: Fathers, sons, and the search for masculinity.* New York: Putnam.

Plutchik, R. (1980). *Emotions: A psychoevolutionary synthesis.* New York: Harper & Row.

Pollack, L., & Thoits, P. (1989). Processes in emotional socialization. *Social Psychological Quarterly, 52,* 22–34.

Potter, S. H. (1988). The cultural construction of emotion in rural Chinese social life. *Ethos, 16,* 181–208.

Pulkkinen, L. (1983). Finland: The search for alternatives to aggression. In A. Goldstein & M. Segal (Eds.), *Aggression in global perspective.* New York: Pergamon.

Putnam, F., & Trickett, P. (1991, May). *Dissociation in sexually abused girls.* Paper presented at the annual meeting of the American Psychiatric Association, New Orleans, LA.

Ratner, H., & Stettner, L. (1991). Thinking and feeling: Putting Humpty Dumpty together again. *Merrill–Palmer Quarterly, 37,* 1–26.

Reik, T. (1949). *Listening with the third ear.* New York: Farrar, Straus.

Reimer, M. (1996). "Sinking into the ground:" The development and consequences of shame in adolescence. *Developmental Review, 16,* 321–363.

Reissland, N. (1994). The socialisation of pride in young children. *International Journal of Behavioral Development, 17,* 541–552.

Richard, B. A., & Dodge, K. (1982). Social maladjustment and problem solving in school-aged children. *Journal of Consulting and Clinical Psychology, 50,* 226–233.

Ridgeway, D., Waters, E., & Kuczaj, S. A. (1985). Acquisition of emotion-descriptive language: Receptive and productive vocabulary norms for ages 18 month to 6 years. *Developmental Psychology, 21,* 901–908.

Rimé, B. (1995). The social sharing of emotion as a source for the social knowledge of emotion. In J. A. Russell, J. Fernandez-Dols, A. Manstead, & J. Wellenkamp (Eds.), *Everyday conceptions of emotion: An introduction to the psychology, anthropology and linguistics of emotion* (pp. 475–489). Hingham, MA: Kluwer.

Roberts, T., & Pennebaker, J. (1993). *Toward a his and her model of perceptual cue use.* Unpublished manuscript, Department of Psychology, Colorado College, Colorado Springs.

Roberts, W., & Strayer, J. (1987). Parents' responses to the emotional distress of their children: Relations with children's competence. *Developmental Psychology, 23,* 415–422.

Roecker, C., Dubow, E., & Donaldson, D. (1996). Cross-situational patterns in children's coping with observed interpersonal conflict. *Journal of Clinical Child Psychology, 25,* 288–299.

Rose-Krasnor, L. (1997). The nature of social competence: A theoretical review. *Social Development, 6,* 111–135.

Rosenberg, M. (1987). Children of battered women: The effects of witnessing violence on their social problem-solving abilities. *Behavior Therapist, 4,* 85–89.

Rosenthal, R., & DePaulo, B. (1979). Sex differences in accommodation in nonverbal communication. In R. Rosenthal (Ed.), *Skill in nonverbal communication* (pp. 68–103). Cambridge, MA: Oelgeschlager, Gunn, & Hain.

Rothbart, M., & Bates, J. E. (1997). Temperament. In N. Eisenberg (Ed.), *Handbook of child psychology* (5th ed.): *Vol. 3. Social, emotional and personality development* (pp. 105–176). New York: Wiley.

Rothbart, M., Ziaie, H., & O'Boyle, C. (1992). Self-regulation and emotion in infancy. *New Directions for Child Development, 55,* 7–23.

Rubin, K., Chen, X., McDougall, P., Bowker, A., & McKinnon, J. (1995). The Waterloo Longitudinal Project: Predicting internalizing and externalizing problems in adolescence. *Development and Psychopathology, 7,* 751–764.

Ruble, D., Boggiano, A., Feldman, N., & Loebl, J. (1980). A developmental analysis of the role of social comparison in self-evaluation. *Developmental Psychology, 16,* 105–115.

Ruble, D., & Martin, C. L. (1998). Gender development. In N. Eisenberg (Ed.), *Handbook of child psychology* (5th ed.): *Social, emotional and personality development* (pp. 933–1016). New York: Wiley.

Russell, J. A. (1991). Culture and the categorization of emotion. *Psychological Bulletin, 110,* 426–450.

Russell, J. A., & Bullock, M. (1985). Multidimensional scaling of emotional facial expressions: Similarities from preschoolers to adults. *Journal of Personality and Social Psychology, 48,* 1290–1298.

Russell, J. A., Fernandez-Dols, J. M., Manstead, A., & Wellenkamp, J. (Eds.). (1996). *Everyday conceptions of emotion: An introduction to the psychology, anthropology and linguistics of emotion.* Hingham, MA: Kluwer.

Russell, J. A., & Ridgeway, D. (1983). Dimensions underlying children's emotion concepts. *Developmental Psychology, 19(6),* 795–804.

Rutter, M., Izard, C., & Read, P. (Eds.). (1986). *Depression in young people.* New York: Guilford Press.

Ryan, G. (1989). Victim to victimizer: Rethinking victim treatment. *Journal of Interpersonal Violence, 4,* 325–341.

Saarni, C. (1978). Cognitive and communicative features of emotional experience, or do you show what you think you feel? In M. Lewis & L. Rosenblum (Eds.), *The development of affect* (pp. 361–375). New York: Plenum.

Saarni, C. (1979a). Children's understanding of display rules for expressive behavior. *Developmental Psychology, 15,* 424–429.

Saarni, C. (1979b, April). *When not to show what you feel: Children's understanding of the relations between emotional experience and expressive behavior.* Paper presented at the meeting of the Society for Research in Child Development, San Francisco.

Saarni, C. (1982). Social and affective functions of nonverbal behavior: Developmental concerns. In R. S. Feldman (Ed.), *Development of nonverbal behavior in children* (pp. 123–143). New York: Springer Verlag.

Saarni, C. (1984). An observational study of children's attempts to monitor their expressive behavior. *Child Development, 55,* 1504–1513.

Saarni, C. (1985). Indirect processes in affect socialization. In M. Lewis & C. Saarni (Eds.), *The socialization of emotions* (pp. 187–209). New York: Plenum.

Saarni, C. (1987, April). *Children's beliefs about parental expectations for emotional-expressive behavior management.* Paper presented at the biennial meeting of the Society for Research in Child Development, Baltimore.

Saarni, C. (1988). Children's understanding of the interpersonal consequences of dissemblance of nonverbal emotional–expressive behavior. *Journal of Nonverbal Behavior, 12*(4, Pt. 2), 275–294.

Saarni, C. (1989a). Children's beliefs about emotion. In M. Luszez & T. Nettelbeck (Eds.), *Psychological development: Perspectives across the life-span* (pp. 69–78). Amsterdam: Elsevier.

Saarni, C. (1989b). Children's understanding of strategic control of emotional expression in social transactions. In C. Saarni & P. L. Harris (Eds.), *Children's understanding of emotion* (pp. 181–208). New York: Cambridge University Press.

Saarni, C. (1990a). Emotional competence: How emotions and relationships become integrated. In R. A. Thompson (Ed.), *Nebraska Symposium on Motivation: Vol. 36. Socioemotional development* (pp. 115–182). Lincoln: University of Nebraska Press.

Saarni, C. (1990b). *Psychometric properties of the Parent Attitude toward Children's Expressiveness Scale.* (Available from ERIC, No. 317–301)

Saarni, C. (1991, April). *Social context and management of emotional-expressive behavior: Children's expectancies for when to dissemble what they feel.* Paper presented at the biennial meeting of the Society for Research in Child Development, Seattle.

Saarni, C. (1992). Children's emotional-expressive behaviors as regulators of others' happy and sad states. *New Directions for Child Development, 55,* 91–106.

Saarni, C. (1993). Socialization of emotion. In M. Lewis & J. Haviland (Eds.), *Handbook of emotions* (pp. 435–446). New York: Guilford Press.

Saarni, C. (1997). Coping with aversive feelings. *Motivation and Emotion, 21,* 45–63.

Saarni, C., & Harris, P. L. (Eds.). (1989). *Children's understanding of emotion.* New York: Cambridge University Press.

Saarni, C., & Lewis, M. (1993). Deceit and illusion in human affairs. In M. Lewis & C. Saarni (Eds.), *Lying and deception in every day life* (pp. 1–29). New York: Guilford Press.

Saarni, C., Mumme, D. L., & Campos, J. (1998). Emotional development: Action, communication, and understanding. In N. Eisenberg (Ed.), *Handbook of child psychology* (5th ed.): *Vol. 3. Social, emotional and personality development* (pp. 237–309). New York: Wiley.

Saarni, C., & von Salisch, M. (1993). The socialization of emotional dissemblance. In M. Lewis & C. Saarni (Eds.), *Lying and deception in everyday life* (pp. 106–125). New York: Guilford Press.

Salladay, R. (1997, November 9). Unabomber journal—how victims got chosen. *San Francisco Examiner,* pp. A-1, A-21.

Salovey, P., & Sluyter, D. (Eds.). (1997). *Emotional development and emotional intelligence.* New York: Basic Books.

Sarbin, T. (1989). Emotions as narrative emplotments. In M. Packer & R. Addison (Eds.), *Entering the circle: Hermeneutic investigation in psychology* (pp. 185–201). Albany: State University of New York Press.

Sarbin, T. (1990). The narrative quality of action. *Theoretical and Philosophical Psychology, 10,* 49–65.

Satir, V. (1967). *Conjoint family therapy*. Palo Alto, CA: Science & Behavior Books.

Saunders, D., Lynch, A., Grayson, M., & Linz, D. (1987). The inventory of beliefs about wife beating: The construction and initial validation of a measure of beliefs and attitudes. *Violence and Victims, 2,* 39–55.

Seligman, M. (1975). *Helplessness: On depression, development, and death.* San Francisco: Freeman.

Seligman, M., Peterson, C., Kaslow, N., Tanenbaum, R., Alloy, L., & Abramson, L. (1984). Explanatory style and depressive symptoms among school children. *Journal of Abnormal Psychology, 93,* 235–238.

Selman, R. (1981). What children understand of intrapsychic processes. In E. Shapiro & E. Weber (Eds.), *Cognitive and affective growth* (pp. 187–215). Hillsdale, NJ: Erlbaum.

Selman, R., Beardslee, W., Schultz, L., Krupa, M., & Podorefsky, D. (1986). Assessing adolescent interpersonal negotiation strategies: Toward the integration of structural and functional models. *Developmental Psychology, 22,* 450–459.

Selman, R., & Demorest, A. (1984). Observing troubled children's interpersonal negotiation strategies: Implications for a developmental model. *Child Development, 55,* 288–304.

Selman, R., & Demorest, A. (1987). Putting thoughts and feelings into perspective: A developmental view on how children deal with interpersonal disequilibrium. In D. Bearison & H. Zimiles (Eds.), *Thought and emotion* (pp. 93–128). Hillsdale, NJ: Erlbaum.

Shantz, C. U. (1993). Children's conflicts: Representations and lessons learned. In R. Cocking & K. A. Renninger (Eds.), *The development and meaning of psychological distance* (pp. 185–202). Hillsdale, NJ: Erlbaum.

Shaver, P., Schwartz, J., Kirson, D., & O'Connor, C. (1987). Emotion knowledge: Further exploration of a prototype approach. *Journal of Personality and Social Psychology, 52,* 1061–1086.

Shelton, M., & Rogers, R. (1981). Fear-arousing and empathy-arousing appeals to help. The pathos of persuasion. *Journal of Applied Social Psychology, 11,* 366–378.

Shennum, W. A., & Bugental, D. B. (1982). The development of control over affective expression in nonverbal behavior. In R. S. Feldman (Ed.), *Development of nonverbal behavior in children* (pp. 101–118). New York: Springer Verlag.

Schibuk, M., Bond, M., & Bouffard, R. (1989). The development of defenses in childhood. *Canadian Journal of Psychiatry, 34,* 581–588.

Shields, S. A. (1984). Reports of bodily change in anxiety, sadness and anger. *Motivation and Emotion, 8,* 1–21.

Shigaki, I. S. (1983). Child care practices in Japan and the United States: How do they reflect cultural values in young children? *Young Children, 38,* 13–24.

Shore, B. (1996). *Culture in mind: Cognition, culture, and the problem of meaning.* New York: Oxford University Press.

Shweder, R. (1993). The cultural psychology of the emotions. In M. Lewis & J. Haviland (Eds.), *Handbook of emotions* (pp. 417–431). New York: Guilford Press.

Shweder, R., Goodnow, J., Hatano, G., LeVine, R., Markus, H., & Miller, P. J. (1998). The cultural psychology of development: One mind, many mentalities. In R. Lerner (Ed.), *Handbook of child psychology* (5th ed.): *Vol. 1. Theoretical models of human development* (pp. 865–937). New York: Wiley.

Sigman, M., Kasari, C., Kwon, J., & Yirmiya, N. (1992). Responses to the negative emotions of others by autistic, mentally retarded, and normal children. *Child Development, 63,* 796–807.

Sigmon, S., & Snyder, C. R. (1993). Looking at oneself in a rose-colored mirror: The role of excuses in the negotiation of a personal reality. In M. Lewis & C. Saarni (Eds.), *Lying and deception in every day life* (pp. 148–165). New York: Guilford Press.

Slade, A. (1986). Symbolic play and separation-individuation: A naturalistic study. *Bulletin of the Menninger Clinic, 50,* 541–563.

Slade, A. (1994). Making meaning and making believe. In A. Slade & D. Wolf (Eds.), *Children at play: Clinical and developmental approaches to meaning representation* (pp. 81–107). New York: Oxford University Press.

Smiley, P., & Huttenlocher, J. (1989). Young children's acquisition of emotion concepts. In C. Saarni & P. Harris (Eds.), *Children's understanding of emotion* (pp. 27–49). New York: Cambridge University Press.

Snary, J., & Keljo, K. (1991). In a Gemeinschaft voice: The cross-cultural expansion of moral development theory. In W. Kurtines & J. Gewirtz (Eds.), *Handbook of moral behavior and development* (Vol. 1, pp. 395–424). Hillsdale, NJ: Erlbaum.

Sodian, B., Taylor, C., Harris, P. L., & Perner, J. (1991). Early deception and the child's theory of mind: False trails and genuine markers. *Child Development, 62,* 468–483.

Sonkin, D. (1988). The male batterer: Clinical and research issues. *Victims and Violence, 3,* 65–79.

Sorce, J., Emde, R., Campos, J., & Klinnert, M. (1985). Maternal emotional signaling: Its effect on the visual cliff behavior of 1-year-olds. *Developmental Psychology, 21,* 195–200.

Sorensen, E. S. (1993). *Children's stress and coping.* New York: Guilford Press.

Southam-Gerow, M., & Kendall, P. C. (1997). *Emotion and child psychopathology: Developmental and clinical considerations.* Unpublished manuscript, Temple University, Philadelphia.

Spencer, P. A., & Deyo, D. (1993). Cognitive and social aspects of deaf children's play. In M. Marschark & M. D. Clark (Eds.), *Psychological perspectives on deafness* (pp. 65–91). Hillsdale, NJ: Erlbaum.

Sperry, L. L., & Sperry, D. (1996). The early development of narrative skills. *Cognitive Development, 11,* 443–465.

Staub, E. (1991). Psychological and cultural origins of extreme destructiveness and extreme altruism. In W. Kurtines & J. Gewirtz (Eds.), *Handbook of moral behavior and development* (Vol. 1, pp. 425–446). Hillsdale, NJ: Erlbaum.

Stein, N., & Trabasso, T. (1989). Children's understanding of changing emotional states. In C. Saarni & P. Harris (Eds.), *Children's understanding of emotion* (pp. 50–80). New York: Cambridge University Press.

Stein, N., & Trabasso, T. (1993). The representation and organization of emotional experience: Unfolding the emotion episode. In M. Lewis & J. Haviland (Eds.), *Handbook of emotions* (pp. 279–300). New York: Guilford Press.

Steinberg, S., & Laird, J. (1989). Parent attributions of emotion to their children and the cues children use in perceiving their own emotions. *Motivation and Emotion, 13,* 179–191.

Stern, D. (1985). *The interpersonal world of the infant.* New York: Basic Books.

Stipek, D. (1995). The development of pride and shame in toddlers. In J. P. Tangney & K. W. Fischer (Eds.), *Self-conscious emotions: The psychology of shame, guilt, embarrassment, and pride* (pp. 237–252). New York: Guilford Press.

Stipek, D., Recchia, S., & McClintic, S. (1992). Self- evaluation in young children. *Monographs of the Society for Research in Child Development, 57*(Serial No. 226), 1–83.

Straus, M. B. (1994). *Violence in the lives of adolescents.* New York: Norton.

Strayer, J. (1986). Children's attributions regarding the situational determinants of emotion in self and other. *Developmental Psychology, 22,* 649–654.

Strayer, J. (1987). Affective and cognitive perspectives on empathy. In N. Eisenberg & J. Strayer (Eds.), *Empathy and its development* (pp. 218–244). New York: Cambridge University Press.

Strayer, J. (1989). What children know and feel in response to witnessing affective events. In C. Saarni & P. Harris (Eds.), *Children's understanding of emotion* (pp. 259–292). New York: Cambridge University Press.

Strayer, J., & Roberts, W. (1989). Children's empathy and role-taking: Child and parental factors and relations to prosocial behavior. *Journal of Applied Developmental Psychology, 10,* 227–239.

Strayer, J., & Roberts, W. (1997). Children's personal distance and their empathy: Indices of interpersonal closeness. *International Journal of Behavioral Development, 20,* 385–403.

Strayer, J., & Schroeder, M. (1989). Children's helping strategies: Influences of emotion, empathy, and age. In N. Eisenberg (Ed.), *New directions for child development: No. 44. Empathy and related emotional responses.* San Francisco: Jossey-Bass.

Swann, W. B. (1987). Identity negotiation: Where two roads meet. *Journal of Personality and Social Psychology, 53,* 1038–1051.

Tangney, J. P., & Fischer, K. W. (Eds.). (1995). *Self-conscious emotions: The psychology of shame, guilt, embarrassment, and pride.* New York: Guilford Press.

Taylor, M. (1997, November 9). A trail of bombs. *San Francisco Chronicle,* pp. 1, 4–5.

Taylor, S. E. (1989). *Positive illusions: Creative self-deception and the healthy mind.* New York: Basic Books.

Taylor, S. E., & Brown, J. D. (1988). Illusion and well-being: A social psychological perspective on mental health. *Psychological Bulletin, 103,* 193–210.

Tedeschi, J. (1981). *Impression management theory and social psychological research.* New York: Academic Press.

Tedeschi, J., & Norman, N. (1985). Social power, self-presentation, and the self.

In B. Schlenker (Ed.), *The self and social life* (pp. 293–322). New York: McGraw-Hill.

Terwogt, M. M., & Olthof, T. (1989). Awareness and self-regulation of emotion in young children. In C. Saarni & P. Harris (Eds.), *Children's understanding of emotion* (pp. 209–237). New York: Cambridge University Press.

Teyber, E. (1985). *Interpersonal process in psychotherapy.* Pacific Grove, CA: Brooks/ Cole.

Thompson, R. A. (1989). Causal attributions and children's emotional understanding. In C. Saarni & P. Harris (Eds.), *Children's understanding of emotion* (pp. 117–150). New York: Cambridge University Press.

Thompson, R. A. (1990). Emotion and self-regulation. In R. A. Thompson (Ed.), *Nebraska Symposium on Motivation: Vol. 36. Socioemotional development* (pp. 367–467). Lincoln: University of Nebraska Press.

Thompson, R. A. (1991). Emotional regulation and emotional development. *Educational Psychology Review, 3,* 269–307.

Thompson, R. A. (1994). Emotion regulation: A theme in search of definition. In N. Fox (Ed.), The development of emotion regulation: Behavioral and biological considerations. *Monographs of the Society for Research in Child Development, 59*(Serial No. 240), 25–52.

Trepper, T., & Niedner, D. (1996). Intrafamily child abuse. In F. Kaslow (Ed.), *Handbook of relational diagnosis* (pp. 394–406). New York: Wiley.

Trickett, P., & Kuczynski, L. (1986). Children's misbehaviors and parental discipline strategies in abusive and nonabusive families. *Developmental Psychology, 22,* 115–123.

Trickett, P., & Putnam, F. (1991, August). *Patterns of symptoms in prepubertal and pubertal sexually abused girls.* Paper presented at the annual meeting of the American Psychological Association, San Francisco.

Turiel, E. (1998). The development of morality. In N. Eisenberg (Ed.), *Handbook of child psychology* (5th ed.): *Vol. 3. Social, emotional and personality development* (pp. 863–932). New York: Wiley.

Underwood, B., & Moore, B. S. (1982). Perspective-taking and altruism. *Psychological Bulletin, 91,* 143–173.

Underwood, M. K. (1997). Peer social status and children's choices about the expression and control of positive and negative emotions. *Merrill–Palmer Quarterly, 43*(4), 610–634.

Underwood, M. K., Coie, J., & Herbsman, C. (1992). Display rules for anger and aggression in school-age children. *Child Development, 63,* 366–380.

Underwood, M., Hurley, J., Johanson, C., & Mosley, J. (in press). An experimental, observational investigation of children's responses to peer provocation: Developmental and gender differences in middle childhood. *Child Development.*

Underwood, M. K., Kupersmidt, J. B., & Coie, J. D. (1996). Childhood peer sociometric status and aggression as predictors of adolescent childbearing. *Journal of Research on Adolescence, 6*(2), 201–223.

Unks, G. (Ed.). (1995). *The gay teen: Educational practice and theory for lesbian, gay, and bisexual adolescents.* New York: Routledge.

van der Kolk, B., & Fisler, R. (1994). Childhood abuse and neglect and loss of self-regulation. *Bulletin of the Menninger Clinic, 58,* 145–168.

von Salisch, M. (1991). *Kinderfreundschaften.* Göttingen, Germany: Hogrefe.

von Salisch, M. (1993, April). *To show or not to show it: Self-worth and the dilemma of anger expression.* Paper presented at the biennial meeting of the Society for Research in Child Development, Washington, DC.

von Salisch, M. (1996a). Relationships between children: Symmetry and asymmetry among peers, friend, and siblings. In A. E. Auhagen & M. von Salisch (Eds.), *The diversity of human relationships* (pp. 59–77). New York: Cambridge University Press.

von Salisch, M. (1996b). What boys and girls expect when they express their anger toward a friend. In N. Frijda (Ed.), *Proceedings of the biennial meeting of the Society for Research on Emotions* (pp. 169–173). Toronto: ISRE.

Vuchinich, S., Emery, R. E., & Cassidy, J. (1988). Family members as third parties in dyadic family conflict: Strategies, alliances and outcomes. *Child Development, 59,* 1293–1302.

Walbott, H., & Scherer, K. (1995). Cultural determinants in experiencing shame and guilt. In J. P. Tangney & K. W. Fischer (Eds.), *Self-conscious emotions: The psychology of shame, guilt, embarrassment, and pride* (pp. 465–487). New York: Guilford Press.

Walden, T. (1991). Infant social referencing. In J. Garber & K. Dodge (Eds.), *The development of emotion regulation and dysregulation* (pp. 69–88). Cambridge, UK: Cambridge University Press.

Walden, T., & Field, I. (1988). *Preschool children's social competence and production and discrimination of affective expressions.* Unpublished manuscript, Vanderbilt University, Nashville, TN.

Walden, T., & Knieps, L. (1996). Reading and responding to social signals. In M. Lewis & M. W. Sullivan (Eds.), *Emotional development in atypical children* (pp. 29–42). Hillsdale, NJ: Erlbaum.

Walden, T., & Smith, M. C. (1997). Emotion regulation. *Motivation and emotion, 21,* 7–25.

Walker, E. (1981). Emotion recognition in disturbed and normal children: A research note. *Journal of Child Psychology and Psychiatry, 22,* 263–268.

Walker, L. J., & Hennig, K. (1997). Moral development in the broader context of personality. In S. Hala (Ed.), *The development of social cognition* (pp. 297–327). East Sussex, UK: Psychology Press.

Walker, L. J., Pitts, R., Hennig, K., & Matsuba, M. (1995). Reasoning about morality and real-life moral problems. In M. Killen & D. Hart (Eds.), *Morality in everyday life and developmental perspectives* (pp. 371–407). Cambridge: Cambridge University Press.

Walker, L. J., & Taylor, J. H. (1991). Family interactions and the development of moral reasoning. *Child Development, 62,* 264–283.

Watson, A. J., & Valtin, R. (1997). Secrecy in middle childhood. *International Journal of Behavioral Development, 21,* 431–452.

Watzlawick, P., Beavin, J., & Jackson, D. (1967). *Pragmatics of human communication: A study of interactional patterns, pathologies, and paradoxes.* New York: Norton.

Weber, H., & Laux, L. (1993). Presentation of emotion. In G. Van Heck, P. Bonaiuto, I. Deary, & W. Nowack (Eds.), *Personality psychology in Europe* (Vol. 4, pp. 235–255). Netherlands: Tilburg University Press.

Weeks, S., & Hobson, R. (1987). The salience of facial expression for children with autism. *Journal of Child Psychology and Psychiatry, 28,* 137–151.

Weiner, B. (1985). An attributional theory of achievement motivation and emotions. *Psychological Review, 92,* 548–573.

Weiner, B., & Graham, S. (1984). An attributional approach to emotional development. In C. Izard, J. Kagan, & R. Zajonc (Eds.), *Emotions, cognition, and behavior* (pp. 167–191). New York: Cambridge University Press.

Weiner, B., & Handel, S. J. (1985). A cognition–emotion–action sequence: Anticipated emotional consequences of causal attributions and reported communication strategy. *Developmental Psychology, 21,* 102–107.

Weiss, B., Dodge, K., Bates, J., & Pettit, G. (1992). Some consequences of early harsh discipline: Child aggression and maladaptive social information processing style. *Child Development, 63,* 1321–1335.

Weissberg, R., & Greenberg, M. T. (1998). School and community competence-enhancement and prevention programs. In I. Sigel & K. A. Renninger (Eds.), *Handbook of child psychology* (5th ed.): *Vol 4. Child psychology in practice* (pp. 877–954). New York: Wiley.

Weissman, M. M., Gammon, G., John, K., Merikangas, K., Warner, V., Prusoff, B., & Sholomskas, D. (1987). Children of depressed parents: Increased psychopathology and early onset of major depression. *Archives of General Psychiatry, 44,* 847–853.

Weisz, J., Sigman, M., Weiss, B., & Mosk, J. (1993). Parent reports of behavioral and emotional problems among children in Kenya, Thailand, and the United States. *Child Development, 64,* 98–109.

Wellman, H., & Banerjee, M. (1991). Mind and emotion: Children's understanding of the emotional consequences of beliefs and desires. *British Journal of Developmental Psychology, 9,* 191–214.

Wellman, H., Harris, P. L., Banerjee, M., & Sinclair, A. (1995). Early understanding of emotion: Evidence from natural language. *Cognition and Emotion, 9,* 117–149.

Wellman, H., & Wooley, J. (1990). From simple desires to ordinary beliefs: The early development of everyday psychology. *Cognition, 35,* 245–275.

White, G. M. (1994). Affecting culture: Emotion and morality in everyday life. In S. Kitayama & H. Markus (Eds.), *Emotion and culture* (pp. 219–239). Washington, DC: American Psychological Association.

White, R. W. (1959). Motivation reconsidered: The concept of competence. *Psychological Review, 66,* 297–333.

Whitesell, N. R., & Harter, S. (1996). The interpersonal context of emotion: Anger with close friends and classmates. *Child Development, 67,* 1345–1359.

Whiting, B. B., & Edwards, C. P. (1988). *Children of different worlds.* Cambridge, MA: Harvard University Press.

Wierzbicka, A. (1992). *Semantics, culture and cognition.* New York: Oxford University Press.

Wierzbicka, A. (1994). Emotion, language, and cultural scripts. In S. Kitayama &

H. Markus (Eds.), *Emotion and culture* (pp. 133–196). Washington, D.C.: American Psychological Association.

Wiggers, M., & C. van Lieshout. (1985). Development of recognition of emotions: Children's reliance on situational and facial expressive cues. *Developmental Psychology, 21,* 338–349.

Wilson, J. Q. (1993). *The moral sense.* New York: Free Press.

Wintre, M., & Vallance, D. (1994). A developmental sequence in the comprehension of emotions: Intensity, multiple emotions, and valence. *Developmental Psychology, 30,* 509–514.

Wolchik, S., & Sandler, I. (Eds.). (1997). *Handbook of children's coping: Linking theory with intervention.* New York: Plenum.

Wolf, D. P. (1990). Being of several minds: Voices and versions of the self in early childhood. In D. Cicchetti & M. Beeghly (Eds.), *The self in transition: Infancy to childhood* (pp. 183–212). Chicago: University of Chicago Press.

Wootton, J. P., Frick, P., Shelton, K., & Silverthorn, P. (1997). Ineffective parent and childhood conduct problems: The moderating role of callous-unemotional traits. *Journal of Consulting and Clinical Psychology, 65,* 301–308.

Yirmiya, N., Kasari, C., Sigman, M., & Mundy, P. (1989). Facial expressions of affect in autistic, mentally retarded and normal children. *Journal of Child Psychology and Psychiatry, 30,* 725–735.

Yirmiya, N., & Weiner, B. (1986). Perceptions of controllability and anticipated anger. *Cognitive Development, 1,* 273–280.

Zabel, R. (1979). Recognition of emotions in facial expressions by emotionally disturbed and nondisturbed children. *Psychology in the Schools, 16,* 119–126.

Zahn-Waxler, C. (1991). The case for empathy: A developmental review. *Psychological Inquiry, 2,* 155–158.

Zahn-Waxler, C., Cole, P. M., & Barrett, K. C. (1991). Guilt and empathy: Sex differences and implications for the development of depression. In J. Garber & K. Dodge (Eds.), *The development of emotion regulation and dysregulation* (pp. 243–272). New York: Cambridge University Press.

Zahn-Waxler, C., & Kochanska, G. (1990). The origins of guilt. In R. Thompson (Ed.), *Nebraska Symposium on Motivation: Vol. 36. Socioemotional development* (pp. 183–258). Lincoln: University of Nebraska Press.

Zahn-Waxler, C., & Radke-Yarrow, M. (1982). The development of altruism: Alternative research strategies. In N. Eisenberg (Ed.), *The development of prosocial behavior* (pp. 109–137). New York: Academic Press.

Zahn-Waxler, C., Radke-Yarrow, M., & King, R. (1979). Child rearing and children's prosocial initiations toward victims of distress. *Child Development, 50,* 319–330.

Zahn-Waxler, C., & Robinson, J. (1995). Empathy and guilt: Early origins of feelings of responsibility. In J. P. Tangney & K. W. Fischer (Eds.), *Self-conscious emotions: The psychology of shame, guilt, embarrassment, and pride* (pp. 143–173). New York: Guilford Press.

Zeman, J., & Garber, J. (1996). Display rules for anger, sadness, and pain: It depends on who is watching. *Child Development, 67,* 957–973.

Zeman, J., & Shipman, K. (1996). Children's expression of negative affect: Reasons and methods. *Developmental Psychology, 32,* 842–849.

Zeman, J., & Shipman, K. (1997). Social–contextual influences on expectancies for managing anger and sadness: The transition from middle childhood to adolescence. *Developmental Psychology, 33,* 917–924.

Zivin, G. (1985). Separating the issues in the study of expressive development: A framing chapter. In G. Zivin (Ed.), *The development of expressive behavior* (pp. 3–22). New York: Academic Press.

Zivin, G. (1986). Processes of expressive behavior development. *Merrill–Palmer Quarterly, 32,* 103–140.

Zuckerman, M., & Przewuzman, S. (1979). Decoding and encoding facial expressions in preschool-age children. *Environmental Psychology and Nonverbal Behavior, 3,* 147–163.

Author Index

369

Subject Index